# Magnetic Source Imaging
# of the Human Brain

# Magnetic Source Imaging of the Human Brain

*Edited by*

### Zhong-Lin Lu
*University of Southern California*

### Lloyd Kaufman
*New York University*

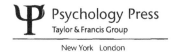

Psychology Press
Taylor & Francis Group

New York   London

First Published by Lawrence Erlbaum Associates, Inc., Publishers
10 Industrial Avenue
Mahwah, New Jersey 07430

Reprinted 2008 by Psychology Press

Cover design by Kathryn Houghtaling Lacey

**Library of Congress Cataloging-in-Publication Data**

Magnetic source imaging of the human brain / edited by Zhong-Lin Lu, Lloyd Kaufman.
       p. cm.
Includes bibliographical references and index.
ISBN 0-8058-4511-9 (cloth : alk. paper)
ISBN 0-8058-4512-7 (pbk. : alk. paper)
1. Magnetoencephalography.  I. Lu, Zhong-Lin.  III. Kaufman, Lloyd.
RC386.6.M36 M34   2003
616.8'047548—dc21                                    2002029734
                                                         CIP

Printed in the United States of America
10  9  8  7  6  5  4  3  2  1

# Contents

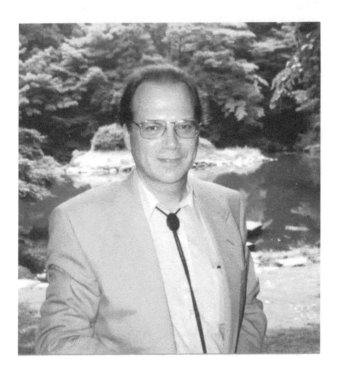

Samuel J. Williamson at the Sanshiro Pond, University of Tokyo, July, 1996
(photo courtesy of Professor Shoogo Ueno).

# Preface

Very faint magnetic fields are now routinely detected outside the human scalp. These fields result from flow of ionic currents within the neurons of the brain and are undistorted by the intervening skull and other tissues. They were first detected more than 25 years ago, and the technology associated with these *neuromagnetic* fields has since grown enormously. The first superconducting devices used to measure the field detected it at a single point in space outside the head. Today, hundreds of exquisitely sensitive devices operating at the temperature of liquid helium measure the field at many places at once, thus making it possible to determine the configuration of neuronal currents that give rise to the detected fields. These currents vary with voluntary motor activity, sensory stimulation, and mental activity of various kinds. They also betray the presence of many pathological states and processes. Properly interpreted, the *magnetoencephalogram* is a functional imaging modality that enables a scientist or clinician to literally view the workings of the brain with a temporal resolution measured in milliseconds. Logically this *magnetic source imaging* (MSI) is an ideal complement to functional magnetic resonance imaging (MRI), positron emission tomography, and other functional imaging modalities. It is surprising that this is not yet widely recognized.

Perhaps the lack of recognition is related to the pre-eminent role played by low-temperature physics in much of the early literature and the abstract concepts underlying more recent efforts to convert measures of the extracranial magnetic field to images of the brain in action. Insufficient attention has been paid to communicating the essence of MSI to a wider scientific audience. It seems fairly easy to grasp the significance of readily interpreted functional MRI images colored or shaded to reveal the regions of the brain that were apparently more or less active during the performance of some mental task. By contrast, current dipole moments, current source distributions, and isofield contour plots seem to communicate little to the unprepared reader. This situation cannot be remedied by referring interested scientists to an extensive but highly specialized literature, written in a language recognized by a relatively few specialists. Hence, this book is designed to acquaint serious students and scientists with MSI.

On September 24, 1999, a group of prominent scientists gathered to honor Professor Samuel J. Williamson, one of the most influential early pioneers of MSI. This conference at New York University was entitled *"Neuromagnetism at the Millennium."* The speakers were physicists, engineers, physicians, cognitive scientists, neural scientists, and psychologists. They discussed the history of the field as well as the current state of the art. Some dealt with near-term and therefore predictable future developments of the technology. All in attendance agreed that a similarly full treatment in the form of a book would go a long way toward filling the need described earlier.

Although this book originated as the proceedings of a conference, it has been organized and expanded to cover the field in a coherent manner. We solicited new chapters from outstanding scholars and prepared an introductory tutorial chapter. Contributors include distinguished scientists from many different countries, including Canada, Japan, Finland, Germany, Italy, the Netherlands, Turkey, and, of course, the United States. Some are widely known outside the field of MSI. The list of authors includes many who are members of their nation's academies of science, recipients of prestigious scientific prizes, and authors of some of the most widely cited articles in their own special fields. Most of the authors have made pioneering contributions to the field of MSI and, obviously, all recognize the potential importance of this field. We are extremely pleased that this distinguished group agreed to participate in the conference to honor Professor Williamson and to contribute chapters to this book.

This book is self-contained. It covers MSI from beginning to end. The first sections review the principles and methodology, and the remainder reviews the results obtained by the most important laboratories worldwide. As indicated earlier, to prepare the readers, we wrote chapter 1 to introduce the field and to provide a framework for the rest of the book. We think this volume would be a suitable textbook for upper-level undergraduate and graduate courses on brain imaging (in fact, several authors have been using their own chapters in graduate courses). However, the book is primarily intended for scientists, graduate and postdoctoral students working in areas of biomagnetism, brain imaging, and cognitive neuroscience.

All the contributors and many other people have given us a great deal of help in producing this book. In particular, we thank George Sperling for his advice and Bill Webber for his encouragement and cooperation. We are very grateful to Sara Scudder and Janet Lincoln for their careful and thoughtful assistance. We also thank New York University and its Department of Physics for sponsoring the conference that led to this book. Biomagnetic Technologies, Inc. (now 4D Neuromagnetic Imaging, Inc.) provided some additional financial support. We are especially grateful to those who came from as far away as Finland, Japan, Italy, and many other places to make their contributions. These many scholars came because of Samuel J. Williamson's scientific and personal contributions to their work. We dedicate this book to Sam Williamson, a true pioneer who played a major role in creating the field of MSI of the human brain.

—*Zhong-Lin Lu, Irvine, California*
—*Lloyd Kaufman, Roslyn Heights, New York*

# 1

# Basics of Neuromagnetism and Magnetic Source Imaging

Lloyd Kaufman
*New York University*

Zhong-Lin Lu
*University of Southern California*

This chapter provides an overview of *neuromagnetism,* which is defined as the study of magnetic fields associated with the electrical activity of neurons. Like the other chapters in this volume, this chapter especially emphasizes the magnetic fields generated by the human brain. In view of this emphasis, we introduce the reader to *magnetoencephalography*, a technique that measures the external magnetic field, near the scalp, of the intact human brain. This general overview is designed to help newcomers appreciate the more technical chapters. It provides a relatively nontechnical description of the physical basis of the neuromagnetic field, the different methods used to detect it, and how the magnetoencephalogram complements the *electroencephalogram*. We explain how analysis of MEG data can yield high temporal and reasonable spatial resolution "representations" of current distributions on the cerebral cortex. These magnetic source images complement the other functional imaging modalities. Furthermore, we describe some typical uses of *magnetic source imaging* in medicine and in cognitive neural science. Finally, we briefly discuss complementary modes of functional brain imaging, such as *positron emission tomography* and *functional magnetic resonance imaging,* as well as recent attempts to combine multiple imaging modalities to achieve high spatiotemporal resolution functional images of the human brain.

One goal of this chapter is to acquaint readers with areas of research that are awaiting the attention of creative scientists. To achieve this goal, we must make a seemingly esoteric subject accessible. Hence, this chapter does not provide an exhaustive review of the literature; instead, we attempt to elucidate relevant principles, methods, and results in as simple a manner as possible and point the way so that even beginners will recognize opportunities to make advances in the field. The other chapters in this volume cite the relevant literature and describe historical precedents in great detail and can serve as a basis for further study and research. Thus, one of our major goals is to prepare beginners to read these chapters.

## THE NEUROGENESIS OF MAGNETOENCEPHALOGRAPHY

In chapter 2 of this volume, Yoshio Okada provides a detailed discussion of how neurons give rise to magnetic fields. In this section we offer a brief and simplified account.

### Primary and Volume Currents

Neurotransmitters crossing a synapse produce local changes in the electric potential across the target membrane. This postsynaptic potential tends to be either excitatory or inhibitory; that is, it either reduces or increases the polarization of the target membrane, depending on the nature of the neurotransmitter. The interior resting voltage of the cell is normally negative with respect to its exterior. As the polarization of the membrane is reduced, or even reversed, near the synapse the internal potential of the cell membrane becomes less negative relative to that of more distant regions of the membrane. This difference in potential between one region of the cell's inner wall and that of more distant regions results in current flow. Conversely, when the local transmembrane potential is increased (hyperpolarized) so that negativity of the interior of the membrane is greater near the synapse relative to more distant regions, negative ions will tend to flow away from that region toward more distant portions of the cell. This intracellular ionic current flow may persist for a relatively long time. The entire neuron can be thought of as a very small battery and a resistor connected to its positive pole. The battery–resistor combination is immersed in a saline solution. Because the solution is a conductor, it completes the circuit between the (positive) end of the resistor and the negative pole of the battery. This allows ionic current to flow widely throughout the solution from the positive end of the resistor to the opposite (negative) pole of the battery. The positive end of the resistor tends to lose charge as negative ions flow from it into the saline medium. This charge is replaced by ions from within the battery. These negative ions inside the battery are replenished in turn by inflowing ions from the medium. As a consequence, charge is conserved, because there is a continuous flow of current around the complete battery–resistor–medium circuit. We refer to the intracellular current, within the battery and resistor, as the *primary current*. The primary current represents the ionic currents flowing within elongated processes of neurons, for example, dendrites of pyramidal cells of the cerebral cortex. Alternatively, the currents flowing outward from the battery–resistor circuit into the saline solution and inward from that solution toward the circuit's opposite pole are referred to as the *volume currents*. These currents correspond to extracellular currents that flow within the cerebrospinal fluid throughout the intracranial space. Because the skull has very high electric resistance, volume currents flow through the orbits of the eyes and other openings in the skull into the scalp, where they create the potential differences that underlie the electroencephalogram (EEG). The magnetic fields surrounding the neurons pass undisturbed through the skull to produce the magnetoencephalogram (MEG).

Both the volume currents and the intracellular ionic currents are depicted schematically in Fig. 1.1. In this instance, we assume that the source of the magnetic field **B** is a segment of current that is very small relative to the distance at which the field is measured. Hence, it is possible to model it as an *equivalent current dipole* (ECD). Because magnetic fields are superimposable (i.e., they are additive and do not interact with each other), extracranial fields do not arise from a single neuron but actually represent the sum of the fields of many similarly oriented hypercolumns of concurrently active cortical cells.

In Fig. 1.1, $\mathbf{Q} = I \times \vec{L}$, where $I$ is the amplitude of the current and $\vec{L}$ is the length and direction of the current segment. Because the dipole has both direction and strength, **Q** is a vector quantity representing the strength of the dipole in ampere–meters (the dipole's *moment*). The volume current also varies in strength and direction. The symbol $\mathbf{J^V}$ indicates that the value of the direction and strength of the volume current depends on the position at which it is measured.

All moving electric charges are accompanied by magnetic fields. Because the volume currents are composed of moving electric charges, these too must be accompanied by magnetic fields. However, when the dipole is immersed in an infinitely large volume (or in a finite sphere), the direc-

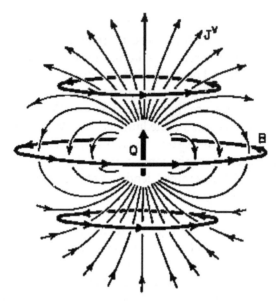

FIG. 1.1.   A current dipole immersed in a homogeneous conducting medium. The magnetic field (**B**) is due solely to the current dipole (moment = Q), with the volume currents (represented by the thin lines [J$^v$]) making no contribution to the field.

tion of the field associated with an ion at one place and time is opposite from that associated with ions at other places at the same time. Therefore, the fields of these oppositely directed moving charges cancel each other out, that is, the sum of the fields of the volume current measured at some distant point is effectively zero. Thus, the field measured at a distance is due solely to the net primary current, which is largely associated with postsynaptic dendritic potential changes.

A distinction is often made between *open-field* and *closed-field* neurons. The latter are so designated because their dendritic trees are approximately symmetrical in three dimensions. Because of their morphological symmetry, these cells are presumed to contribute little to either electric or magnetic fields detected some distance away, because the net electric and magnetic fields produced by symmetric current distributions are zero. For example, basket cells are sometimes described as closed-field cells. On the other hand, pyramidal cells are prototypical open-field neurons, because their apical dendrites incorporate one-dimensional elongated processes. Ionic currents within these dendrites are excellent candidate sources of external fields and potentials. However, one must bear in mind that cell morphology alone does not determine whether a cell's magnetic field is detectable at a distance. For a cell with a symmetric dendritic tree, there could still be an asymmetric distribution of primary current (e.g., due to asymmetric presynaptic activities) and therefore a field that can be detected at a distance. Thus, although the literature often implies that pyramidal cells are the sole sources of external fields, this claim has not been proved. For example, stellate cells do not have elongated dendrites. They, and not pyramidal cells, are predominant in the visual cortex. Yet some of the strongest MEG (and EEG) signals arise from the visual cortex.

As already noted, the volume currents flowing in the dermis of the scalp create the potential differences that underlie the EEG. Brain tissue and the fluid filling the subarachnoid space are relatively good conductors, especially as compared with the skull, which is highly resistive. These anisotropies in conductivity must be taken into account in attempts to identify the neural sources of scalp-detected potentials (Nunez, 1981). The difficulties in locating neural sources of EEG/event-related potential (ERP) are further compounded by the fact that the skull and other tissues are relatively asymmetrical, so that the paths of flowing volume currents are also asymmetrical. Finally, in measuring the EEG (as well as the ERPs considered later), one must use a reference or ground electrode. This is never a truly indifferent electrode, as it is affected by activity of the brain at regions that may be far from the "active" electrode. One must take this into account in interpreting a pattern of potentials across the scalp. Despite these factors, the EEG is capable of providing vital information regarding the linkage between particular scalp-detected phenomena and underlying process. For example, the presence of the classic spike and wave in the EEG may be diagnostic of epilepsy, even though sometimes it is not possible to accurately determine the location of the lesion responsible for seizures. To take another example, despite early controversy regarding the source of the N100 component of the *auditory-evoked potential* (AEP), this component proved to be a useful candidate for the study of attention.

To summarize, the scalp is "transparent" to magnetic fields (see chap. 2, this volume) but not to the electric potential produced by the brain. This makes interpretation of MEG a much simpler problem than that of EEG. Even though many recent ERP localization methods attempt to take account of these conductivity problems by using sophisticated volume conductor models of the head, ERP source localization is still a very difficult problem. A good example is in the study of N100, a relatively negative voltage peak (component) in the AEP that occurs about 100 msec after the onset of an acoustic stimulus. (In the MEG literature, the magnetic counterpart to N100 is often referred to as *M100*.) The AEP is normally detected at a midline electrode (at the vertex). As explained in chapter 9 of this volume, the sources of this component lie within the auditory cortex of each of two hemispheres. MEG experiments have revealed that at least two (and probably more) sources in each hemisphere underlie N100. The sources in the two hemispheres differ in strength and are affected somewhat differently by attention to tonal stimuli (Curtis, Kaufman, & Williamson, 1988). The many published AEP studies do not report this asymmetry. Similarly, auditory evoked fields (AEFs) in response to tones of different pitch have sources that occupy different positions along the auditory cortex. The tonotopic organization of the human auditory cortex was first revealed in MEG experiments (Romani, Williamson, & Kaufman, 1982). The tonotopic organization of the human auditory cortex is described by Cosimo Del Gratta and Gian Luca Romani in chapter 10. Other imaging modalities have confirmed this finding. For example, single photon emission tomography has revealed a similar organization of the human auditory cortex (Ottaviani et al., 1997). Similar findings were obtained using functional magnetic resonance imaging (fMRI; Wessinger, Buonocore, Kussmaul, & Mangun, 1997).

Thus far, even after 20 years, this property of the auditory cortex has not been revealed in any AEP study, although an experiment with indwelling electrodes has confirmed the finding (Liegeois-Chauvel et al., 2001). So, even though the ultimate sources of the AEP and the AEF are the same, the two types of measures (MEG and EEG) differ in certain vital respects. We now make these differences clear.

## Effect of Source Orientation

For the present it is useful to represent the sources of the MEG and EEG as equivalent current dipoles. Let us assume that the volume currents associated with an ECD underlie the EEG, and the field surrounding the ECD is a source of the MEG.

Many early MEG studies made the simplifying assumption that the head may be represented by a sphere the radius of which is approximately the same as the radius of curvature of the skull over which neuromagnetic measurements are made. As we shall see, this practice is beginning to give way to one in which more realistic head shapes are used (see chap. 3). For the sake of clarity, however, we stay with the older and still widely applied practice.

The sphere in Fig. 1.2a is 20 cm in diameter, and a current dipole is located 4 cm beneath its surface. It is very important to note that the current dipole is oriented at a right angle to a radius, that is, it is oriented tangentially with respect to the surface of the sphere. In practice, the field is measured simultaneously at many points about the sphere's surface. Each pickup coil of the *neuromagnetometer* used to detect the field is also oriented tangentially with respect to the surface. Therefore, it senses the radial component of the field, not its tangential component. Note that the radial component of the field is associated with the tangential component of the dipole moment; the tangential component of the field is associated with the radial component of the dipole moment. It is customary to project these measurements onto a planar surface, which in this example has an area of 22.4 cm × 22.4 cm.

The radial component of the field is directed either outward or inward with respect to the surface of the sphere and does not include the component tangential to the surface. The strength of this radial component of the field varies with the place of measurement and is represented by the *isofield contours* shown in Fig. 1.2b. These isofield contours form a typical *dipolar field pattern*. It contains one region where the emerging field is at its maximum and another where the re-entering field is at its maximum. The centers of these regions are labeled *field extrema*. As one moves along a line defining the shortest path connecting these two extrema, a point is reached where the strength of the radial component of the field is zero. This zero point is precisely halfway between the field extrema. Moreover, the ECD lies directly under this point. Because our hypothetical

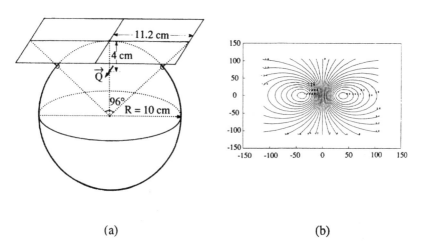

(a)                                    (b)

FIG. 1.2.    Panel (a): schematic of a current dipole 4 cm beneath the surface of a 10-cm radius sphere. The radial component of the field is projected onto the surface of a rectangle tangential to the sphere. The center of the rectangle is directly over the point dipole. Panel (b): the isofield contour plot on the surface of the rectangle. The contours represent the relative radial field strengths in arbitrary units.

measurements are restricted to the radial component of the field, the radial component has a value of zero halfway between the two extrema. As a matter of fact, the depth of an ECD lying directly beneath this halfway point is easily computed from the distance separating the field extrema on the surface of the scalp and the radius of the sphere that best fits the scalp on which those extrema are found. This insight made it possible to establish the tonotopic progression of sources along the auditory cortex (Romani et al., 1982).

Assuming that an ECD is 4 cm beneath the surface of a 10-cm radius sphere and oriented tangentially with respect to its surface (Fig. 1.2A), the relative strengths of the emerging and re-entering components of the field were computed. The isofield contours of Fig. 1.2B were then plotted. The computation is based on Equations 1.1 and 1.2.

$$\overrightarrow{B_{\vec{r}}} = \frac{\mu_0}{4_\pi} \frac{\vec{Q} \times (\vec{r} - \vec{r_0})}{|\vec{r} - \vec{r_0}|^3} \tag{1.1}$$

where $\overrightarrow{B\vec{r}}$ = the field at a point $\vec{r}$ in space, $\vec{r}_0$ = the vector from the center of the sphere to the dipole, $\vec{Q}$ = the current dipole moment, and $\mu_0$ = the permeability of free space. Because the isofield contours of Fig. 1.2 represent only the strengths of the radial component of the field at the surface of the sphere, that component, $\vec{B}$ $(\overrightarrow{B_n})$, is simply the dot product

$$\overrightarrow{B_n} = \vec{B} \cdot \vec{r} / |\vec{r}| . \tag{1.2}$$

If the dipole shown inside the sphere of Fig. 1.2 were tilted so that it is no longer tangential to the surface of the sphere, it could be described as being composed of two components, one oriented tangentially and the other radially. Ultimately, as the tilt increases, the dipole has no tangential component, because it is aligned with a radius extending from the center of the sphere to its surface. As the ECD is tilted from its initial tangential orientation, the dipolar field pattern at the surface simply diminishes in intensity. When the dipole's orientation is entirely radial, no radial field can be detected at the sphere's surface. It is interesting to note that the field pattern does not shift in position even as its intensity diminishes throughout the time that the dipole is rotating. The dipole would still lie directly beneath the point bisecting the distance between the field extrema. In other words, if the conductive volume is perfectly spherical, then measures at the surface of the sphere are sensitive only to the tangential component of the current dipole moment and not to the radial component of the current dipole moment.

The electric potential distribution across the spherical surface has different properties. As already indicated, the volume currents that accompany the current dipole produce potential differences across the surface of the sphere. These may be represented by *isopotential* contours similar in appearance to the dipolar pattern of the isofield contours described earlier. (In attempts to achieve a more realistic model of the human head, three or four concentric spheres representing layers of different conductivity replace the single sphere shown in Fig. 1.2. These different layers result in a spreading or blurring of the isopotential contours, but it remains essentially dipolar when the underlying dipole is tangential to the scalp.) The most significant difference between the isofield and isopotential contours in this simple example is that the latter are rotated 90° on the projection plane with respect to the former. However, as the dipole is tilted from its tangential orientation, the positions of the isopotential contours shift and become asymmetrical. The potential at the extremum associated with the more distal (deeper) end of the underlying dipole grows weaker, while the extremum associated with the opposite pole (which is closer to the surface) grows stronger. The latter extremum migrates toward a point directly over the dipole, while the opposed extremum moves away from that point. Finally, when the dipole is oriented along a radius of the sphere, there is only one extremum on the surface. Of course, asymmetrical differences in conductivity within the head would result in greater differences between the patterns of isofield and isopotential contours.

The distinction between radial and tangential ECDs is important. For example, if the MEG represents tangential sources and the EEG represents both tangential and radial sources, it may be possible to subtract MEG data from some transform of EEG data and obtain an "image" of the radial sources. It is widely accepted that the radial sources dwell in the gyri of the cortex, while the tangential sources are to be found in the sulci. This could have obvious advantages.

Despite widespread recognition of this possibility, one must be circumspect with regard to its actual promise. For one thing, real sources of electric and magnetic fields in the brain are not point current dipoles; they are assemblies of many concurrently active neurons. Lu and Williamson (1991) estimated that the typical cortical area involved in coherent sensory-evoked responses is about 80–100 $mm^2$. A hypercolumn is composed of about 30,000 neurons, and several of these hypercolumns must be active if they are to produce a detectable field or a detectable difference in scalp potential. All neurons are bent, so any hypercolumn, even if it is largely normal to the surface of a gyrus, contains both radial and tangential components. Consequently, neurons in gyri will produce extracranial dipolar field patterns, although these are likely to be very much weaker than if the same arrays of neurons were in the walls of a sulcus. Similarly, columns of neurons oriented approximately normal to the surface of a sulcus will have radial as well as tangential components. Hence, neurons in a sulcus may well contribute to the ostensibly "monopolar" isopotential patterns on the scalp associated with radially oriented sources. Hence, with sufficiently sensitive instruments, sources in gyruses would be detected in extracranial fields.

Although we emphasize that the skull is not a sphere, some truly remarkable results were achieved with the skull modeled as a best-fitting sphere (e.g., Romani et al., 1982). It is worthwhile to consider why this is the case.

The early assumption that the skull and scalp do not distort magnetic fields is now confirmed. The fields that emerge from and re-enter the skull are not altered by the presence of the skull and scalp (see chap. 2). Hence, one can effectively ignore the physical skull and scalp when measuring the radial component of the neuromagnetic field. Today, large arrays of detectors are usually arranged to fit the spherical surface of the tail section of the cryogenic dewars of neuromagnetometers. The fields penetrate this tail section without distortion. The surface of the tail section of the dewar is placed so that it is concentric with a sphere that best fits the head. The skull may not be perfectly concentric with the spherical array of sensors; hence, the measured field may include some contribution by the tangential field component. In effect, this introduces an error in the measured magnitude of the field. However, the position of a virtual current dipole placed at a known location in a model of a head can be determined with an accuracy of about 2 mm (Yamamoto, Williamson, Kaufman, Nicholson, & Llinas, 1988). Apparently, assuming that the head is spherical is not necessarily a major source of error in evaluating MEG data. This is not the case for the EEG, and one should consider this potential mismatch when attempting joint use of EEG and MEG data.

In a real head, a sphere with a particular radius of curvature may be a nearly perfect match to the curvature of the skull lying immediately above a current dipole source. The source may be radially oriented with respect to that particular sphere. However, the radii of curvature of adjacent regions of the skull may be different; hence, the same dipole is not exclusively radial in orientation with respect to those segments of the skull. It is obvious that a realistic head shape makes the distinction between radially and tangentially oriented dipoles somewhat ambiguous. Therefore, it is important to evaluate how realistic head shapes affect the measured electric and magnetic fields (see chap. 3).

## MEASURING THE NEUROMAGNETIC FIELD

Ions flowing within neurons are surrounded by magnetic fields. Thus, intracellular ionic currents result in magnetic fields that surround neurons. Fields of different neurons do not interact with each other. Therefore, the measured field at a point in space is simply the sum of the fields contributed by each neuron. Because the field strength varies inversely with the square of the distance from a small (current dipole) source, a field measured at a point outside the human scalp would reflect the activity of relatively nearby neurons and be largely uncontaminated by fields of very distant neurons. As we shall see, suitably sensitive instruments make it possible to detect such fields of the brain. Thus far we have discussed fields associated with very simple sources, that is, ECDs immersed in a conducting solution enclosed by a nonconducting spherelike skull. Before turning to more realistic situations, we should introduce the methods used to measure the neuromagnetic field.

Fig. 1.3 is a schematic representation of a single-channel system that was used to measure the brain's neuromagnetc field. (It is important to note that existing systems use a very large number of sensors, and the single-channel shown here corresponds to only one of those sensors [see chaps. 7 and 8].) In Fig. 1.3, a magnetic field is shown emerging from one region of of a subject's skull and re-entering a nearby region. The isofield contours represent those places where the emerging and re-entering fields have lesser values than the fields at the two extrema. The purpose is to measure the component of the field normal to the scalp at each of many positions.

The fields in question are extremely weak (about 50 femto Tesla), being on the order of 1 billionth the strength of the earth's steady field ($= 50$ micro Tesla), which is weaker than the fields of manmade magnets and motors as well as those associated with vibrating steel building frames and other urban sources of electromagnetic fields. This requires the use of an exquisitely sensitive instrument with a low intrinsic noise level and also capable of discriminating against extraneous magnetic fields. The sensitivity is provided by a device known as a *SQUID* (*superconducting*

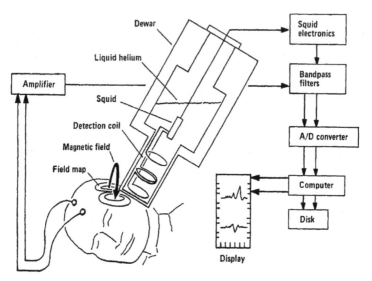

FIG. 1.3. Schematic of a single-channel neuromagnetometer measuring the brain's magnetic field. SQUID = superconducting quantum interference device.

*qu*antum *i*nterference *d*evice), which operates at the temperature of liquid helium (4.2° K). Fig. 1.3 depicts a SQUID contained within a cryogenic *dewar* where it is immersed in liquid helium, along with other components. The field emerging from and re-entering the skull is undistorted as it passes through the bottom of the tail section of the dewar.

In Fig. 1.3 the field from the brain is sensed by the bottom-most (detection) coil of a set of coils within the tail section of the dewar. The complete set of coils (sometimes referred to as a *flux transporter*) is composed of a superconducting material such as niobium, which, at very low temperatures, has no resistance at all to the flow of an electric current. This particular configuration of coils is referred to as a *second-order gradiometer.* Roughly, this is how it works: Assume that we have a single coil of superconducting material in the dewar. If a magnet is nearby when liquid helium is poured over the coil (so that the loop enters the superconducting state), a current will continue to flow in the coil even after the magnet is removed. This current traps the enclosed magnetic flux (the *Meisner effect*). When the external magnetic field is changed, the current changes as well, to keep the trapped flux constant. Hence, the single coil may function as a *magnetometer* in the sense that monitoring the current flow is equivalent to measuring the applied magnetic field. However, since the magnetometer measures field per se, it is affected by fields from distant as well as nearby sources. The multiple coils shown in Fig. 1.3 are wound in series with each other and also act to keep the trapped flux constant. However, this configuration is relatively insensitive to changes in fields from distant sources.

When a field is stronger near the bottom-most detection coil, the current flow will change in the entire gradiometer. In this case the detection coil is wound clockwise, while the next higher coil is wound counterclockwise. In fact, all adjacent coils are wound in opposition to each other. Thus, when placed in a uniform field the currents made to flow in these coils would cancel each other out. Because this gradiometer is composed of four loops (to form a *second-order gradiometer*), the application of a field with a uniform gradient would also result in self-cancellation of any effect. By contrast, the magnetometer (sometimes referred to as a *zero-order gradiometer*) responds to both uniform fields and fields with uniform spatial gradients. Fields of distant sources tend to have uniform spatial gradients. However, a nonuniform field (one with high spatial derivatives, as shown in the figure) has a stronger effect on the bottom-most coil, and this leads to a net change in current flow within the entire gradiometer.

This property of second-order gradiometers makes them relatively insensitive to fields associated with distant sources. In effect, the operation of a gradiometer (as opposed to a simple *magnetometer,* which is composed of a single coil of superconducting material) is analogous to the common-mode rejection of noise that is made possible by bipolar electrodes in EEG recordings. A *third-order gradiometer*, which is composed of even more coils, is even less sensitive to uniform fields as well as fields with moderate spatial gradients. In fact, a well-balanced second- or third-order gradiometer makes it possible to measure weak neuromagnetic fields in many unshielded environments despite the presence of ambient magnetic fields (see chap. 7). However, to gain maximum sensitivity to signals of interest, for some purposes the dewar and the human subject or patient are usually placed within a magnetically shielded room.

The SQUID never "sees" the external field it is trying to measure. It is isolated within a superconducting shield inside the dewar, effectively isolating it from the environment. However, the gradiometer includes a very small *signal coil* wound in series with all of the other coils. Unlike the other coils, the signal coil is located inside the superconducting shield along with the SQUID. In fact, the only contact the SQUID has with the outside world is through the signal coil. Whenever a field is applied to the detection coil so that current flows throughout the gradiometer, the

SQUID detects the current flowing in the signal coil, because that current is accompanied by its own magnetic field.

To describe this in more detail would distract us from our main objective. It suffices to say that the detection coils "sense" the magnetic field near the scalp, the signal coils "transmit" the currents in the detection coils to the SQUID, and the SQUID "converts" the currents in the signal coils to voltages that can be amplified and recorded by conventional electronic devices. The voltages are directly proportional to the magnetic field strength near the scalp. The single-channel system described here is based on the system designed and constructed by Brenner, Williamson, and Kaufman (1975) and used to detect the first evoked neuromagnetic field in an unshielded environment. However, as intimated earlier, this has been superseded by systems containing 200 or more SQUIDs. Also, the SQUIDs in use today are far more sensitive than the original SQUID and may be used with very different gradiometer configurations. For example, a gradiometer composed of several superconducting coils in a single plane may be used to sample differences in the radial field across the surface of the scalp. Such a configuration is described in some detail in chapter 9. Also, today sophisticated software is used to process signals from simple magnetometers to emulate different gradiometer configurations. Various whole-head systems are described in chapters 7–9.

Measuring the field at many places simultaneously permits identification of sources of neuromagnetic fields within the brain, thus overcoming one major problem. Early investigators had to assume that the source does not change from one measurement to another as a single-channel system is moved to sample the field at many different positions above the scalp. It is no longer necessary to make such an assumption.

## EVENT-RELATED BRAIN ACTIVITY

It is obvious that the signals actually detected by neuromagnetometers are not produced by isolated current dipoles floating around in conducting solutions within spherical heads. However, in keeping with the didactic motive of this chapter, we approach more realistic situations slowly and in the process show why an elementaristic approach using spherical head models and point current dipoles has real value. We begin by considering Fig. 1.4.

It has been known for many years that activity in the brain stem may be evoked by acoustic stimuli and picked up by scalp electrodes. The ex-

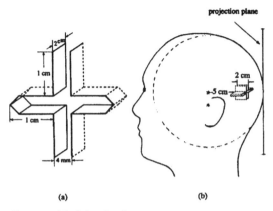

FIG. 1.4.   Cruciform model of the visual cortex.

tremely weak auditory brain stem evoked responses begin to appear about 2 msec after the onset of stimulation and run their courses before much stronger responses of the auditory cortex are picked up. On occasion, the latter are seen after a single stimulus event and are certainly strong enough to be detected reliably after averaging a few dozen trials. However, the brain stem activity must be averaged over several thousand trials to be detected. With the exception of this type of brain stem activity, most brain activity seen in the EEG or the MEG originates in the dendrites of cells of the cerebral cortex—in the gray matter of the brain (see chap. 12 for examples of signals that may well be attributable to fields associated with spike potentials). As we shall see, this is enormously helpful in determining the approximate location in the brain of the sources of observed evoked magnetic fields.

The cortex of each hemisphere may be thought of as a two-dimensional but highly rumpled (convoluted) sheet of neural tissue. Although it is about 2 mm thick, this thickness is negligible when fields are measured at a distance. It is useful to think of this two-dimensional sheet as populated by a very large number of dipolar sources, all oriented normal to its surface. (We conducted computer simulations in which the individual dipoles of a large array are randomly tilted by as much as 45° from the normal. The summed isofield contours describing the radial component of magnetic fields at the surface of a spherical skull are essentially the same as when all of the dipoles are normal to the surface.) Of course, the dipoles represent aggregates of cells.

The cerebral cortex contains approximately 10 billion cells. Even if the cells were independent of each other, on occasion, by chance alone, ionic currents within significant numbers of them would flow in the same direction at the same time. We refer to this as *synchronization*. In many instances this synchronization is initiated by some external or internal event. Where the initiating external event is a sensory stimulus—for example, a flash of light—we refer to a *sensory-evoked response*. Where the sensory stimulus results in the flow of current within a sufficient number of neighboring columns of cells within the same window of time (the activity need not start or end at precisely the same time), then it may be possible to pick up either an evoked potential or an evoked field. It has been estimated that something on the order of 100,000 concurrently active cells may be sufficient to produce a detectable extracranial neuromagnetic field. The visual cortex is a useful example. The central $2°$ of the retina (the *fovea*) is known to affect roughly 25% of the entire primary visual cortex (Brodmann's area 17). It is worth noting that the diameter of the entire fovea corresponds to a ~0.5-mm diameter image of a disk on the retina. This small patch of light centered on the retina could affect much of the occipital pole as well as a large area extending deeply into the longitudinal fissure, including the calcarine fissure. If the same small patch of light were moved away from the fovea and into the peripheral visual field, it would affect a very rapidly decreasing proportion of the cortex extending into the longitudinal fissure. The shape of the visual cortex is schematized in Fig. 1.4. This crosslike shape is sometimes referred to as the *cruciform model* of visual cortex. The calcarine fissure represents the arms of the cross, and the longitudinal fissure is the space between the two halves of the cross. Real brains lack this degree of symmetry, but the model is useful in several respects. First, it helps in explaining the retinotopic organization of the visual cortex and, second, it clearly illustrates how the shape of the brain might affect its observed neuromagnetic field.

Figure 1.5 illustrates how different regions of the visual cortex are excited when appropriate stimuli are placed in different quadrants of the visual field. The neurons of the cerebral cortex are arranged in columns oriented normally to its surface, so activation of the lower left quadrant of the cruciform model must result in a net flow of current either inward (away from the surface) or outward. Thus, it is possible to activate a rather large area of the cortex merely by presenting a moving or flashing pattern in an appropriate retinal location. The vast majority of columns of cells in these activated areas may be conducting current in the same direction at more or less the same time. Intuitively, this source of evoked activity is a far cry from a point current dipole.

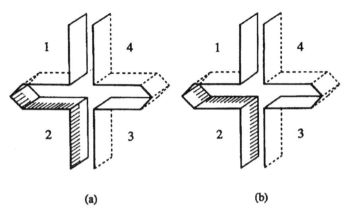

FIG. 1.5. A simulation in which the upper right quadrant of the visual field activates cortical cells of the lower left quadrant of the cruciform visual cortex. The shaded region in Panel (a) lies closer to the occipital pole and illustrates a possible distribution of activity evoked by stimulation in the upper right quadrant of the fovea. As the stimulus is moved away from the fovea and farther into the peripheral field, the depth of activity along the cortex shifts inward, as indicated by the greater depth of activity signified by the shaded area of Panel (b). The dipoles (columns of cells) in the shaded areas are oriented normal to the surface of the cortex.

The unshaded areas of cortex are also active. The cells in the unshaded areas are synchronized with each other by chance alone. For our purposes we may assume that the columns of cells filling the unshaded regions are randomly active; that is, the direction and magnitude of net current flow in one column cannot be predicted from that of its near neighbors. In point of fact, at any instant of time this random activity effectively masks the more coherent activity of the columns within the shaded areas. This explains why *signal averaging,* or some other method for enhancing signals relative to "noise," is needed to recover evoked fields and potentials.

Kaufman, Kaufman, and Wang (1991) computed the isofield patterns associated with synchronized activation within the shaded areas shown in Fig. 1.5. Specifically, they assumed that the shaded areas covered many dipoles, all oriented normal to the shaded surface. The only difference between Fig. 1.5a and Fig. 1.5b is that the shaded area in the latter is 1 cm deeper than the similar shaded area of Fig. 1.5a. The magnitudes of these dipoles were randomized, but their directions were the same, signifying that they are all synchronized with each other. In this simulation the large unshaded areas of the entire cruciform cortex were populated by unsynchronized dipoles, that is, dipoles whose moments were all randomized. On average, the magnitude of current flowing in the synchronized dipoles was the same as that in the unsynchronized dipoles, although different values were selected at random every time the field at the surface of the skull was sampled. Overall, in this simulation the cruciform cortex was populated with 1,386 current dipoles. By superposition, the radial component of the field at the surface of the spherical head due to all of the dipoles was computed at 841 points, and these were plotted to form the isofield contour plots projected onto a plane. Several such plots are shown in Fig. 1.6. One hundred plots were computed to illustrate how the pattern of isofield contours changes because of random contributions by the asynchronous dipoles.

The asymmetries of the two lefthand isofield contour plots in Fig. 1.6a and Fig. 1.6b are due to random contributions by the dipoles that populate the unshaded walls of the cruciform cortex. These asymmetries cannot be accounted for by assuming that a single current dipole underlies the ob-

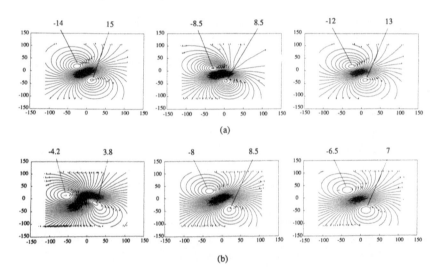

FIG. 1.6.    Isofield contour plots associated with activation of a large number of current dipoles oriented normal to the surface of the cruciform cortex. The three plots in the upper row (Panel [a]) of the figure are based on synchronized activity in the outermost shaded area illustrated in Fig. 1.5. The two plots on the left side of (a) were selected at random from 100 such plots, where each corresponds to a different set of dipole moments. These 100 plots were averaged to produce the third plot on the right of (a). Note that the average values of the field extrema in this plot differ in magnitude from the two to its left. Also, the plots on the left are not as symmetrical as the average plot. The latter is best fit by the field that would be produced by a single equivalent current dipole. The relatively asymmetrical patterns on the left reflect contributions of dipoles dwelling in the unshaded portions of the cortex. Some subset of these dipoles would be synchronized with the evoking stimulus by chance alone. The three lower plots (Panel [b]) are based on synchronization of the (1-cm) deeper shaded area of Fig. 1.5b. Here, too, the single "trial" plots to the left are asymmetrical and differ in orientation and magnitude from each other and from the average plot on the right. Note that the space separating the average field extrema in (b) is wider than that of the righthand plot of (a).

served field. Instead, a much better fit is achieved when one assumes that multiple dipoles contribute to the field. However, this pattern changes from one set of measurements to another. Averaging sharply reduces this variability, because the randomly varying moments of the dipoles that populate the unshaded regions tend to be self-canceling when their fields are averaged, and the resulting plot is a much closer fit to the pattern that would be produced by a single equivalent current dipole. Hence, a field pattern produced by hundreds or even thousands of dipoles can easily be confused with a pattern produced by a single equivalent current dipole.

### Comments on Signal Averaging

Readers who are familiar with signal averaging may choose to skip this section, but several of its passages may prove to be worth scanning. Some subtle and frequently overlooked assumptions underlie this simple procedure for recovering signals from noise, and it is good to keep them in mind. For example, if the so-called "signal" (the event-related response) is not independent of ongoing asynchronous activity of the brain, then averaging can lead one to discard important data along with the noise. This is quite relevant to our discussion of spontaneous brain activity.

Figure 1.6 provides a demonstration of the effects of signal averaging. Isofield contour plots similar to those shown in Fig. 1.6 can be thought of as instantaneous maps of the field obtained by many sensors at once. One hundred such maps were generated as follows: One hundred independent sets of random numbers were generated to represent the current dipole moments (directions of current flow and their magnitudes) of all the dipoles in the unshaded areas of Fig. 1.5. This is the region that is assumed to be unaffected by the presentation of a stimulus. Similarly, the dipoles under the shaded areas were also represented by 100 independent sets of random numbers, but these represent only their magnitudes, as the direction of current flow was the same for all of the dipoles. The commonality of direction of current flow in this region is assumed to be due to the action of a stimulus or event that has the effect of synchronizing the neurons within the shaded regions. All of these values were used to compute the fields represented by 100 different isofield contour maps, represented by the samples in Fig. 1.6. The 100 contour maps derived from the more shallow shaded area were then averaged to create the plot on the upper right side of the figure. Similarly, another 100 maps were averaged to create the lower plot on the same side of the figure. This averaging process reveals a contour plot largely due to the synchronized activity of the neurons under the shaded patch of the cortex. The cortex is normally active, regardless of whether a stimulus is present. Therefore, a sensor placed above the occipital cortex will detect a magnetic field at all times. Because of the asynchronous activity of the neurons that contribute to this field, its direction and strength will be different from time to time. However, when the field is repeatedly measured at a fixed time after the presentation of a stimulus, the field due to asynchronous activity will tend to be self-canceling, whereas averaging will reveal the synchronized activity evoked by the stimulus. Activity time-locked to the stimulus will increase arithmetically with the number of samples taken, whereas the presumably Gaussian background noise (due to the asynchronous activity, instrumentation noise, and ambient noise) will increase only as the square root of the number of samples. Although in realistic situations the background noise on a single trial is much greater in magnitude than the evoked response, when a sufficient number of samples enter the average, the evoked response ultimately becomes significantly larger in amplitude than the noise. All of this assumes that the noise is independent of the evoked response. Much of the literature tacitly assumes that a change in voltage or field that is time locked to the evoking event is the only relevant consequence of stimulation. As we shall see, this assumption is often invalid.

## Are Event-Related Voltages and Fields Independent of Brain Noise?

The logic underlying this section is quite simple. We begin by assuming that neural tissue is active regardless of whether a particular external stimulus is presented. The activity may be due to intrinsic biochemical changes, activity originating in the thalamus and transmitted to the cortex, or any of several possible conditions. The external stimulus, on reaching the cortex, may well interrupt or alter this ongoing activity. Hence, if the stimulus causes the current flow within a neuronal population to be synchronized, it may also either add to (or subtract from) the ongoing activity. If the evoked activity merely adds linearly to the ongoing activity, then, in effect, it is independent of that activity, and the time-locked response is the only consequence of stimulation. However, if the level of activity of the affected neurons is not the linear sum of the ongoing activity and of the evoked activity, then consequences of stimulation may not be detectible in the averaged response.

***Linear and Nonlinear Systems.***    Any system, whether it is an electronic circuit or a portion of the nervous system, can be described as being either a *linear system* or as a *nonlinear system*. If two signals are applied concurrently to a linear system, the output of that system is equal to the sum of the outputs of the same system to the same inputs presented at different times. In this case, we say that the *superposition principle* applies to the system. When the superposition principle does not apply, we say that the system is nonlinear.

If a sinusoidally varying signal is applied to a linear system, then its output will be a sinusoid at the same frequency as the input. Although the amplitude of the output may not be uniform for inputs of different frequency, a linear system always responds at the same frequency as that of the input. It has been known for some time that visual responses evoked by sinusoidally modulated light often occur at twice the frequency of the stimulus. Any system that responds to an input of one frequency with an output of another frequency is necessarily nonlinear.

Figure 1.7 explains how frequency doubling occurs in the case of one nonlinear system. In this case, the output of the system is the square of the input. (The same is true if the output is proportional to the square of the input, except that the proportionality constant defines the amplification afforded by the system.) Thus, where the input is $a \sin \omega t$, the output

$$Y_{output} = (a^2 \sin^2 \omega t) \ . \tag{1.3}$$

From elementary trigonometry,

$$A^2 \sin^2 \omega t = a/2 - a/2 \cos 2\omega t \ . \tag{1.4}$$

As in Fig. 1.7, this demonstrates that, when squared by a nonlinear system, a sinusoidal input (frequency $= \omega t$) with amplitude $a$ results in an output at twice the frequency of the input ($2\omega t$) and one half the amplitude of that frequency. Furthermore, the output has a Fourier component which, in this case, has an amplitude $a/2$ and a frequency of zero (a *dc* component).

Squaring is not the only form of nonlinearity. For example, many biological systems transform an input stimulus so that the response of the system is approximately proportional to the logarithm of the stimulus.

The output of such a system to a sinusoidal signal oscillating about an average value of zero (as in Fig. 1.8) contains a *dc* offset and odd harmonics of the frequency of the input. Similarly, systems that clip the

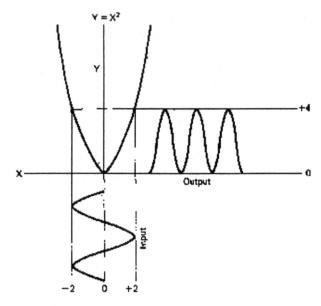

FIG. 1.7.    Effect of applying a sine wave (input) to a device whose output is the square of the input. The graph represents the equation $Y = X^2$. Note that the sinusoidal input has a mean value of zero and, in arbitrary units, its amplitude peaks at 2 and −2. The output amplitude peaks at 4 and 0, so it happens to be the same (4 units) as that of the input. However, the average of the squared output is one half the peak-to-peak amplitude, and the output contains a sine wave.

smoothly varying positive and negative peaks of sine wave inputs also generate odd harmonics.

Half-wave rectifiers are sometimes referred to as *linear rectifiers*. These are not linear at all; rather, their outputs represent only the positive (or negative) peaks of sinusoidal inputs, and these too contain odd harmonics of the input. In general, the relative amplitudes of these harmonics depend on the nature of the nonlinearity and on whether the input signal is a simple sine wave or if it can be represented as the modulation of a steady *dc* signal. In fact, if the *dc* component of the input is large relative to its sinusoidal modulation, the effect of the existing nonlinearity may become negligible. Incidentally, this is one of the main reasons why researchers studying the response of the visual system to sinusoidally modulated light may use a near-threshold degree of modulation of a steady light as a stimulus. Despite its inherent nonlinearity, when presented with such a stimulus the visual system is approximately linear in its behavior. It is said that real eyes evolved to deal with large-scale changes in

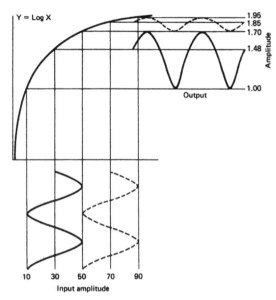

FIG. 1.8. The output of this nonlinear system is proportional to the logarithm of its input. As demonstrated here, a sinusoidal input is distorted by the system so that its output is not a pure sine wave. In this case the distortion is most obvious when the input is low (solid line) and less obvious when the input rides on a high *dc* (dashed line). This is one reason why vision researchers superimpose a sinusoidal variation in light level on a *dc* "pedestal."

visual stimulation, so allowing for effects of nearly pervasive nonlinearity is essential to understanding the perceptual process.

Nonlinearities exemplified by different kinds of rectification—for example, square law—have quite different effects from those attributable to saturation, for example, when a sensory stimulus is so intense that an otherwise linear system ceases to respond to additional increases in its intensity. We do not consider such effects here except to say that in some evoked-response experiments investigators fail to use a range of stimulus intensities—for example, contrast or loudness—that include very low values as well as high ones. This is the only way to determine if the observed responses are influenced by saturation nonlinearities rather than some other ostensible cause.

***Interactions of Signals at Different Frequencies.*** Thus far we have not dealt directly with the interaction between the response of the brain and its ongoing activity. It is easier to understand how such an interaction may come about by describing what happens when two signals of different frequencies are applied concurrently to the same nonlinear system. As stated earlier, in a linear system the response to concurrent stimuli is the same as sum of the responses to the two stimuli applied separately. It is extremely important to note that even if the brain as a whole were essentially nonlinear, if the two stimuli were to affect different regions so that no interaction is possible, then the response would also be the same as the sum of the responses to the two stimuli when applied separately. In chapter 5, Regan and Regan exploit this distinction to gain insight into how signals are parsed by the sensory systems. For now we deal only with the case where two different signals are applied concurrently to the same nonlinear system.

Suppose that lights are modulated at two different frequencies, and the frequency of one is not a harmonic of the other. For example, one light is modulated at 7 Hz and the other at 10 Hz. Both lights are imaged in the same place on the retina. When a signal-averaging computer is time locked to a signal at 7 Hz, then a response is usually recovered at that frequency or, on occasion, at its second harmonic, that is, 14 Hz. Similarly, when time locked to the concurrently presented 10-Hz stimulus, a response is recovered at 10 Hz and at its second harmonic, that is, 20 Hz. It is interesting to note that when the 7-Hz and 10-Hz signals that drive the two stimuli are multiplied, the output of the multiplier does not contain signals at either 10 Hz or 7 Hz. Rather, the output is at 3 Hz (the difference between 7 and 10 Hz—the so-called *difference frequency*) and at 17 Hz (the *sum frequency*). If the output of the multiplier were applied to a signal-averaging computer time locked to either of the original 7- and 10-Hz inputs to the multiplier, the averaging computer would reveal no signals whatsoever. This is because the sum and difference frequencies are not integer multiples of 7 or 10 Hz. Now suppose that when the two stimuli are presented to a subject, some of the affected portions of the nervous system are nonlinear. The result is that the nonlinearities produce sum and difference frequencies, and these cannot be recovered when a signal averager is time locked to either stimulus. It is of some interest to note that Helmholtz (1885/1954) postulated the presence of nonlinearities in the auditory system to account for the so-called *combination tones*. These are perceived when a listener is presented with two different pure tones far enough apart in frequency so that one does not hear ordinary beats. In chapter 5, Regan and Regan describe several kinds of nonlinearity and how it results in the generation of frequencies that are not harmonics of concurrently applied stimuli. Taken together, the bands of frequencies generated by nonlinear interactions are referred to as *sidebands*. Using a very sensitive spectrum analyzer rather than an averaging computer, Regan and Regan were able to discern the presence of sidebands when the subject is stimulated and their absence without stimulation. These sidebands do not contain components that are harmonics of the applied stimuli. As Regan and Regan point out, this information may be invisible to the averaging computer, but it can still be retrieved and used to gain insights into the nature of neural processes underlying sensory phenomena. For example, detecting frequency components that are a consequence of stimulation but are unrelated harmonically to the stimuli is a powerful way to determine where in the brain inputs from different sense modalities produce effects that interact with each other.

We now illustrate this point with a hypothetical experiment. Suppose that a periodic visual stimulus is presented to the eyes and that periodic acoustic stimuli are presented to the ears. If the two types of stimuli are not harmonics of each other, then an averaging computer can easily detect the separate and independent responses they evoke in the visual and auditory parts of the brain. Regan and Regan (1987) used this approach to determine whether independent channels exist within single-sense modalities, for example. In our hypothetical experiment one can set the sweep duration of the averaging computer so that it corresponds to the period of the visual stimulus and then to the period of the acoustic stimulus. The visual and auditory responses would emerge from the background noise. If the neural effects of these stimuli should interact with each other, then a high- resolution spectrum analysis can reveal the presence of the products of the interaction, that is, sidebands. By mapping the fields about the scalp that fluctuate in step with frequency components of the sidebands, it is possible to locate the regions of the brain in which the interactions occur, as these regions may be represented as current dipoles. This appears to be a very promising line of research that should be pursued by researchers working in EEG as well as in magnetic source imaging (MSI).

In this chapter, however, our concern is less with the sidebands generated by concurrently presented stimuli than with the question of the independence (superimposability) of effects of sensory stimuli and the ongoing activity of the brain. However, the same basic principles apply.

Models of cortical circuits may incorporate extracortical oscillators that lead to apparently spontaneous changes in neuronal membrane potentials. So, for example, signals originating in the brain stem activate cortical neurons at the frequencies of the alpha rhythms. Similarly, when a sensory stimulus is applied to the organism, signals travel along thalamocortical pathways to evoke cortical activity. These evoked responses may well interact in the cortical neurons with the effects of signals from the hypothetical extracortical oscillators. In this case the evoked response would modulate the so-called "spontaneous activity" of the affected cortical neurons (Kaufman & Locker, 1970).

***Cross-Modulation of Evoked Response and Spontaneous Brain Activity.*** When a response evoked at one frequency interacts with a concurrent response evoked at some other frequency, one says that each response modulates the other. In fact, this is precisely what happens when an electric signal at acoustic frequencies is used to modulate another electric signal at a radio frequency to produce an amplitude-modulated wave for radio transmission. The modulated wave is composed of the original radio frequency signal plus sidebands composed of the sums and differences of the original acoustic signal and the radio frequency signal. By contrast, ongoing brain activity is not a spectrum of discrete frequency components; rather, the spectrum is continuous. As a result, the sidebands are not composed of discrete spectral lines. They, too, form a continuous spectrum. Despite this difference, we shall see that the ongoing activity of the brain can be altered or modulated in amplitude when a response is evoked by a sensory stimulus.

The presence of this modulation is proof of two things: first, that the brain responds in a nonlinear manner to incoming signals, and second, that the measured activity of the brain is not independent of the so-called noise represented by the brain's spontaneous activity.

Hans Berger, the discoverer of the EEG, also discovered a phenomenon he described as *alpha blockage.* A frequency band ranging from about 8 Hz to 12 Hz predominates in the EEG measured over the occipital region of the brain. This is the so-called *alpha band.* It is strongest when the subject is resting with eyes closed and diminishes dramatically if subjects open their eyes and become alert and attentive. During this state of alpha blockage the EEG is dominated by activity in a band around 20 Hz or, roughly, twice the alpha frequency. This so-called *beta* activity is weaker in amplitude than the alpha activity it purportedly replaces. It should be noted that activity at roughly 8 Hz to 12 Hz tends to be predominant over most of the scalp, but when it appears to arise in the region of motor cortex it is referred to as *mu* activity. For the purposes of this chapter we refer to all activity in this frequency band as alpha. In any event, an early and still widely accepted theory is that activity in the alpha band is due to the synchronization of many cortical neurons whose electric fields tend to oscillate at a frequency in a band surrounding 10 Hz. According to this theory, the replacement of alpha by beta is due to the desynchronization of the neurons, which occurs when the neurons are activated. The ostensible desynchronization implies that the individual neurons still oscillate at alpha frequencies, but the fields of these neurons tend to be self-canceling when they are out of step with each other. So, according to this view, the lesser energy detectable at beta frequencies really means that the neurons are more active, rather than less active, during alpha blockage. On the basis of this, one can claim that alpha blockage is not due to a suppression of alpha activity that goes on independently of any other activity in which the neurons might become engaged. However, when otherwise engaged, the neurons are no longer idling along in a synchronous fashion. Hence, by this theory, the signal (which results in activation) is independent of the noise. However, evidence suggests that this view may not apply.

It seems likely that event-related or -evoked activity modulates ongoing activity of the brain, which implies that the evoked response is not independent of the so-called noise. We should also note that computer simulations of a sheet of asynchronous dipoles oriented normally to the surface of the walls of a sulcus show that more field power may be produced when the dipoles are synchronized than when they are desynchronized (Kaufman et al., 1991). This depends on the geometry of the cortex, especially its symmetry. In the EEG domain, synchronized dipoles located in the gyrus may actually produce higher voltages at the scalp than when they are asynchronous. In any event, it is far from proven that alpha blockage is due solely to desynchronization; it may also be due to some kind interaction of event-related activity and spontaneous activity.

***Measuring the Interaction.***    One way to determine whether evoked activity interacts with spontaneous activity is to examine the entire frequency spectrum of the brain's magnetic or electric fields. This could reveal that energy is added at frequencies that are not harmonics of the fundamental frequency of the stimulus. During signal averaging such frequency components would be discarded along with noise. Thus far, little research has used this straightforward approach. However, an indirect method has revealed the presence of modulation of brain activity by event-related activity.

Kaufman and Price (1967) developed this indirect method to examine high-frequency cortical activity (300 Hz–1000 Hz) associated with visual stimulation. This is the same band of activity that Hashimoto discusses in chapter 12. Kaufman and Price recognized that a 1-msec pulse (as in the action potential) has a frequency spectrum containing energy at frequencies ranging from *dc* to about 1 kHz. As it happens, the frequency spectrum of a single impulse is essentially the same as that of an infinite number of randomly occurring identical impulses. Therefore, if a large number of impulses occur in a more or less random sequence across many neurons within the same interval of time, it is theoretically possible to detect activity at frequencies well above the range of the normal EEG (*dc* – ~60 Hz) with scalp electrodes. The stimulus was a light flashing at 15 Hz. The output of a wide-band amplifier measured the voltage across two scalp electrodes over the occipital cortex. The output of the amplifier was filtered to pass activity between 300 Hz and 1000 Hz. This activity was then squared (rectified) and applied to a low-pass filter. A lock-in amplifier was used to detect activity in the rectified EEG at 15 Hz that was time locked to the stimulus. The presence of such activity would indicate that the high-frequency band was modulated by evoked activity at the frequency of the stimulus. A statistically significant response was found. This indicated that visual stimulation resulted not only in an evoked response at the frequency of the stimulus but also in side bands that were not harmonics of the stimulus. These side bands happened to be in the high-frequency domain. Essentially this same method has revealed that activity in the low-frequency band of the normal EEG and MEG is also modulated by sensory stimulation and other events.

Assuming that a 15-Hz visual stimulus does not evoke responses containing harmonics above 150 Hz, the responses detected after squaring the 300 Hz–1 KHz band can be thought of as the variance about a mean zero response. (Actually, assuming them to be present, Kaufman and Price [1967] undertook to remove such high harmonics, and the remaining noise was still modulated at 15 Hz.) Kaufman and Locker (1970) used this same procedure to demonstrate a similar modulation of harmonically unrelated activity within the normal EEG band by a visual stimulus.

The variance about a mean response of zero is proportional to *power*. Voltage is often expressed in terms of *rms* (root mean square) volts. It should be noted that *rms* voltage is mathematically identical to the familiar *standard deviation* of statistics, which, in turn, is the square root of variance. Hence, *electric power* is the same as variance (voltage squared), whereas *field power* is equivalent to field squared. Several studies have revealed that MEG and EEG power fluctuate during the performance of several different cognitive tasks, for example, memory search for tones and for visual forms, as well as during a mental rotation task (Kaufman, Curtis, Wang, & Williamson, 1991; Kaufman, Schwartz, Salustri, & Williamson, 1990; Michel, Kaufman, & Williamson, 1993; Rojas, Teale, Sheeder, & Reite, 2000). In these studies it was found that the duration of a profoundly reduced level of alpha power was highly correlated with time to scan memory for tones or forms as well as to signal completion of a mental rotation task. The distribution of affected field power across the scalp appeared to differ with the modality involved, and was therefore not a generalized effect of, for example, heightened alertness. The affected activity is not synchronized with any stimulus event, although the modulation of its power is related to the time required to perform the task. ERP and event-related field (ERF) studies of short-term memory search and many other cognitive tasks reveal differences in amplitude of various response components, but in most studies these are not as well correlated with the time required to complete the task.

It is clear that background activity is affected by stimulation and by performance of cognitive tasks. These effects are not mirrored in the standard ERP or ERF. Hence, this is an area that should be explored more extensively. For the present it suffices to stress the following point: The so-called noise rejected during signal averaging may well contain significant information related to sensory responses and cognitive processes. This could involve specific regions of the cortex, depending on the modality and the nature of the task. One way to begin to study the relation between this information and mental processes is simply to compute the variance within different frequency bands about the average response. This is well within the capabilities of modern desktop computers, so researchers no longer need to rely solely on differences between average responses both within and across subjects, which is the traditional way to study response reliability and its inverse, variability.

## LOCATING THE SOURCE

One of the ostensible advantages of MEG is that the radial neuromagnetic field is not distorted by the intervening bone, skin, and other tissues. Hence, in principle it should be simpler to locate the source of the observed field than it is to do so on the basis of EEG measures. Because evidence suggests that spontaneous activity originating in specific regions of the cortex may be differentially affected by cognitive tasks, it is of some interest to inquire as to how well one might locate those regions on the basis of field or field power data. Wang and Kaufman deal with this particular issue in some detail in chapter 4. We shall briefly introduce the same topic here, beginning with the much simpler problem of locating the source of a neuromagnetic field when that source is modeled as an equivalent current dipole.

## The Problem With the Inverse Problem

Brenner, Lipton, Kaufman, and Williamson (1978) stimulated the little finger of one hand with a periodic electric impulse. This evoked a neuromagnetic field in a confined region over the hemisphere contralateral to the stimulated finger. The investigators measured the radial field at many places across the scalp. The same stimulus was applied to the thumb of the same hand, and the field pattern was measured again. As expected, the field pattern associated with the stimulation of the little finger contained a region where the field was directed outward from the head and, at the same time after stimulation, another region where the field was directed inward. The same polarity reversal of the field pattern was associated with the stimulation of the thumb, but one important difference was evident in the empirical isofield contour plots: The field extrema associated with stimulation of the little finger were about 2 cm lower on the scalp than those associated with stimulation of the thumb. Furthermore, these field extrema were located approximately above the projection of the central sulcus onto the scalp. The source of activity evoked by stimulation of the little finger is located along the posterior bank of the central sulcus and about 2 cm lower down than the source of activity evoked by stimulation of the thumb. This was probably the first empirical evidence that it is possible to identify the locations of current dipole sources on the human cerebral cortex, and it led directly to many studies in which ECD localization was based on neuromagnetic field measurements. As Wang and Kaufman discuss in chapter 4, it is possible to compute the field everywhere outside a sphere filled with a conducting fluid and containing a current dipole of a given strength, orientation, and position. One, and only one, field pattern can be attributed to this dipole. Hence, one says that there is a unique solution to the so-called *forward problem*. However, it is not possible to determine the strength, orientation, and position of a current dipole solely on the basis of the observed external field. This follows from the fact that any number of dipoles or combinations of dipoles could produce the same field. When one considers that all actual measurements are accompanied by noise, the uncertainty surrounding the validity of any putative source of the observed field is even greater. Even without this uncertainty, in principle it is impossible to discover a unique solution to the so-called *inverse problem*.

Investigators attempting to identify sources of observed field patterns (such as those associated with the little finger and thumb) resort to different strategies. We do not consider all of them here, but most begin with an informed guess as to the location of the source, for example, normal to the posterior bank of the central sulcus when studying responses to stimulation of a finger. Computer simulations may be used in which a current dipole is placed at a particular location in a sphere that best fits the subject's head, isofield contours plotted on the basis of solutions to the forward problem using Equations 1.1 and 1.2. The fit of these contours to those that were actually observed is tested. The moment, depth, and orientation of the dipole is then altered in an iterative fashion until a best fit (in the least squares sense) is achieved. The computed position of the dipole is then plotted in a magnetic resonance imaging scan. A similar procedure may be used when dealing with pathological states in which particular waveforms recur with some frequency (e.g., interictal spikes in the MEGs of some epileptics). When the computed positions of ostensible dipole sources are plotted in magnetic resonance imaging scans of such patients, the ECDs are often found to be in or near observable lesions. In some cases the lesions cannot be visualized, but surgical procedures have revealed small tumors near the computed sites of the ECDs.

A single equivalent current dipole may well account for an observed field pattern, and, when noise is relatively low, one might achieve an even better fit by assuming contributions of quadrupolar and possibly higher order sources. This alone is a useful but relatively modest accomplishment when compared with a larger goal of MSI. As we have taken pains to point out, the actual sources of observed fields are extended distributions of currents on the cerebral cortex. Many investigators have been tantalized by the possibility of finding a way to describe these extended distributions of current based on measurements of the brain's magnetic field. In chapter 4, Wang and Kaufman cite and briefly describe some of these efforts. They describe one such approach, the *minimum norm least squares* (MNLS) inverse, in some detail, along with results of computer simulations. The simulations were designed to demonstrate that there are circumstances in which it is entirely feasible to find a unique solution to the problem of describing the spatial distribution of currents on the cortex. Solutions to these inverse problems primarily require accurate knowledge of the geometry of the surface of the cortex and also assume that the elements of current that make up the distribution flow normal to the surface of the cortex. In principle, given a properly constrained problem, it is possible to arrive at a unique solution to the inverse problem of describing distributed current sources of observed magnetic fields. The MNLS inverse described by Wang and Kaufman has not yet been tested using real MEG data. Sufficiently large arrays of sensors were not available at the time of its formulation. It is possible to conduct such tests today.

Wang and Kaufman also describe in chapter 4 an extension of the MNLS to deal with incoherent sources of field power. This extension was specifically developed to permit forming images of extended sources associated with data similar to those illustrated by Fig. 1.9. Thus, it is intended to make it possible to delineate regions of cortex that become more active relative to their surroundings as well as regions whose activity is suppressed as subjects engage in various mental tasks. It seems likely that simple ECDs may not be very useful as source models when

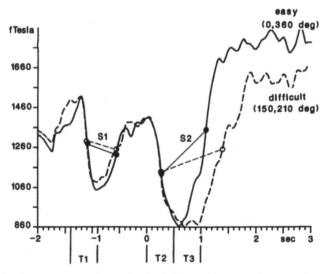

FIG. 1.9.   Average variation in amplitude of alpha activity over a 5-sec epoch as the subject engages in mental rotation tasks. Alpha amplitude (in femtoTesla) is the square root of mean field power in the band of 8 Hz to 12 Hz. Time in seconds is shown along the abscissa. A letter of the alphabet was presented at Time 0, and the subject had to decide if it was the same as a previously seen upright letter (inspection letter) or its mirror image. The letter at Time 0 might be upright or tilted at an angle as well as left–right reversed. The task was more difficult for a large angle of tilt than for a small one. This is reflected in reaction time, which increased with tilt angle. The solid line represents data obtained when the task was easy (no tilt angle) and the dashed line when the task was difficult. Note that the depression in the level of alpha had the same duration (S1) for the inspection letter in both the easy and difficult tasks. However, S2 is markedly different, as it is much longer for the difficult than for the easy tasks. S2 is highly correlated with reaction time for all six subjects in this study. deg = degrees. (Adapted from Michel et al., 1993).

dealing with variations in alpha power. MEG studies have indicated that alpha spindles are generated by time-varying configurations of a large number of discrete sources (Ilmoniemi, Williamson, & Hostetller, 1988; Williamson, Wang, & Ilmoniemi, 1989).

As we note in the last section of this chapter (APPLICATIONS OF MSI), one of the ostensible advantages of MSI is that it is capable of resolving very small differences in time of onset and duration of activity of different cortical regions. Thus, when applied to studying cognitive processes it is capable of determining the temporal order of activation of these regions of cortex. When coupled with images of areas of cortical activation, this fine temporal resolution should be extraordinarily helpful in both basic and clinical research.

## The Spatial Resolution of MSI

The spatial resolution of an instrument may be defined in several different ways. In the field of optics, for example, it was once defined as the minimum angular separation of pairs of points or bars that would permit them to be distinguished from a single point or bar. Thus, the older vision literature refers to the minimum detectable separation of two black bars on a white background, which is sometimes given as 1 arcmin. This measure of resolution proved to be inadequate as it could not predict the detectability of separation of spatial patterns with configurations even slightly different, for example, bars with the same spatial layout but of different contrast. Furthermore, lines, bars, dots, and letters of the alphabet all yielded seemingly incommensurable results. This ambiguity ultimately led to the development of Fourier optics and to the definition of resolution in terms of the spatial modulation transfer function which, in vision, is referred to as the *contrast sensitivity function*. In optics, linear systems analysis based on measured modulation transfer functions predicts the spatial resolution of optical systems for spatial patterns with arbitrary configurations.

The concept of *resolution* is also used to compare functional brain imaging modalities, but similar ambiguities apply here as well. In some cases resolution is defined as the minimum detectable separation of two relatively active regions of cerebral cortex. In positron emission tomography (PET) or fMRI, resolving two regions of active neural tissue is limited in part by physical properties of blood flow in and around the active tissue as well as the physical attributes of the sensor systems. For MSI, the literature sometimes reports that it provides a spatial resolution of about 1 to 2 cm (Committee on the Mathematics and Physics of Emerging Dynamic

Biomedical Imaging, 1996). However, this estimate seems inconsistent with some empirical observations. This inconsistency may be due in part to the ambiguity inherent in the use of the term *resolution*. Unfortunately, as yet there have been no serious efforts to calibrate neuromagnetometers in terms of their actual abilities to resolve sources of extra-cranial magnetic fields. Instead, researchers have focused on the accuracy with which MSI can localize single sources. The accuracy of localizing a single source is affected by many factors, including (a) the signal-to-noise ratio of the MEG recording, (b) the number of and nature of spatial samples of the extracranial magnetic field, (c) the precision of location and orientation of the sensor in three-dimensional space relative to the head, (d) the depth of the source and how close the source is to the center of the best-fitting local sphere, (e) the assumed head model (see chap. 3), (f) prior knowledge of the anatomy of the surface on which the source may exist (see chap. 4), (g) approximations in computation of the forward solution (see chap. 3), and (h) the extent of and variability in the spatial distribution of the source.

Several studies (cf. Barth, Sutherling, Broffman, & Beatty, 1986; Weinberg, Brickett, Coolsma, & Baff, 1986; Yamamoto et al., 1988) have demonstrated an accuracy of ~3 mm in locating a current dipole source, provided that the signal-to-noise ratio is sufficient to permit repeated measures and that the spatial sampling of the field is adequate to permit generating a good fit to a computed isofield contour map. These conditions occurred when the actual source was within 4 cm to 5 cm of the surface of the skull. Barth et al. (1986) found that the accuracy worsened to 8 mm to 9 mm as the source was placed at increasingly greater depths in the head. (In this experiment the source was a virtual current dipole inside a cadaver's skull filled with a conducting gel.) In all of these cases the current dipole was oriented so that it was totally or largely tangential to the overlying skull, for otherwise the strength of its radial field would have been vanishingly small (Cohen, Cuffin, Yunokuchi, Maniewski, Purcell, Cosgrove, et al., 1990; see comments by Williamson, 1991, and by Hari, Hamalainen, Ilmoniemi, & Lounasmaa, 1991).

It is particularly instructive to reconsider the experimental determination of the tonotopic map of the human auditory cortex (Romani et al., 1982). This experiment was conducted using a single-channel neuromagnetometer, but the field was sampled at a very large number of positions in many repeated trials. At each placement of the single-channel neuromagnetometer the stimulus was an amplitude-modulated sinusoidal tone of each of several different carrier frequencies ranging from

100 Hz to 4000 Hz. The isofield contour map obtained at each of these carrier frequencies was not determined until all of the data were collected and sorted by carrier frequency. It is likely that if each stimulus were a complex tone composed of several different carrier frequencies, the resulting map would have been indistinguishable from that generated by a single equivalent current dipole. Yet when the maps were based on separated sets of trials, they differed significantly from each other. In fact, on the basis of the data they obtained, Romani et al. were able to "resolve" sources separated from each other by distances of a few millimeters. Similarly, in studying the organization of the first and second somatosensory cortices, Hari et al. (1984) obtained millimeter accuracy in resolving these sources.

It should be borne in mind that if Romani et al. (1982) had presented two of their stimuli concurrently, the resulting field map is likely to have been similar to one generated by a single dipole. Hence, strictly speaking, they would have been unable to resolve the ostensibly two sources contributing to the net field. However, with precise prior knowledge of the anatomy, along with the assumption that the sources "lived" on the surface of the cortex, then the MNLS inverse—or, possibly, related methods—could have differentiated the multiple sources. Naturally, this would depend on the amount of noise in the data but, thus far, although encouraging, studies of the effect of noise on such computations have been conducted only in computer simulations.

It is rather surprising that research has not yet been conducted using the techniques devised by Regan and Regan (chap. 5) to determine how well MSI can resolve two concurrently activated cortical areas. Consider the following hypothetical experiment: Two tones of different frequency are modulated by two harmonically unrelated low-frequency sinusoids. All of the MEG data collected at a single position are sorted so that the strength of the field fluctuating at the frequency of one of the two sinusoids is averaged separately from that of the field fluctuating at the frequency of the other sinusoid. This may result in two different field maps and permit resolution of two different sources along the surface of the auditory cortex. If the stimuli should produce effects that exhibit nonlinear interactions, then the results could not be predicted from the sum of the results obtained by presenting the two stimuli separately. Even here, however, responses at the frequencies of the sidebands may be detectable as well. In any event, we still do not fully appreciate the ability of MSI to resolve sources. Neither do we yet understand how rich the potential results of such investigations may be.

## COMPLEMENTARY FUNCTIONAL IMAGING MODALITIES

In this section we briefly review several of the most widely cited forms of functional brain imaging. We do this so MSI can be seen in perspective, especially as it is now evident that these different modalities complement each other; that is, their joint use may well yield more information than can be achieved by using any method alone.

The imaging modalities we review here are primarily PET and fMRI. We touch only lightly on EEG, as it was considered extensively earlier in this chapter. We do not deal at all with electrical impedance tomography (cf. Holder, 1993), because it is not yet widely cited. Neither do we discuss single photon emission tomography, as it appears to be waning in importance as a functional imaging modality. It is important to note, however, that some efforts have been made to combine MEG with impedance tomography. The connection seems quite natural, as magnetic field sensors can be used to monitor the flow of currents imposed on the body. In chapter 11, Maclin describes PET and fMRI in some detail, as well as the newly emerging modality of optical (near infrared) spectroscopy and the related evoked optical response. In this section we deal largely with the relation among MSI, PET, and fMRI. We consider the relative advantages and disadvantages of each modality and mention some ostensible advantages associated with combining them.

## PET

PET is based on detection of positron emitting radiotracers (Bohm, Eriksson, Bergstrom, Litton, & Sundman, 1987; Ter-Pogossian, Mullani, Hood, Higgins, & Ficke, 1978; Thompson, Yamamoto, & Meyer, 1979). A PET scanner detects gamma rays from intravenously administered (or inhaled) positron-emitting isotopes. Paired gamma ray detections are computed into functional images. With the radio-labeled tracers in the subject's blood, PET provides an indirect measure of neuronal activity through direct measurements of local blood flow or metabolism change as a function of task performance. In certain clinical applications the concern is with sustained metabolic levels. Deviation from normal is indicative of some disease processes.

A number of positron-emitting radiotracers can be used for PET. The most commonly used are fluorine (F18) and oxygen (O15). Fluorine is normally used to measure glucose metabolic rate. It provides a spatial resolution of about 3.5 mm in a plane but a temporal resolution of about 32 minutes. Attached to water molecules, O15 is used in PET to measure patterns of blood flow. The spatial resolution is not as good as the F18 method; however, the temporal resolution is about 60 sec.

Because fMRI offers better temporal and spatial resolution and does not require injection of radioactive materials, fMRI is preferred by many researchers. However, the diversity of specific brain chemical systems provides PET with a unique advantage over other imaging modalities. For example, PET can be used with other radiolabels (e.g., L-dopa) to image aspects of the dopamine, serotonin, benzodiazapine, N-methyl-D-aspartate, and other neurotransmitter systems.

Ingenious experiments have been performed to determine which regions of the brain become active during performance of different cognitive tasks (cf. Raichle, 1997). However, it is not possible to determine the temporal order in which these regions are activated.

## fMRI

As a relative newcomer in brain imaging, fMRI is rapidly becoming the most popular functional imaging modality for basic research purposes. Many university laboratories devoted to cognitive neuroscience and psychology already have or soon will have installed powerful state-of-the-art fMRI systems. Basically, an fMRI system measures changes in blood oxygenation and blood volume correlated with neural activity (Belliveau et al., 1992; Ogawa et al, 1993; chap. 11, this volume). Consider a working model for one of the most commonly used imaging methods in fMRI: blood oxygenation level dependent fMRI. An increase in neuronal activity causes local vasodilatation, which results in an increased local blood flow. The need for oxygenated hemoglobin generated by neural activity exceeds the need associated with the resting metabolic processes. The locally increased ratio of oxygenated hemoglobin (a diamagnetic substance with low magnetic susceptibility) and deoxygenated hemoglobin (a paramagnetic substance with high magnetic susceptibility) reduces the microscopic magnetic field in homogeneities in the neighborhood of venules, veins, and red blood cells within veins. This leads to increased image intensity in MRI.

Using strong magnetic fields and the principle of nuclear resonance, fMRI, like PET, provides an indirect measure of neuronal activity through direct measurements of local blood oxygenation level or flow as a function of task performance. At the time of this writing, the state-of-the-art fMRI systems typically provide approximately $3 \times 3 \times 4$ mm spatial resolution. The temporal resolution of fMRI, however, is on the order of seconds, limited by the slowness of the hemodynamics.

## EEG

Three major advantages of EEG are (a) high temporal resolution (up to millisecond accuracy), (b) direct measurement of postsynaptic potential, and (c) relatively inexpensive instrumentation (a high-density EEG system costs about $100–200K). However, it suffers from ambiguities in source localization. The spatial resolution of EEG is estimated to be a couple of centimeters.

MEG shares the two advantages with EEG: (a) high temporal resolution and (b) direct measurement of postsynaptic potential. However, as we pointed out early in this chapter, a major additional advantage of MEG lies in the transparency of intervening tissue to magnetic fields and, consequently, much simpler magnetic inverse solutions. The spatial resolution of MEG is estimated to be 2 mm to 5 mm (a figure that depends on the depth of the source). On the other hand, MEG is about one order of magnitude more expensive than EEG.

Assuming that cortical regions involved in mental tasks can be identified, it is possible to determine the order of activation using either EEG or MEG.

## Combining the Modalities

MRI as a method for imaging anatomical structures is also of great potential use, especially in identifying the structures where current dipole sources computed from MEG and EEG data may lie. As described in chapter 4, accurate information as to the geometry of the cerebral cortex is central to achieving reasonable inverse solutions for imaging current distributions. So it is now obvious that whenever extensive EEG or MEG mapping is conducted to reveal the locations of lesions or places at which various mental processes are implemented, high-resolution MRI scans are required.

Whereas both PET and fMRI offer excellent spatial resolution (e.g., Belliveau et al., 1992; Raichle, 1997), EEG and MEG offer very good temporal resolution (e.g., Kaufman & Williamson, 1980; Regan, 1989). As a consequence, it is widely recognized that the optimal brain imaging strategy for cognitive neuroscience is a combination of different imaging modalities (Belliveau et al., 1993; Dale & Sereno, 1995; George et al., 1995; Heinze et al., 1994; Korvenoja et al., 1999; Mangun, Buonocore, Girelli, & Jha, 1998; Menon, Ford, Lim, Glover, & Pfefferbaum, 1997; Simpson et al., 1995). This includes joint spatiotemporal analyses of simultaneous recordings of two imaging modalities—for example, fMRI and EEG—as well as MRI/fMRI constrained EEG/MEG source localization.

It is important to recognize that different imaging modalities measure different physical phenomena and do not necessarily provide a direct measure of neural activity. Hence, the measures obtained using one imaging modality may not necessarily correspond to those registered by another modality. Furthermore, the spatial locations of "neural activity" registered by one modality may not be identical to that obtained via another modality (cf. chap. 11). Put more explicitly, an emerging research problem is that of determining the degree to which regions of altered blood flow are commensurate with regions of enhanced or depressed neural activity, and in identifying whether a change in blood flow represents enhancement or depression in local neural activity. The joint use of MSI and fMRI is essential to resolving this problem.

## APPLICATIONS OF MSI

As described in many of the chapters of this book, MSI is widely applied in medicine; it also finds use as a basic research modality, especially in the field of cognitive neuroscience. In the 1970s, researchers working in what came to be called *biomagnetism* in general, and *neuromagnetism* in particular, focused on developing instruments with sufficient sensitivity to measure the weak fields generated by biological phenomena. Instrumentation based on advances in low-temperature physics was of primary concern, because it enabled detection of exquisitely weak magnetic fields. As this technology improved, it became possible to routinely detect and map neuromagnetic fields. Then, in the 1980s and 1990s, the emphasis shifted to applying the technology to medicine and to cognitive science.

Most of the remaining chapters in this volume provide many instances of how MSI is and has been applied. Clinical applications to stroke and in epilepsy are described in chapters 11 and 14. The systems now being used in clinical settings are described in chapters 7 through 9. In chapter 9, Lounasmaa and Hari also describe many of the results obtained in their Helsinki laboratory that bear on cognitive science. Many other chapters also describe results related to sensory and cognitive processes. In chapter 13, Lu and Sperling examine the way in which the temporal resolution of MEG makes it possible to determine the decay times of neural processes occurring concurrently at different places in the brain. They illustrate how this may help to determine the time courses of iconic and echoic short-term memory as well as clarify the relation between different levels of processing of sensory information. Chapter 13 also contains an excellent introduction to how one might use both MSI and psychophysical strategies in examining issues of central concern to cognitive science. This is an area that is ripe for major discoveries.

## REFERENCES

Barth D. S., Sutherling W., Broffman, J., & Beatty, J. (1986). Magnetic localization of a dipolar current source implanted in a sphere and a human cranium. *Electroencephalography & Clinical Neurophysiology, 63,* 260–262.

Belliveau, J. W., Baker, J. R., Kwong, K. K., Rosen, B. R., George, J. S., Aine, C. J., Lewine, J. D., Sanders, J. A., Simpson, G. V., & Foxe, J. J. (1993). Functional neuroimaging combining fMRI, MEG, and EEG. *Proceedings of the International Society of Magnetic Resonance Medicine, 1,* 6.

Belliveau, J. W., Kwong, K. K., Kennedy, D. N., Baker, J. R., Stern, C. E., Benson, R., Chesler, D. A., Weisskoff, R. M., Cohen, M. S., Tootell, R. B. H., Fox, P. T., Brady, T. J., & Rosen, B. R. (1992). Magnetic Resonance Imaging Mapping of Brain Function—Human Visual Cortex. *Investigative Radiology, 27*(S2), S59–S65.

Bohm, C., Eriksson, L., Bergstrom, M., Litton, J., & Sundman, R. (1978). A computer assisted ring detector positron camera system for reconstruction tomography of the brain. *IEEE Transactions on Nuclear Science, NS, 25,* 624–636.

Brenner, D., Lipton, J., Kaufman, L., & Williamson, S. J. (1978). Somatically evoked fields of the human brain. *Science, 199,* 81.

Brenner, D., Williamson, S. J., & Kaufman, L. (1975, October). Visually evoked magnetic fields of the human brain *Science, 190,* 480–482.

Cohen, D., Cuffin, B. N., Yunokuchi, K., Maniewski, R., Purcell, C., Cosgrove, R., Ives, J., Kennedy, J. G., & Schomer, D. L. (1990). MEG versus EEG localization test using implanted sources in the human brain. *Annals of Neurology, 28,* 811–817.

Committee on the Mathematics and Physics of Emerging Dynamic Biomedical Imaging. (1996). *Mathematics and physics of emerging biomedical imaging.* National Academy Press: Washington, DC.

Curtis, S., Kaufman, L., & Williamson, S. J. (1988). Divided attention revisited: Selection based on location or pitch. In K. Atsumi, M. Kotani, S. Ueno, T. Katila, & S. J. Williamson (Eds.), *Biomagnetism, 87* (pp. 138–141). Tokyo: Denki University Press.

Dale, A. M., & Serena, M. I. (1995). Improved localization of cortical activity by combining EEG and MEG with MRI cortical surface reconstruction: A linear approach. *Journal of Cognitive Neuroscience, 5*(2), 162–176.

George, J. S., Aine, C. J., Mosher, J. C., Schmidt, D. M., Ranken, D. M., Schlitt, H. A., Wood, D. C., Lewine, J. D., Sanders, J. A., & Belliveau, J. W. (1995). Mapping function in the human brain with magnetoencephalography, anatomical magnetic resonance imaging, and functional magnetic resonance imaging. *Journal of Clinical Neurophysiology, 12*(5), 406–431.

Hari, R., Hamalainen, M., Ilmoniemi, R., & Lounasmaa, O. V. (1991). MEG versus EEG localization test. *Annals of Neurology, 30,* 222–223.

Hari, R., Reinikaninen, K., Kaukoranta, E., Hämäläinen, M., Ilmoniemi, R., Penttinen, A., Salminen, J., & Teszner, D. (1984). Somatosensory evoked cerebral magnetic fields from SI and SII in man. *Electroencephalography & Clinical Neurophysiology, 57,* 254–263.

Heinze, H. J., Mangun, G. R., Burchert, W., Hinrichs, H., Scholz, M., Munte, T. F., Gos, A., Scherg, M., Johannes, S., Hundeshagen, H., Gazzaniga, M. S., & Hillyard, S. A. (1994). Combined spatial and temporal imaging of brain activity during visual selective attention in humans. *Nature, 372,* 543–546.

Helmholtz, H. von. (1885) *On the sensations of tone,* From 4th German ed. A. J. Ellis (Trans.), New York, Dover, 1954. (Original work published 1885)

Holder, D. (Ed.). (1993). *Clinical and physiological applications of electrical impedance tomography.* London: UCL Press Limited.

Ilmoniemi, R. J., Williamson, S. J., & Hostetler, W. E. (1988). New method for the study of spontaneous brain activity. In K. Atsumi, K. Kotani, S. Ueno, T. Katila, & S. J. Williamson (Eds.), *Biomagnetism, 87* (pp. 182–185). Tokyo: Tokyo Denki University Press.

Kaufman, L., Curtis, S., Wang, J. Z., & Williamson, S. J. (1991). Changes in cortical activity when subjects scan memory for tones. *Electroencephalography & Clinical Neurophysiology, 82,* 266–284.

Kaufman, L., Kaufman, J. H., & Wang, J. Z. (1991). On cortical folds and neuromagnetic fields. *Electroencephalography & Clinical Neurophysiology, 79,* 211–226.

Kaufman, L., & Locker, J. (1970). Sensory modulation of the EEG. *Proceedings of the 78th Annual Convention of the American Psychological Association, 1,* 79–80.

Kaufman, L., & Price, R. (1967). The detection of cortical spike activity at the human scalp. *IEEE Transactions on Bio-Medical Engineering. BME-14,* 84–90.

Kaufman, L., Schwartz, B. J., Salustri, C., & Williamson, S. J. (1990). Local inhibition of spontaneous brain activity during mental imagery. *Journal of Cognitive Neuroscience, 2,* 124–132.

Kaufman, L., & Williamson, S. J. (1980). The evoked magnetic field of the human brain. In F. L. Denmark (Ed.), *Psychology: The leading edge.* New York: New York Academy of Sciences, 45–65.

Korvenoja, A., Huttunen, J., Salli, E., Pohjonen, H., Martinkauppi, S., Palva, L. M., Lauronen, L., Virtanen, J., Ilmoniemi, R. J., & Aronen, H. J. (1999). Activation of multiple cortical areas in response to somatosensory stimulation: Combined magnetoencephalographic and functional magnetic resonance imaging. *Human Brain Mapping, 8,* 13–27.

Liegeois-Chauvel, C., Giraud, K., Badier, J.-M., & Marquis, P. (2001). Intracerebral evoked potentials in pitch perception reveal a functional asymmetry of the human auditory cortex. In R. J. Zatorre & I. Peretz (Eds.), *The biological foundations of music.* New York: New York Academy of Sciences.

Lu, Z.-L., & Williamson, S. J. (1991). Spatial extent of coherent sensory-evoked cortical activity. *Experimental Brain Research, 84,* 411–416.

Mangun, G. R., Buonocore, M. H., Girelli, M., & Jha, A. P. (1998). ERP and fMRI measures of visual spatial selective attention. *Human Brain Mapping, 6,* 383–389.

Menon, V., Ford, J. M., Lim, K. O., Glover, G. H., & Pfefferbaum, A. (1997). Combined event-related fMRI and EEG evidence for temporal-parietal cortex activation during target detection. *Neuroreport, 8,* 3029–3037.

Michel, C., Kaufman, L., & Williamson, S. J. (1993). Duration of EEG and MEG alpha suppression increases with angle in a mental rotation task, *Journal of Cognitive Neuroscience, 6*(2), 139–150.

Nunez, P. L. (1981). *Electric fields of the brain: The neurophysics of EEG.* New York: Oxford University Press.

Ogawa, S., Menon, R. S., Tank, D. W., Kim, S.-G., Merkle, H., Ellermann, J. M., & Ugurbil, K. (1993). Functional brain mapping by blood oxygenation level-dependent contrast magnetic resonance imaging: A comparison of signal characteristics with a biophysical model. *Biophysics Journal, 64,* 803–812.

Ottaviani, F., Di Girolamo, S., Briglia, G., De Rossi, G., Di Giuda, D., & Di Nardo, W. (1997, September–October). Tonotopic organization of human auditory cortex analyzed by SPECT. *Audiology, 36,* 241–248.

Raichle, M. E. (1997). Functional brain imaging and verbal behavior. In J. W. Donahoe & V. P. Dorsel (Eds.), *Neural-network models of cognition: Biobehavioral foundations* (pp. 438–454). Amsterdam: North-Holland/Elsevier Science.

Regan, D. (1989). *Human brain electrophysiology: Evoked potentials and evoked magnetic fields in science and medicine.* New York: Elsevier.

Regan, D., & Regan, M. P. (1987). Nonlinearity in human visual responses and a limitation of Fourier methods. *Vision Research, 27,* 2181–2183.

Rojas, D. C., Teale, P. D., Sheeder, J. L., & Reite, M. L. (2000). Neuromagnetic alpha suppression during an auditory Sternberg task. Evidence for a serial, self-terminating search of short-term memory. *Cognitive Brain Research, 10,* 85–89.

Romani, G. L., Williamson, S. J., & Kaufman, L. (1982, June). Tonotopic organization of the human auditory cortex. *Science, 216,* 1339–1340.

Simpson, G. V., Pflieger, M. E., Foxe, J. J., Ahlfors, S. P., Vaughan, H. G., Hrabe, J., Ilmoniemi, R. J., & Lantos, G. (1995). Dynamic neuroimaging of brain function. *Journal of Clinical Neurophysiology, 12*(5), 432–449.

Ter-Pogossian, M. M., Mullani, N. A., Hood, J. T., Higgins, C. S., & Ficke, D. C., (1978). Design considerations for a positron emission transverse tomograph (PETT V) for imaging of the brain. *Journal of Computer Assisted Tomography, 2,* 539–544.

Thompson, C. J., Yamamoto, Y. L., & Meyer, E. (1979). Positome II: A high efficiency positron imaging device for dynamic brain studies. *IEEE Transactions on Nuclear Science, NS, 26,* 583–389.

Weinberg, H., Brickett, P., Coolsma, F., & Baff, M. (1986). Magnetic localization of intracranial dipoles: Simulation with a physical model. *Electroencephalography & Clinical Neurophysiology, 64,* 159–170.

Wessinger, M. C., Buonocore, M. H., Kussmaul, C. L., & Mangun, G. R. (1997). Tonotopy in human auditory cortex examined with functional magnetic resonance imaging. *Human Brain Mapping, 5,* 18–25.

Williamson, S. J. (1991). MEG versus EEG localization test. *Annals of Neurology, 30,* 222–222.

Williamson, S. J., Wang, J. Z., & Ilmoniemi, R. (1989). Method for locating sources of human alpha activity. In S. J. Williamson, M. Hoke, G. Stroink, & M. Kotani (Eds.), *Advances in biomagnetism* (pp. 257–260). New York: Plenum.

Yamamoto, T., Williamson, S. J., Kaufman, L., Nicholson, C., & Llinas, R. (1988). Magnetic localization of neuronal activity in the human brain. *Proceedings of the National Academy of Sciences (USA), 85,* 8732–8736.

# 2

# Toward Understanding the Physiological Origins of Neuromagnetic Signals

Yoshio Okada
*University of New Mexico School of Medicine*

A systematic study on the physiological study of magnetoencephalography (MEG) and electroencephalography (EEG) carried out since 1984 is described. The results obtained from the turtle cerebellum *in vitro,* hippocampus slices *in vitro,* the somatosensory cortex of the pig *in vivo,* and several other preparations provided concrete empirical support for many of the basic assumptions used in interpreting MEG and EEG signals from the humans. They have also provided insights on the physiological bases of pathophysiological events such as migraine and stroke.

This chapter describes results of a systematic study of the physiological basis of magnetoencephalography (MEG) and electroencephalography (EEG) that has been carried out from the spring of 1984 in my laboratory. As I show, this line of study has provided a concrete empirical basis for the basic assumptions that have been used in the biomagnetism community to interpret MEG and EEG data from humans. The study is described in a chronological order as this permits me to describe the development of magnetophysiology.

## TURTLE CEREBELLUM STUDIES

### First Measurements

In the spring of 1984, Charles Nicholson and I carried out the first measurements of the magnetic field from an *in vitro* brain preparation in order
to show that our theoretical calculations based on the theories of
Geselowitz (1970) and others provide correct predictions of the magnitude of magnetic field from a neuronal tissue of a unit volume. As is the
case for any completely new investigation, this study was improvised in
many ways. We used the isolated *in vitro* preparation of the whole cerebellum of turtle for this initial study because of the unique ability of the turtle brain to withstand long periods of anoxia. This property eliminated
one source of uncertainty in our attempt to detect the magnetic field
from a brain tissue for the first time. Figure 2.1 shows the experimental
setup. The nonmagnetic micromanipulators were constructed in house.
They were used to hold the stimulating and recording electrodes. A simple platform was fabricated and placed into the beaker to hold the cerebellum. The caudal portion of the turtle brain was placed on an isotonic
agar block situated on the platform. The stimulating electrodes were
placed onto the dorsal surface of the cerebellum to stimulate the parallel
fibers. To measure the evoked magnetic field, the detection coil of a single-channel MEG system was placed above the cerebellum. Because the
MEG sensor was designed for human studies, it was not optimal for this
*in vitro* study. The detection coil could not be placed closer than about 2
cm above the cerebellum.

We predicted that the magnetic field from a neuronal tissue with 2 to 4
mm$^2$ in active surface area with dipolar current elements perpendicular
to the surface should be about 200 femto Tesla at a height of 2 cm. The
field was scanned above the cerebellum to look for two locations with a
maximum field intensity but of opposite polarity. The mapping revealed
that there were indeed such field extrema with a magnitude of approximately 200 fT along the direction perpendicular to the surface of the
Ringer solution. After determining the field extrema, the detection coil
was placed at one of the extrema, and the field was measured before and
after applying 10 mM $MnCl_2$, which blocks synaptic transmission. The
results are shown in Fig. 2.1B. The stimulus artefact was quite large (with
an additional comb-filter artefact at around 16.7 msec). Nevertheless, we
obtained the first evidence showing that a magnetic field can be measured from this neuronal preparation. Traces **a** and **b** are replications in

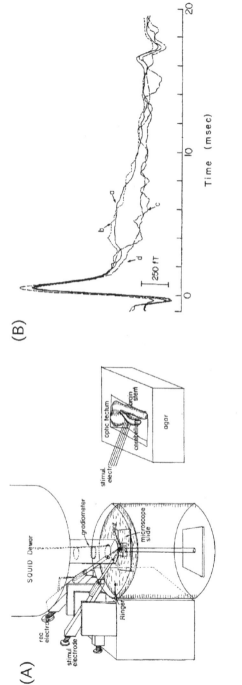

FIG. 2.1. Experimental arrangement of the first magnetoencephalography (MEG) study of the magnetic field from an *in vitro* brain preparation (turtle cerebellum). Panel A: the caudal portion of the turtle brain beyond the optic tectum was removed from the rest of the brain and placed in a well of an isotonic agar block that sat upon a glass platform. The beaker was filled with physiological Ringer solution at room temperature. The dorsal cerebellar surface was electrically stimulated with an array of electrodes (electr). The evoked field potential was recorded from the dorsal surface with a wire electrode. The evoked magnetic field was recorded (rec) above the preparation with a single-channel MEG sensor originally built for human studies. Panel B: an example of the magnetic field from a turtle cerebellum. Traces a and b are replications in normal Ringer; Traces c and d are replications in Ringer with 10 mM $MnCl_2$. Although the stimulus artefact is large in this first measurement, there was a component starting 3 msec poststimulus that was abolished by $Mn^{2+}$, which blocks neurotransmission, among other effects (unpublished). SQUID = superconducting quantum interference device.

45

normal Ringer. They contained a deflection starting at about 3 msec after stimulation. Traces **c** and **d** were obtained after adding $MnCl_2$ to the bath. Bath application of $Mn^{2+}$ completely abolished this component, demonstrating that the signal with a magnitude of about 200 fT was neural in origin.

## Tests of Basic Assumptions of MEG

The quality of the data improved once we became successful in routinely collecting the signals. This allowed us to test some of the basic assumptions in the field of MEG. Figure 2.2 shows an evoked magnetic field from an isolated cerebellar preparation over the surface of the bath (Okada, Nicholson, & Llinás, 1989). The cerebellum was removed from the rest of the brain and suspended by nylon nets in a bath of Ringer solution. The cerebellar peduncle was stimulated with a bipolar electrode. The evoked field potential was recorded within the cerebellum with a glass micro-pipette. The component of the evoked magnetic field normal to the bath surface was recorded at a distance of 17 mm above the center of the cere-bellum with a single-channel second-order gradiometer similar to the one used in the initial pilot study. The recordings were done in a magnetically shielded, two-layer cylindrical chamber. The evoked fields shown on the right side of Fig. 2.2 first demonstrated that we improved our experimen-tal techniques to the point where the stimulus artefact was virtually eliminated. The artefact within the first 0.5 msec after stimulus onset was removed digitally. Second, the field distribution demonstrated that it was dipolar with the field extrema on the rostral and caudal sides of the cerebellum. The field was centered above the cerebellum located at the origin with its dorsal surface facing + y-axis. In a related study (Okada & Nicholson, 1988b), we showed that this field was dipolar by fitting a the-oretical dipolar function to the data and by determining that the field amplitude decreased as an inverse square of the distance between the center of the cerebellum and height of the field extrema above the cere-bellum. Third, it showed that the field during the initial response was produced by currents directed from the ventral to the dorsal surface of the cerebellum, because the field was directed outward on the rostral side and inward into the bath on the caudal side. This direction of current was parallel to the longitudinal axis of the Purkinje cells which was tangential to the surface of the bath.

In another series of experiments we tested one of the basic assumptions in MEG, namely, that the signal is due to currents tangential to the bath

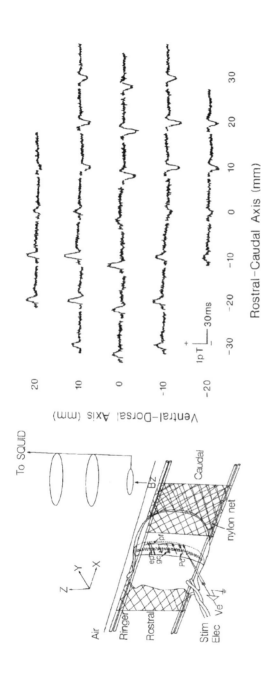

FIG. 2.2. Left panel: the entire cerebellum isolated from the turtle brain was suspended by a pair of nylon nets in a bath of Ringer solution. The cerebellar peduncle was stimulated briefly with a bipolar electrode. The magnetic field due to the evoked neuronal responses was measured at a height of 17 mm from the center of the cerebellum. Right panel: spatial distribution of the component of the magnetic field normal to the bath surface produced by an isolated turtle cerebellum located at the origin. The stimulus artefacts were experimentally reduced and did not distort the signals produced by the cerebellum. Artefacts within the first 0.5 msec after stimulation were digitally removed in this display. SQUID = superconducting quantum interference device; Bz = bath surface; Ve = evoked field potential; Stim Elec = stimulating electrode. From "Magnetoencephalography (MEG) as a New Tool for Non-Invasive Realtime Analysis of Normal and Abnormal Brain Activity in Humans" by Y. C. Okada, C. Nicholson, and R Llinás, in *Visualization of Brain Functions*, D. Ottoson and W. Rostene (Eds.), 1989. Copyright 1989 by Stockton Press. Adapted by permission.

surface (Geselowitz, 1970). This assumption was previously tested in a physical model with an artificial dipolar in a large saline bath (Cohen & Hosaka, 1976). In our study (see Fig. 2.3), we rotated the cerebellum in the y–z plane with the x-axis as its axis of rotation. Unlike the design shown in Fig. 2.2, the dorsal surface along the midline of the cerebellum was stimulated with a pair of silver wires at each angle of rotation. The top of Fig. 2.3 shows the raw waveforms of the magnetic field as a function of orientation of the cerebellum. The field amplitude was maximum, but of opposite polarity at 0 and 180°, that is, when the current along the longitudinal axis of the Purkinje cells was tangential to the bath surface. As the direction of the current became more vertical, the field decreased in amplitude, reaching the reversal point at the orientation of 90°. The bottom part of Fig. 2.3 shows the amplitude of the three components at latencies of 1.2, 3.0, and 5.4 msec as a function of orientation. The smooth curves are the cosine of the angle of orientation. The good fit in all cases showed that the field was produced by the tangential component of the current perpendicular to the cerebellar surface.

We carried out a series of field potential measurements with the preparation shown in Fig. 2.2 to determine the currents responsible for the magnetic fields found in Figs. 2.2 and 2.3; that is, we determined the nature of the currents along the longitudinal axis of the Purkinje cells responsible for the magnetic fields such as the one presented in Fig. 2.2. The lefthand side of Fig. 2.4 shows the field potentials measured at a fixed depth of 250 μm from the ventral surface that were evoked by stimulations of the cerebellar peduncle (Okada et al., 1989). The righthand side of Fig 2.4 shows the isopotential profile at the peak latencies of the various components between 2.8 and 24.4 msec. These data were collected from the same preparations in which the magnetic fields were measured as in Fig. 2.2. Thus, we could conclude that the magnetic field with a magnitude on the order of 1 pT shown in Fig. 2.2 was produced by activity within a tissue with a volume of about 10 mm³; that is, the cerebellum is capable of producing 100 fT/mm³ at a distance of about 2 cm. This corresponds to a current dipole moment density of 1 nA·m/mm³ or 1 nA·m/mm² in active surface area, because the cerebellum is about 1 mm thick.

We have furthermore determined that the magnetic fields such as those shown in Figs. 2.2 and 2.3 were produced by the Purkinje cells. The laminar field potential profiles were determined at the center of activity shown in Fig. 2.4. Figure 2.5 shows examples of such a profile obtained as the microelectrode was pushed into the cerebellum from the ventral side (A) and as it was pulled out (B; Okada & Nicholson, 1988a). The current

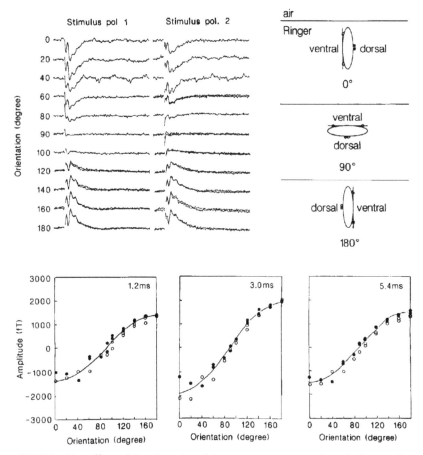

FIG. 2.3.   Top: effects of the orientation of the current generator on the evoked magnetic fields. Waveforms of the evoked magnetic field normal to the bath surface as a function of orientation of the cerebellum are shown in the inset. Bottom: the data are shown separately for two polarities (pol) of the stimulation. Amplitude of the three components of the evoked magnetic fields is a function of angle of the cerebellum. The smooth curves are the cosines of the angle of orientation. The good fits show that the magnetic field was produced by the component of the generator tangential to the bath surface. Adapted from Okada and Nicholson (1988b).

source density (CSD) analysis (Freeman & Nicholson, 1975; Nicholson & Freeman, 1975) was applied to the data. The CSD analysis showed that the extracellular current sink (upward in this case) was located near the Purkinje cell layer (most likely in the dendritic trunk) and the current source about 150 μm toward the distal apical dendrites, suggesting that

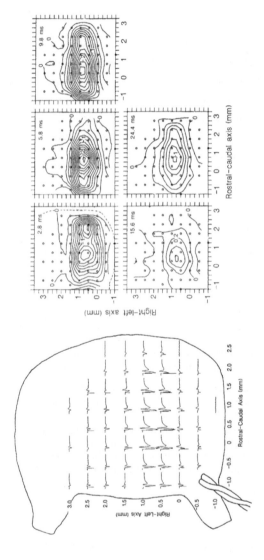

FIG. 2.4. Left panel: evoked field potentials at a depth of 250 μm from the ventral surface from the same cerebellum in which magnetic fields such as those shown in Fig. 2.2 were obtained. Right panels: isopotential maps of five components of the evoked potentials. This type of data was used to estimate the size of active tissue (7–10 mm² in surface area) underlying the magnetic fields such as those in Fig. 2.2. Based on Fig. 9 of Okada et al. (1989) and Okada and Nicholson (1988a).

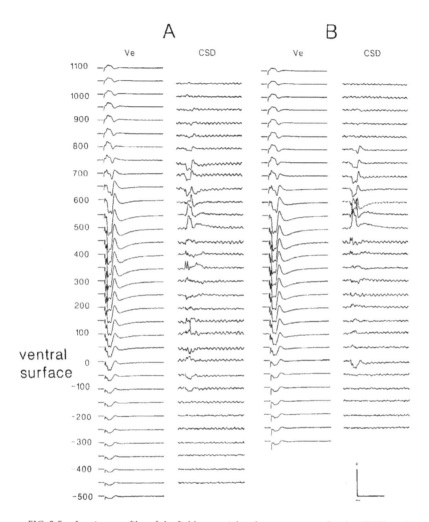

FIG. 2.5. Laminar profiles of the field potential and current source density (CSD) at the center of activity in the turtle cerebellum in the experiments such as those shown in Figs. 2.2 and 2.4 A and B were obtained during the penetration and withdrawal of the recording glass micropipette from the ventral surface of the cerebellum. Current sink was up in this display. Calibration 2 mV/3mA/mm$^3$/20 ms. Extracellular conductivity was assumed to be 0.5 S/m based on the study published by Okada et al. (1994, Okada & Nicholson, 1988a). Ve = evoked field potential.

the currents were predominantly due to the climbing fibers that make strong monosynaptic excitatory connections onto the proximal third of the apical dendrites. This CSD pattern is consistent with the fact that the peduncle contains not only the mossy fibers but also the climbing fibers. This result indicated that the cellular currents responsible for the magnetic fields shown in Fig. 2.2 were produced by the Purkinje cells.

The cellular currents estimated with the CSD analysis were used to predict the magnetic field (Okada, 1989). Figure 2.6 shows the predicted and measured magnetic fields in the cerebellar preparation. According to Plonsey (1981), the neuromagnetic field is due to a sum of intra- and extracellular currents. Our CSD analysis showed that the intracellular currents responsible for the magnetic field were directed toward the distal apical dendrites. The extracellular currents associated with these currents complete the current loop and are directed toward the soma. The external magnetic field is produced not by the intra- and extracellular currents within the volume of the intra- and extracellular spaces but by the surface currents on both sides of the cellular membrane. The cross-product of this surface current vector and the surface element determines the direction of the current. Because the surface elements are directed toward the opposite directions on the surfaces of the membrane, the magnetic fields due to intra- and extracellular currents flow in the

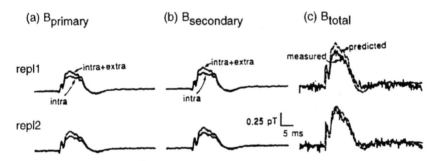

FIG. 2.6.  Predicted and measured evoked magnetic fields from the isolated turtle cerebellum (Okada, 1989). The predictions were obtained from the current source density (CSD) estimates along the direction perpendicular to the cerebellar surface at the center of activity as determined in experiments such as that shown in Fig. 2.4. The estimates are given separately for the magnetic fields that would be produced by the intra- and extracellular currents. The calculations were done for the primary currents produced by neurons in the cerebellum ($B_{primary}$) and for the secondary currents produced by the currents at the boundary between the cerebellum and the Ringer solution ($B_{secondary}$). The total predicted fields were compared with the measured magnetic fields obtained from the same cerebellum in which the CSD measurements were carried out. No free parameters were used for the calculated waveforms. repl = replication.

same direction, that is, their magnetic fields add rather than subtract. We calculated the intracellular currents from the CSD profile and estimated the extracellular currents by assuming a conservation of currents. The calculation showed that the observed magnetic field should be mostly due to intracellular currents (a, $B_{primary}$). We also estimated the magnetic fields due to the secondary current sources at the boundary of the cerebellum and saline medium (b, $B_{secondary}$). We added the magnetic fields from the primary and secondary sources to calculate the predicted magnetic fields. A comparison of the prediction against the measured signals showed an excellent agreement, thus demonstrating that the magnetic field pattern in Fig. 2.2 was produced by intracellular and associated extracellular currents.

## MAMMALIAN (GUINEA PIG) HIPPOCAMPAL SLICE STUDIES

### Motivation

As we studied the magnetic fields of the turtle cerebellum, it became clear to us that we needed to establish a fundamental understanding of the relation between cellular currents and the associated magnetic fields if we were to advance the field of biomagnetism study. One option was to stay with this cerebellar preparation and carry out a detailed series of pharmacological studies. However, we recognized that a well-developed mathematical model is necessary to interpret such data, because the interpretation of such experimental results would be far from being straightforward. Roger Traub suggested using the hippocampal slice preparation of the guinea pig, as he was already developing mathematical models needed for such an analysis. Also, it was clear that we needed to study the magnetic fields produced by a mammalian brain tissue if we were to relate our studies to human MEG studies.

### High-Resolution MEG Facility

The first step in carrying out such an analysis was to develop an instrument capable of yielding data from slice preparations with signal-to-noise ratios that would be sufficiently high for quantitative analyses. The one-channel MEG sensor used for the turtle study was inadequate. Thus, we applied for funds from the National Science Foundation to purchase a micro superconducting quantum interference device (microSQUID) that was being developed by John Wikswo and Biomagnetic Technologies (Buchanan, Crum, Cox, & Wikswo, 1989). The microSQUID II became available in the fall of 1991 (Okada, Shah, & Huang, 1994). The microSQUID enabled us to measure magnetic fields at a distance of as little as 1.2 mm from the outside world. Its detection coils are placed in vacuum just inside the outer tail section of the dewar. This short distance increases the measured signal strength by as much as a factor of 100 in comparison to the conventional MEG sensors such as our original one-channel sensor or the whole-head MEG systems being used today for human studies. The microSQUID became part of a new high-resolution MEG facility at the Veterans Affairs Medical Center in Albuquerque, New Mexico. This facility houses the microSQUID in a two-layer magnetically shielded room that was designed and constructed in house (Okada et al., 1994).

## Characteristics of Neuromagnetic Signals From the Hippocampal Slices

In our study, we initially used a transverse slice preparation (Kyuhou and Okada, 1993) and subsequently switched to longitudinal preparations. Figure 2.7 shows a longitudinal preparation and our general experimental setup. The hippocampus was cut along the plane shown in Panel A, and the CA3 region of the slice was isolated from the rest of the tissue and placed onto a nonmagnetic perfusion chamber (Panel B). We developed this chamber specifically for our MEG study. Unlike the chambers used for conventional electrophysiology, this chamber design enabled us to measure magnetic fields from a slice at a distance of 2 mm between the detection coils and the center of the slice. The strip near the pyramidal cell layer was stimulated with an array of bipolar electrodes to synchronously activate the pyramidal cells, and evoked responses were recorded simultaneously with an array of field potential electrodes along the longitudinal axis of the pyramidal cells and with the four detection coils of the microSQUID arranged as shown in Panel C.

We had now developed our experimental techniques to the point where it is possible to obtain high-quality MEG signals from these preparations, even though the slices were only 1 to 3 $mm^3$ in volume. Figure 2.8 shows single-epoch, unaveraged signals from a CA3 longitudinal slice (Okada & Xu, 1996) . The slice was immersed in Ringer solution with 0.1 mM picrotoxin and 0.2-mM 4-aminopyridine. The block of fast inhibition and voltage-sensitive, repolarizing potassium channels resulted in hyperexcitability of the slice, leading to spontaneously occurring syn-

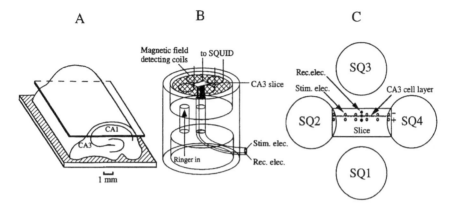

FIG. 2.7.   Experimental arrangement of the hippocampal slice studies. Panel A: geometry for obtaining longitudinal slices from the hippocampus. Panel B: nonmagnetic slice
chamber indicating the placement of the slice, stimulating (stim.) and recording (rec.)
electrodes (elec.) from below the slice and the four detection coils of the microSQUID
sensor. Panel C: arrangement of the stimulating and recording electrodes and the magnetic field detection coils relative to the slice viewed from above. The coils and the slice are
shown in their correct relative sizes (Wu & Okada, 1999). SQUID = superconducting
quantum interference device. SQ1-4 = SQUID pickup coils 1–4.

chronized population spikes that could be measured with the micro-
SQUID without signal averaging. The examples on the left side of Fig. 2.8
consisted of a train of spikes with the upward spikes in SQUID channel 2
due to currents directed from the basal to apical dendrites and the downward spikes in the same record due to currents directed from the apical to
basal dendrites. A steady current was seen after a series of four spikes, indicating a depolarization of the apical dendrites. A 10-Hz, 1-sec train of
stimulations produced a stimulus-locked train of spikes followed by a
train of after-discharges lasting more than 1 sec.

Mapping of the magnetic field above the slice (e.g., Fig. 2.9; Okada et
al., 1997) showed a field distribution similar to the one found above the
cerebellum (Fig. 2.2). The inset shows the measurement positions relative to the longitudinal CA3 slice. The slice was oriented as shown in Fig.
2.7C. Depolarizing stimuli were applied in the stratum radiatum. The resulting magnetic fields could be recorded clearly with 40 epochs/average.
The field pattern was in this case dipolar with both the initial spike and
the subsequent wave due to currents directed from the apical to basal
dendrites of the pyramidal cells.

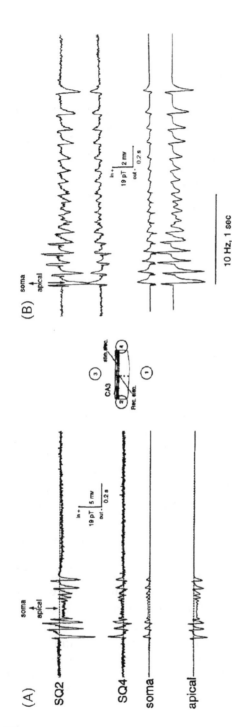

FIG. 2.8.    Panel A: spontaneous multiple population bursts in 0.1-mM picrotoxin and 0.2-mM 4-aminopyridine. Note a *dc* shift during the quiescent period. Panel B: stimulus-locked evoked magnetic fields and afterdischarges in response to a 10-Hz, 1-sec stimulation of the pyramidal cell layer with 1-mM, 50-μs pulses. stim. elec. = stimulating electrode; rec. elec. = recording electrode. From "Single-Epoch Neuromagnetic Signals During Eleptiform Activities in Guinea Pig Longitudinal CA3 Slices" by Y. C. Okada and C. Xu, 1996, *Neuroscience Letters, 211*, p. 157. Copyright 1996 by Elsevier Science. Adapted by permission.

As in our turtle study, we identified the principal neurons in the hippo-campus capable of producing the magnetic fields based on the laminar profile of the field potentials along the longitudinal axis of the pyramidal cells in the transverse CA1 slice (see Fig. 2.10A) and in the longitudinal CA1 slice (Fig. 2.10B; Okada et al., 1997). In both cases the initial spikes in the magnetic fields measured at SQ1 and SQ3 positions were due to action potentials in the apical dendritic trunk and soma of the pyramidal cells, whereas the subsequent wave was due to current sinks in the apical dendrites.

## Relationship Between Cellular Currents and MEG/EEG Signals

The development of a high-resolution MEG facility and improvements in experimental techniques have enabled us to now address the fundamental question of the relation between cellular currents and MEG and EEG signals. Here we illustrate our strategy in our current program of research to

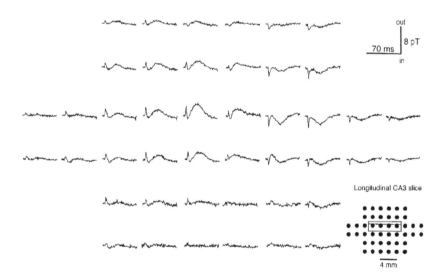

FIG. 2.9. Topography of the magnetic field produced by a longitudinal CA3 slice in Ringer solution with 0.1-mM picrotoxin (37° C). Measurement positions relative to the slice are indicated in the inset. The cell layer is shown by a straight line. The stratum radiatum is below the cell layer. The measurement distance was 2 mm above the slice. The field distribution is antisymmetrical relative to the longitudinal axis of the pyramidal cells, indicating that longitudinal currents were responsible for the signal. 40 epochs/ave. Stim.: 0.5 Hz, 50 μs, 1.2 mA pulses (Okada et al., 1997).

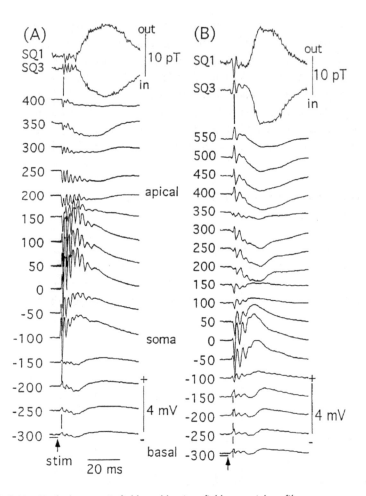

FIG. 2.10. Evoked magnetic fields and laminar field potential profiles were measured along the longitudinal axis of the pyramidal cells in a transverse CA1 slice (Panel A) and in a longitudinal CA1 slice (Panel B). In Panel A represents field potentials were averaged across 20 epochs and the magnetic fields were averaged across 90 epochs. In Panel B field potentials were averaged across 20 epochs; magnetic fields across 60 epochs. Stimulation: 1.0 mA, 50 μs, 2s/stimulus. Ringer solution contained 0.1-mM picrotoxin and 0.05 mM 4-aminopyridine. Spikes in the magnetic field were due to the spikes produced by the soma and apical dendritic trunk of the pyramidal cells, whereas the subsequent slow wave was due to a current sink in the apical dendrites and a current source in the soma and basal dendrite areas (Okada et al., 1997).

address this important question. We obtain three types of data from our experimental analysis. (Fig. 2.11; Wu & Okada, 1998). The magnetic field is measured simultaneously with the field potentials along the longitudinal axis of the pyramidal cells which, as we showed earlier, are the principal neurons producing the signals (see Fig. 2.11A). This allows us to compare these two sets of data from same slices. We also measure the field potentials simultaneously with intracellular potentials from the pyramidal cells in another set of experiments in otherwise identical settings (Fig. 2.11B). Thus, we can use the field potentials as the bridge to relate the magnetic fields to the intracellular activity of the pyramidal cells. Using these three sets of measurements, we have recently identified the characteristic waveforms associated with the depolarizing stimulations of the soma (left side of Fig. 2.11) and apical dendrites (right side of Fig. 2.11).

Our experimental strategy is to characterize the waveforms of the three types of signals before and after various ligand- and voltage-sensitive channels are selectively blocked with appropriate antagonists (Wu & Okada, 1998, 1999, 2000). Figure 2.12 shows such an example in which a calcium- and voltage-sensitive potassium channel of C type is blocked with tetraethylammonium (TEA). This channel type is activated by an increase in intracellular calcium concentration and by membrane depolarization to help repolarize the membrane potential. Tetraethylammonium did not have a strong effect on the initial spike activity, but it increased the slow wave of the magnetic field. This was also seen in the field potential recording. The increase in the slowly varying current directed from the apical to basal dendrites of the pyramidal cells was due to the prolonged membrane depolarization during the calcium spikes as seen in the intracellular records. This type of experiment has been carried out using blockers of various types of potassium conductances (i.e., gK(AHP)—afterhyperpolarization current, gK(C)—C current, gK(A)—A current, gK(DR)—delayed rectifier, gK(D)— D current, gCa—calcium channel, gNa—sodium channel, gNMDA— NMDA channel, gAMPA—AMPA channel).

Most recently, we have started our attempts to understand these data with the help of mathematical models. The 1991 Traub model (Traub, Wong, Miles, & Michelson, 1991) has served as our basic model in comparing theoretical predictions against empirical results. This model represents each pyramidal cell as a single cylinder with compartments for the basal and apical dendrites and soma. It also includes inhibitory cells and excitatory and inhibitory interconnections among these cells in a way that is consistent with known empirical facts. The model represents all the major ligand- and voltage-sensitive channels in each cell. We have extended this

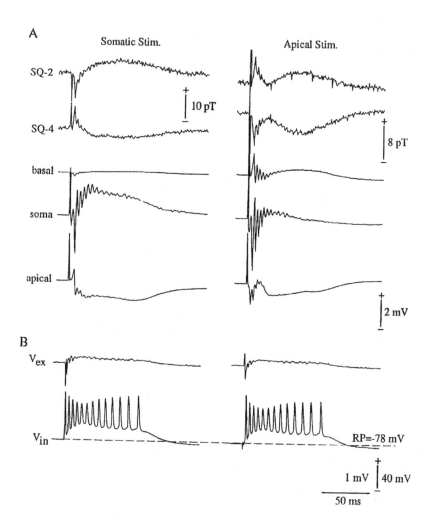

FIG. 2.11. Magnetic fields, field potentials, and intracellular potentials in pyramidal cells produced by a longitudinal CA3 slice. Left side of figure: somatic stimulation. Right side of figure: apical dendritic stimulation. Top two rows: magnetic fields; middle three rows: field potentials. These five traces were recorded simultaneously, 30 epochs/ave. Bottom two rows: field potential in the soma area and simultaneously recorded intracellular potential from the soma of a pyramidal cell (Wu & Okada, 1998). $V_{ex}$ = Extracellular potential; $V_{in}$ = Intracellular potential; RP = resting membrane potential.

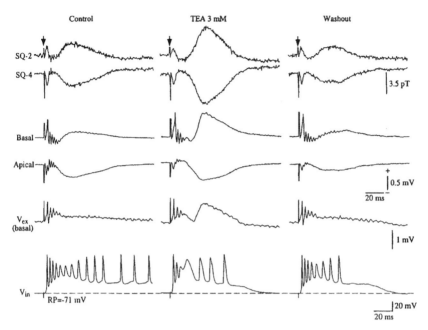

FIG. 2.12.   Effects of tetraethylammonium (TEA) in presence of 0.1-mM picrotoxin on apical stimulation-evoked magnetic fields measured at SQUID channels 2 and 4, field potentials in the basal and apical dendrite areas, and on intracellular potential in a pyramidal cell ($V_{in}$) and simultaneously measured field potential in the basal area ($V_{ex}$ - unaveraged). The magnetic field and field potentials in the top four traces were recorded simultaneously. Arrow indicates stimulus onset. Stimulus artefacts were not removed. The magnetic and $V_{ex}$ recordings are averages of 30 responses. (Wu & Okada, 2000). SQUID = superconducting quantum interference device.

model in two ways. The 1991 model assumes that the extracellular space is isopotential (Traub and Miles, 1991). Also, it does not include the axon for each cell and the axo–axonal gap junctions that are now known to be important for synchronizing the population activity (Traub, Jefferys, & Whittington, 1999). Thus, in one extension of the basic model we explicitly took into account the extracellular potentials to evaluate the role of extracellular currents in synchronization of population activity. In the second extension, we represented the proximal segment of the axon of each pyramidal cell and included the axo–axonal gap junction, with the help of Roger Traub, who kindly supplied us with the basic codes. We are currently in the process of testing the model predictions.

## *IN VIVO* PORCINE SOMATOSENSORY SYSTEM STUDIES

### Comparison of MEG and EEG

Our long-term aim is to help interpret human MEG and EEG signals. Thus, it is necessary to study the characteristics of these signals not only in *in vitro* preparations but also in *in vivo* preparations. Daniel Barth and his colleagues have made important contributions in this respect by looking at the rat preparation (Barth & Di, 1990a, 1990b, 1991; Barth & Sutherling, 1988). Unlike the human brain, which is gyrencephalic, the rat brain is lissencephalic (smooth brain). Thus, we felt that it was important to compare capabilities of MEG and EEG in an animal model whose brain resembles the human brain in many respects. The piglet preparation was not used previously for this purpose, but we have found out from our experience that it is quite useful. The piglet's brain is quite large (about 6 cm along the anterior–posterior axis) and has a well-developed convolution pattern in the cerebral cortex, with deep sulci (Craner & Ray, 1991a, 1991b). Using this *in vivo* piglet preparation, we have evaluated some of the basic assumptions in MEG and EEG research.

Figure 2.13 shows our general experimental arrangement (Okada, Lähteenmäki, & Xu, 1999a). The microSQUID is placed above the somatosensory cortex (Panel A). Depending on the purpose of our study, the sensors are directly above the scalp, the exposed skull, or the dura. The snout is electrically stimulated, and the evoked magnetic field is mapped with the detection coils on a field plane 2 mm above the exposed surface. As shown in Fig. 2.13B, the snout is represented within the large rostrum area (shaded area) of the primary somatosensory cortex (SI) as well as in three other regions of the cortex in each hemisphere. In addition to somatic evoked magnetic fields (SEFs), we measured somatic evoked potentials (SEPs) either on the scalp, skull, dura, or exposed cortex. Fig. 2.13B shows the placement of the electrodes on the exposed skull.

Figure 2.14 shows that both MEG and EEG may provide an accurate localization of the active tissue giving rise to the initial cortical response evoked by snout stimulations (Okada et al., 1999a). The isofield map of the 20-msec component (largest initial cortical response) of the SEF (top left panel) showed an active tissue on the posterior, lateral sulcus of the rostrum area in SI. The arrow indicates the location and orientation of the equivalent current dipole explaining the isofield pattern. The SEF on the dura was similar in isofield pattern and yielded a dipolar generator close to this generator, as shown by the two arrows in the isopotential

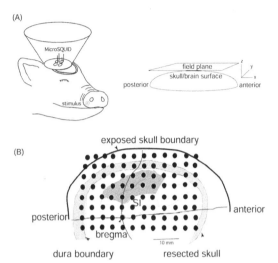

FIG. 2.13.    Experimental arrangement for magnetoencephalography and electroencephalography studies of the somatosensory cortex of the piglet *in vivo*. (A) The microSQUID was placed above the scalp, exposed skull, or exposed dura; the snout was stimulated with a bipolar electrode, and somatic evoked magnetic fields were measured with the detection coils on the field plane about 2 mm above the surface. Panel B: Somatic evoked potentials (SEPs) were measured from the same animals either on the scalp, exposed skull, or cortex with an array of 16 electrodes spaced 1 mm or 4 mm apart. Filled circles show the electrode locations on the exposed skull (Okada et al., 1999a).

map on the top right of the figure. The isopotential map of the 20-msec SEP component measured on the exposed skull was consistent with these two dipole locations estimated from the SEF data. The isopotential map showed a positive area lateral to the sulcus and a negative area medial to the sulcus. The reversal of the potential occurred close to the dipole locations indicated by the two arrows. The locations of the active area determined with the SEF on the dura and skull and with the SEP on the skull were consistent with the electrocorticogram (SEP on cortex) and with intracortical field potential recordings. The electrocorticogram showed a dipolar positive–negative profile centered around the locations of active tissue determined with SEF and SEP. The intracortical measurements showed polarity reversal along track 2, indicating activity at this location, but did not show such polarity reversals along the other tracks.

MEG and EEG produced similar localizations in this example, but in general they revealed different but complementary information. MEG showed activity near the sulci of the SI cortex, whereas EEG showed ac

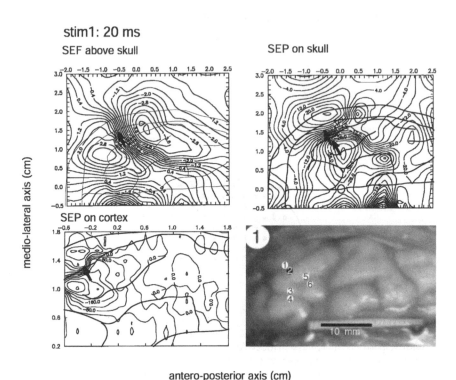

FIG. 2.14. Comparison of somatic evoked magnetic field (SEF) and somatic evoked potential (SEP) distributions on the exposed skull of the piglet elicited by snout stimulations. SEF above the skull: The isofield contour map of the 20-msec (initial cortical) component of the SEF is shown superimposed on an outline of the sulcal pattern of the pig cortex. The negative field was directed into the brain. Arrows indicate the location and direction of the equivalent current dipole representing the active tissue. The source was located on the lateral, posterior sulcal portion of the rostrum area in the primary somatosensory cortex. SEP on skull: The isopotential map of the corresponding 20-msec component of the SEP was measured on the exposed skull shown with the two dipole sources (arrows) determined from the SEF on the skull and on the dura in the same animal. The difference between the two arrows is within the error of estimates. The isopotential map was oriented nearly 90° to the isofield map, with the positivity in front of the arrows and negativity on the back, indicating that both magnetoencephalography and electroencephalography revealed the active tissue in the same area. SEP on cortex: The accuracy of localization was verified with electrocorticographic measurements of the SEP. The SEP pattern on the cortical surface was more restricted than the pattern on the skull, with a positive area in front and a negative area on the back of the arrow, which is the average of the two arrows estimated from SEF data shown for "SEP on skull" (top right panel). Intracortical SEP recordings along Track 2 showed polarity reversal, whereas the recordings along the other five tracks did not show such a reversal, confirming that the active area giving rise to the 20-msec component was correctly localized by the SEF and SEP measured on the skull. In general, however, the active areas identified with SEF were close to the sulcal area, and those identified with SEP were both on the sulcal and gyral area of the SI representing the snout. (Okada et al., 1999a). stim = stimulus; SI = primary somatosensory cortex.

tivity in both the sulcal and gyral portions of the cortex. In some cases, as in this example (Fig. 2.14), the SEP showed activity predominantly in the sulcus, whereas in other cases the SEP showed activity predominantly in the gyrus, and still in other cases the SEP was seen in both areas. This study thus confirmed one of the basic assumptions in MEG and EEG, namely, that MEG is due to currents in the sulci and EEG is due to currents in both the sulci and gyrii.

In another study, Okada, Lähteenmäki, and Xu (1999b) experimentally demonstrated the validity of another major assumption in MEG: that MEG is not distorted by the skull. Figure 2.15 shows the SEF measured on a field plane above the skull (Panel A, skull on), on the same field plane after the skull is removed (Panel B, skull off), and again on the same field plane after the skull is replaced (Panel C, skull on again). The inset shows the measurement locations relative to the cortex of this animal. The measurement area was centered over the anterior region of rostrum area 1 of the SI (Craner & Ray, 1991a). Figure 2.15D shows the SEFs from these three conditions superimposed on each other. The waveforms were virtually identical, independently of whether the skull was on or off the dura. A quantitative analysis of the skull effect showed that there were some distortions in the MEG signal as the generator became deeper. However, the distortion was small for cortical generators.

My colleagues and I are now currently evaluating the accuracy of spatiotemporal multiple dipole localization algorithms in this preparation because the accuracy can be directly verified. Some preliminary results (Okada, Papuashvili, & Xu, 1996) show that such an algorithm may be surprisingly accurate for localizing earlier cortical activities.

## APPLICATIONS OF MEG IN THE STUDY
## OF CNS PATHOPHYSIOLOGY

### Migraine

A phenomenon called *Leâo's spreading depression* (SD) has been considered as the basis of the aura experienced during the prodrome phase of classic migraine (Lauritzen, 1994). SDs produce a very large extracellular negativity (of up to –40 mV) over a period of about 1 min in mammalian brains (Bures, Buresova, & Krivanek, 1974). Thus, we felt that it should also produce a strong MEG signal. We initially verified this prediction in the *in vitro* isolated turtle cerebellar preparation (see Fig. 2.16). Using the same preparation shown in Fig. 2.2, we evoked SDs in the cerebellum

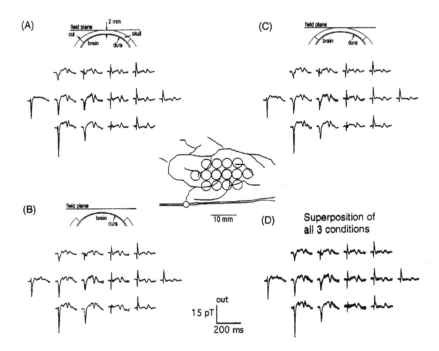

FIG. 2.15.    Effects of the skull on somatic evoked magnetic fields (SEFs). SEFs were measured directly above the primary somatosensory cortex at the locations shown in the inset. Panel A: SEFs on the field plane 1.2 mm above the 2 mm-thick skull (skull on). Panel B:
SEFs on the same field plane with the skull removed (skull off). Panel C: SEFs on the same
field plane with the skull replaced (skull on again). In Panels A–C two replications are
shown at the central two locations to illustrate the reliability of the measurements. Panel
D: superimposition of the signals from Panels A–C. The SEFs were virtually identical,
showing little effects of the skull (Okada et al., 1999b).

with peduncular stimulations after conditioning the tissue with a modified Ringer solution in which 80% of NaCl was replaced by sodium propionate (Okada, Lauritzen, & Nicholson, 1987a, 1987b). The stimulation
produced SDs with similar field potential waveforms as we measured the
magnetic fields at different positions relative to the center of the cerebellum. The numbers in parenthesis indicate the x, y, and z coordinates of
the measurement positions. Unlike the field potentials, however, the
magnetic field was near the baseline along the y-axis at $x = 0$, whereas it
was reversed in polarity along the x-axis. This pattern indicated that cur-

rents perpendicular the cerebellar surface were capable of producing magnetic fields of several picoTeslas at a height of 17 mm.

In isolated chick retina, we found that currents perpendicular to the retinal surface were capable of producing magnetic fields of more than 50 picoTeslas at a height of 3–4 mm (Fig. 2.17; Okada, Kyuhou, & Xu, 1993). In this series of experiments (Okada, do Carmo, Martins-Ferreira, & Nicholson, 1992; Okada et al., 1993), a rectangular retinal tissue from the chick was prepared and placed in a bath of Ringer solution with either el-

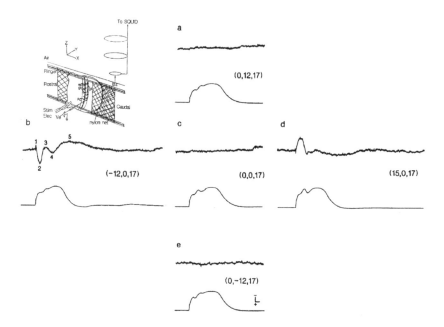

FIG. 2.16.  Magnetic signals of spreading depression (SD) produced by the isolated turtle cerebellum. The inset shows the arrangement. The cerebellum was conditioned for SD by reducing the chloride ion (by substituting 80% of NaCl with sodium propionate) in the Ringer solution bathing the cerebellum, and each episode of SD was elicited by an electrical (Elec) stimulation (stim) of the cerebellar peduncle with a 5-sec, 20-Hz train of 50-µs pulses. Dc signals were recorded at the locations shown by the x–y–z coordinates next to each record (in millimeters) relative to the center of the cerebellum. Dc-field potentials were recorded simultaneously with each magnetic field measurement to ascertain that comparable SDs were elicited across the sequential measurements of the magnetic field with a single-channel MEG sensor. Calib.: 1 pT/10 mV/20s. SQUID = superconducting quantum interference device. Bz = component of the magnetic field along the z-direction normal to the bath surface. See Fig. 2.2 for the other abbreviation. From "Magnetic Field Associated With Spreading Depression: A Model for the Detection of Migraine" by Y. C. Okada, M. Lauritzen, and C. Nicholson, 1987, *Brain Research, 442.* Copyright 1987 by Elsevier Science. Adapted by permission.

evated potassium or reduced chloride ion used to condition the tissue for SD. Each episode of SD was elicited mechanically, by pricking the retina with a glass micropipette. One advantage of this preparation was that the SD could be seen visually with the naked eye as an expanding circular pattern of gray color in a darker background. When the center of the retina was stimulated (Fig. 2.17B), the propagation was symmetrical and circular until the SD hit the top and bottom edges of the rectangular tissue and then propagated to the left and right with a circular wavefront. The SD pattern over the bath was antisymmetrical, as should be the case for a symmetrical current distribution. When one edge of the tissue was stimulated (in this case, the right edge, shown in Panel C), the SD propagated from the right to the left. Thus, the MEG signal was not seen at channel 0 above the initiation site but was present on the other three channels. As the SD moved to the left of channel 0, this channel detected the downward field. A detailed analysis of the field pattern such as the one shown in Fig. 2.17C reveals a propagation of SD to the left. We estimated the location of the center of SD as a function of time from the location of the equivalent current dipole along the surface of the tissue. Figure 2.17D shows that for two replications the dipole was located 4 mm at the initiation of SD, which corresponds to the center of channel 0, and moved at a uniform velocity to the left edge with a velocity of 3 mm/min. This implies that the velocity of the left wavefront was approximately 6 mm/min because the right wavefront was stationary.

These analyses based on *in vitro* studies have suggested that MEG may be useful in characterizing the prodrome phase of migraine if it is accompanied by an SD. MEG might provide new insights into the genesis of migraine by revealing the properties of SD during this period. Thus, we have extended our work to *in vivo* studies. Rabbits have been classically used for SD studies. Thus, we initially studied MEG signals of SD in a rabbit preparation (Bowyer, Okada, et al., 1999). Here, we were able to elicit SDs by electrically stimulating the cortex after conditioning the cortex with modified Ringer solution containing elevated potassium and reduced chloride ions. The SD initiated on the left lateral cortex near electrode 1 propagated toward the midline and into the longitudinal fissure, because SD was successively registered by electrodes 1–4, with electrode 4 located within the fissure. We found that an MEG signal was seen as the SD reached the corner of the longitudinal fissure and propagated downward into the fissure, because the signal started as the SD reached electrode 3, which was located at the corner, and became maximum at about the same time the SD signal became maximum at electrode 4. We thus

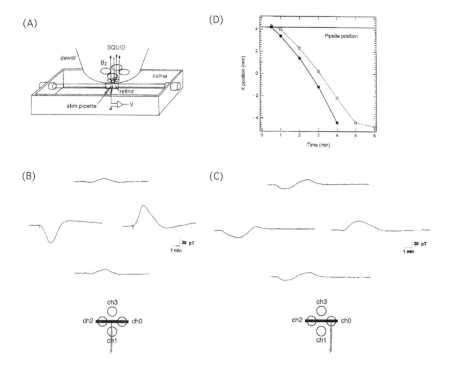

FIG. 2.17. Magnetic signals of spreading depression (SD) in the avian retina *in vitro*. Panel A: experimental arrangement; a rectangular piece of avian retina was mechanically stimulated with a glass micropipette in a conditioning medium to initiate SDs. Panel B: magnetic field of SD initiated at the center of the tissue. SD visible with the naked eye propagated circularly until it reached the top and bottom edge of the tissue, then expanded to the left and right with a circular wavefront. The symmetrical current directed perpendicular to the retinal surface produced the antisymmetrical magnetic field. Panel C: magnetic field of SD initiated at the right edge of the tissue. SD propagated to the left. The component of the field normal to the bath surface was thus zero at channel 0, but it was seen in channels 1–3 immediately after an SD was initiated. As the SD propagated to the left, channel 0 saw an upward field while the remaining channels saw a downward field. Panel D: location of an equivalent current dipole representing the current at the center of the SD as a function of time from the moment of initiation. The dipole moved from near the starting location (the stimulating [stim] pipette was located 4.2 mm to the right) to the terminal location (5 mm to the left) at a uniform speed of 3 mm/min. This implies that the propagation velocity of the left wavefront was approximately 6 mm/min, because the right wavefront was stationary. SQUID = superconducting quantum interference device. From "Tissue Current Associated With Spreading Depression Inferred From Magnetic Field Recordings" by Y. C. Okada, S. Kyuhou, and C. Xu, in A. Lehmenkuhler et al. (Eds.), *Migraine: Basic Mechanisms and Treatments*, 254, 257, 259, 260. Copyright 1993 by Urban and Schwarzenberg. Adapted by permission.

concluded that MEG signals in the rabbit cortex were produced by currents perpendicular to and directed from superficial to deeper layers of the sulcal portion of the cortex.

In the piglet study (Bowyer, Papuashvili, et al., 1999), we found that the MEG signal of SD was more complex than in the rabbit because of the convolutions of the neocortex. We also found that the velocity of propagation was not uniform as in the lissencephalic rabbit cortex. The velocity was about three to four times faster in the gyrus than in the sulcus.

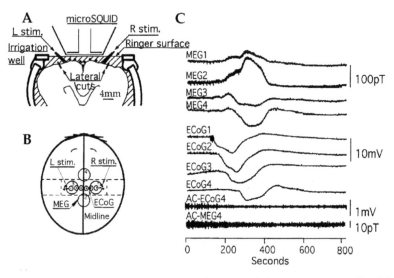

FIG. 2.18.    Magnetic field and simultaneously measured electrocorticograms (EcoGs) of spreading depression (SD) from the cerebral cortex of the rabbit. Panel A: A strip was cut in the cortex, and SDs were elicited wither from the left or right of the strip in order to simplify the path of propagation. The cortex was conditioned for SD with a modified Ringer solution (in which 70% of NaCl was replaced by sodium isethionate and KCl was elevated to 7 mM) in the well. SDs were initiated with a tetanic stimulation of the cortex (in this case, at the location of the left stimulus [L stim.]). SDs were recorded with an array of silver ball electrodes placed along the middle of the strip and with a four-channel microSQUID sensor. Panel B: locations of the magnetic field detectors and electrodes. Panel C: simultaneously measured magnetic fields and ECoG signals during an SD elicited at the left, lateral position. Note that a mirror-image SD pattern was seen at channels 2 and 4 starting at about the time SD was seen by Electrode 3, which was located at the corner of the longitudinal fissure and became maximum in amplitude at about the same time it reached the maximum at Electrode 4 located in the middle of the longitudinal fissure, indicating that currents in sulci and fissures produce magnetic signals during SDs. Because magnetic fields are due to currents tangential to the brain surface, it is concluded that a strong current perpendicular to the cortical surface accompanies episodes of SD (Bowyer, Okada, et al., 1999). SQUID = superconducting quantum interference device; R stim = right stimulation; MEG = magnetoencephalography; AC = alternating current.

We do not yet know whether this result is peculiar to the way we conditioned the cortex or whether it holds generally for gyrencephalic species. These animal studies are quite useful for migraine studies, because they provide crucial information for modeling the generators of SD. If the propagation is nonuniform, then we can use two different velocities in the model. Together with a three-dimensional volumetric information regarding the cortical shape, it should be possible to model the propagation of SD in the human brain. A comparison of the prediction with the data may provide clues as to whether the initiation starts at a focal site or from multiple foci. Such an analysis should also reveal the relation between the electrophysiological activity and the prodrome, such as visual scintillations important for understanding the genesis of migraine.

## Stroke

We have also started to examine whether MEG is potentially useful for characterizing the sequela of various forms of stroke in human patients. In our ongoing study we have been studying the sequela of a hemorrhagic stroke model in the piglet preparation. In this study, an intracortical hemorrhage (ICH) is produced by cortical injection of a small amount of collagenase, which breaks the blood brain barrier and causes slow bleeding. Collagenase is injected into a projection area of the snout. The effects of the injection are monitored by measuring the intracortical somatic evoked potential (cSEP) within the projection area and surrounding area of the rostrum area. As shown in Fig. 2.19, the cSEP in the projection area is rapidly abolished by collagenase (Mun-Bryce, Wilkerson, Papuashvili, & Okada, 2001). Figure 2.19A shows the cSEPs from the projection area of the snout in the SI cortex recorded over a period of about 3 hr after the collagenase injection. The amplitude of the first component decreased, as shown in Panel B. The rate of amplitude decrease was dose dependent. It is interesting that the hemorrhage alters the cSEP not only in the hemisphere ipsilateral to the injury but also in the uninjured opposite hemisphere (S Mun-Bryce, L. Roberts, & Y. Okada, unpublished). We are currently in the process of characterizing this remote effect during the acute and chronic stages after an ICH so that the results may be used to help interpret MEG signals from stroke patients in the future.

We also discovered that an ICH produces recurring episodes of SD (Mun-Bryce et al., 2001). SDs are known to occur after focal ischemia, but this had not been observed after a hemorrhage. Figure 2.20 shows an example of SDs observed after a collagenase injection into the snout area

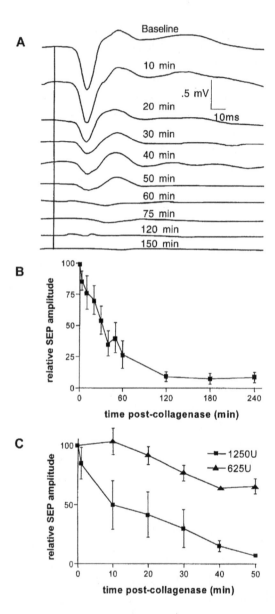

FIG. 2.19. A decrease in intracortical somatic evoked potential (SEP) recorded within the projection area of the snout in the primary somatosensory cortex of the piglet as a function of time after collagenase injection. Panel A: averaged waveforms as a function of time. Panel B: relative amplitude of the first negative component as a function of time after collagenase injection. Panel C: dose-dependent effects on the rate of amplitude decrease (Mun-Bryce et al., 2001).

of the SI. SDs were found to occur initially around the hemorrhagic core; that is, SDs during the "early period" were seen at first at electrodes closest to the injection site and propagated to the surrounding electrodes. With time, SDs ceased to appear near the hemorrhagic core, but they were seen at surrounding locations, suggesting that the initiation sites were located around the periphery of the expanding hemorrhagic core. The discovery of SD in a hemorrhagic stroke model suggests that recurring episodes of SD may be produced in stroke patients as well.

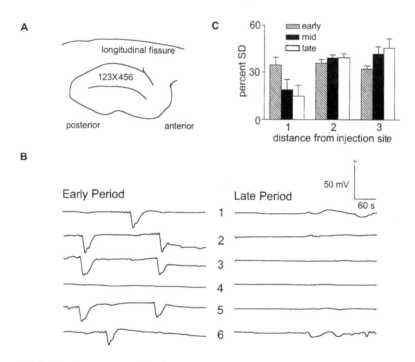

FIG. 2.20.  Recurring episodes of spontaneously produced spreading depression (SD) in the primary somatosensory cortex after collagenase injection at location *x*, indicated in Panel A. Panel B: The SDs recorded at six electrode locations surrounding the injection site during the early period (left) and at a later point in time (right) were seen initially near the injection site and propagated outward and later only at remote locations. Panel C: percentages of SD seen at electrode locations 1 mm (Electrodes 3 and 4), 2 mm (Electrodes 2 and 5) and 3 mm (Electrodes 1 and 6) away from the injection site during early, middle, and late periods. This graph supports the conclusion that the SDs were produced by the expanding peri-injury region of the intracortical hemorrhage (Mun-Bryce et al., 2001).

## CONCLUSION

Researchers are certainly far from being able to provide a comprehensive picture of the foundation of MEG and EEG; however, the research my colleagues and I have conducted during the past 16 years provides some empirical underpinnings of the basic assumptions in interpreting MEG and EEG signals. It is also beginning to provide a new picture on the genesis of MEG and EEG signals within the modern framework of central nervous system physiology. Two examples of applications described here illustrate how an understanding of the physiological origin of neuromagnetic signals may be helpful in CNS pathophysiology research.

## ACKNOWLEDGMENTS

I thank Samuel Williamson, Lloyd Kaufman, Charles Nicholson, and Rodolfo Llinás and all the postdoctoral scientists who have contributed to this program of research. I also acknowledge the support from the National Institutes of Health, which has supported my research without interruption over the last 16 years (Grants NS21149 and NS30968).

## REFERENCES

Barth, D. S., & Di, S. (1990b). Three-dimensional analysis of auditory-evoked potentials in rat neocortex. *Journal of Neurophysiology, 64,* 1527–1536.

Barth, D. S., & Di, S. (1990a). The electrophysiological basis of epileptiform magnetic fields in neocortex. *Brain Research, 530,* 35–39.

Barth, D. S., & Di, S. (1991). The electrophysiological basis of epileptiform magnetic fields in neocortex: Spontaneous ictal phenomena. *Brain Research, 557,* 95–102.

Barth, D., & Sutherling, W. W. (1988). Current-source density and neuromagnetic analysis of the direct cortical responses in rat cortex. *Brain Research, 450,* 280–294.

Bowyer, S. M., Okada, Y. C., Papuashvili, N., Moran, J. E., Barkley, G. L., Welch, K. M. A., & Tepley, N. (1999). Analysis of MEG signals of spreading cortical depression with propagation constrained to a rectangular cortical stri: I. Lissencephalic rabbit model. *Brain Research, 843,* 71–78.

Bowyer, S. M., Papuashvili, N., Kato, S., Moran, J., Barkley, G. L., Welch, K. M. A., Tepley, N., & Okada, Y. C. (1999). Analysis of MEG signals of spreading cortical depression with propagation constrained to a rectangular cortical strip: II. Gyrencephalic swine model. *Brain Research, 843,* 79–86.

Buchanan, D. S., Crum, D. B., Cox, D., & Wikswo, J. P. Jr. (1989). MicroSQUID: A close-spaced four channel magnetometer. In S. J. Williamson, M. Hoke, G. Stroink & M. Kotani, (Eds.), *Advances in biomagnetism* (pp. 677–679). New York: Plenum.

Bures, J., Buresova, O., & Krivanek, J. (1974). *The mechanisms and applications of Leão's spreading depression of electroencephalographic activity.* Prague: Academia.

Cohen, D., & Hosaka, H. (1976). Magnetic field produced by a current dipole. *Journal of Electrocardiology, 9,* 409–417.

Craner, S. L., & Ray, R. H. (1991a). Somatosensory cortex of the neonatal pig: I. Topographical organization of primary somatosensory cortex. (SI). *Journal of Comparative Neurology, 306,* 24–38.

Craner, S. L., & Ray, R. H. (1991b). Somatosensory cortex of the neonatal pig: II. Topographical organization of secondary somatosensory cortex. (SII). *Journal of Comparative Neurology, 306,* 39–48.

Freeman, J. A., & Nicholson, C. (1975). Experimental optimization of current source-density technique for anuran cerebellum. *Journal of Neurophysiology, 38,* 369–382.

Geselowitz, D. B. (1970). On the magnetic field generated outside an inhomogeneous volume conductor by internal current sources. *IEEE Transaction Magnetism, 6,* 346–347.

Kyuhou, S., & Okada, Y. C. (1993). Detection of magnetic signals from isolated transverse CA1 hippocampal slice of the guinea pig. *Journal of Neurophysiology, 70,* 2665–2668.

Lauritzen, M. (1994). Pathophysiology of the migraine aura: The spreading depression theory. *Brain, 117,* 199–210.

Mun-Bryce, S., Wilkerson, A., Papuashvili, N., & Okada, Y. C. (2001). Recurring episodes of spreading depression are spontaneously elicited by collagenase-induced intracerebral hemorrhage in the swine. *Brain Research, 888,* 248–255.

Nicholson, C., & Freeman, J. A. (1975). Theory of current source-density analysis and determination of conductivity tensor for Anuran cerebellum. *Journal of Neurophysiology, 38,* 356–368.

Okada, Y. C. (1989). Recent developments on the physiological basis of magnetoencephalography. In S. J. Williamson (Ed.), *Biomagnetism* (pp. 273–278). New York: Plenum.

Okada, Y. C., do Carmo, R., Martins-Ferreira, H., & Nicholson, C. (1992). Detection of the magnetic fields from isolated avian retina during spreading depression. *Experimental Brain Research, 23,* 89–97.

Okada, Y. C., Kyuhou, S., & Xu, C. (1993). Tissue current associated with spreading depression inferred from magnetic field recordings. In A. Lehmenkuhler et al. (Eds.), *Migraine: Basic mechanisms and treatment* (pp. 249–265). München, Germany: Urban and Schwarzenberg.

Okada, Y. C., Lähteenmäki, A., & Xu, C. (1999a). Comparison of MEG and EEG on the basis of somatic evoked responses elicited by stimulation of the snout in the juvenile swine. *Clinical Neurophysiology, 110,* 214–229.

Okada, Y. C., Lähteenmäki, A., & Xu, C. (1999b). Experimental analysis of distortion of MEG signals by the skull. *Electroencephalography and Clinical Neurophysiology, 110,* 230–238.

Okada, Y. C., Lauritzen, M., & Nicholson, C. (1987a). Magnetic field associated with spreading depression: A model for the detection of migraine. *Brain Research, 442,* 185–190.

Okada, Y. C., Lauritzen, M., & Nicholson, C. (1987b). Source models and physiology. *Physics in Medicine and Biology, 32,* 43–51.

Okada, Y. C., & Nicholson C. (1988a). Currents underlying the magnetic evoked field in the cerebellum. In K. Atsumi, M. Kotani, S. Ueno, T. Katila, & S. J. Williamson (Eds.), *Biomagnetism '87* (pp. 198–201). Tokyo, Japan: Tokyo Denki University Press.

Okada, Y. C., & Nicholson, C. (1988b). Magnetic evoked field associated with transcortical currents in turtle cerebellum. *Biophysical Journal, 53,* 723–731.

Okada, Y. C., Nicholson, C., & Llinás, R. (1989). Magnetoencephalography (MEG) as a new tool for non-invasive realtime analysis of normal and abnormal brain activity in humans. In D. Ottoson & W. Rostene (Eds.), *Visualization of brain functions* (pp. 245–266). New York: Stockton Press.

Okada, Y. C., Papuashvili, N. S., & Xu, C. (1996). What can we learn from MEG studies of the somatosensory system of the swine? In I. Hashimoto, Y. C. Okada, & S. Ogawa (Eds.), *Visualization of information processing in the human brain: Recent advances in MEG and functional MRI (EEG Clin. Neurol. Suppl. 47)* (pp. 35–46). Amsterdam: Elsevier.

Okada, Y. C., Shah, B., & Huang, J.-C. (1994). Ferromagnetic high-permeability alloy alone can provide sufficient low-frequency and eddy-current shieldings for biomagnetic measurements. *IEEE Transaction on Biomedical Engineering, 41,* 688–697.

Okada, Y. C., Wu, J., & Kyuhou, S. (1997). Genesis of MEG signals in a mammalian CNS structure. *Electroencephalography and Clinical Neurophysiology, 103,* 474–485.

Okada, Y. C., & Xu, C. (1996). Single-epoch neuromagnetic signals during epileptiform activities in guinea pig longitudinal CA3 slices. *Neuroscience Letters, 211,* 155–158.

Plonsey, R. (1981). Generation of magnetic fields by the human body (theory). In S. N. Erné, H.-D. Hählbohm, & H. Lübbig (Eds.), *Biomagnetism* (pp. 177–205). Berlin: de Gruyter.

Traub, R. D., Jefferys, J. G. R., & Whittington, M. A. (1999) *Fast oscillations in cortical circuits.* Cambridge, MA: MIT Press.

Traub, R. D., & Miles, R. (1991). *Neuronal networks of the hippocampus.* New York: Cambridge University Press.

Traub, R. D., Wong, R. K. S., Miles, R., & Michelson, H. (1991). A model of a CA3 hippocampal pyramidal neuron incorporating voltage-clamp data on intrinsic conductances. *Journal of Neurophysiology, 66,* 635–650.

Wu, J., & Okada, Y. C. (1998). Physiological bases of the synchronized population spikes and slow wave of the magnetic field generated by a guinea pig longitudinal CA3 slice preparation. *Electroencephalography and Clinical Neurophysiology, 107,* 361–373.

Wu, J., & Okada, Y. C. (1999). Roles of a potassium afterhyperpolarization current in generating neuromagnetic fields and field potentials in longitudinal CA3 slices of the guinea-pig. *Clinical Neurophysiology, 110,* 1858–1867.

Wu, J., & Okada, Y. C. (2000). Ca$^{2+}$- and voltage-activated potassium conductances determine the waveform of neuromagnetic signals from hippocampal CA3 longitudinal slice of guinea-pig. *Clinical Neurophysiology, 111,* 150–160.

# 3

## Forward Problem Solution of Magnetic Source Imaging

N. G. Gençer
C. E. Acar
I. O. Tanzer
*Middle East Technical University*

The representations of the intracellular electric current of the active cell populations in the brain based on the recorded magnetic fields are called *magnetic source images*. For accurate interpretation of the measured data it is necessary to calculate the magnetic fields outside a head model for a known source distribution. In this study, the theory governing the behavior of magnetic field due to current sources in a piecewise conductive body is introduced, and the basic properties are discussed. To localize the sources of the magnetic fields it is essential to develop head models that incorporate the correct geometry and electrical properties of the head. This chapter presents two numerical approaches to develop realistic models: (a) the boundary element method (BEM) and (b) the finite element method (FEM). In the FEM formulation isoparametric quadratic elements are used. In BEM formulations both planar and curved triangles are used. On planar elements the potential function varies linearly, whereas formulations for curved triangles allow quadratic or cubic variation for both the geometry and the potential function. The accuracy in solutions is explored for a tangential dipole source located at different depths in a concentric spherical shell model of the head. The relative difference measures are calculated, and it is shown that the use of higher order elements enhances accuracy in the forward problem solutions.

Magnetic source imaging (MSI) explores the spatiotemporal behavior of electrical sources in the human brain. This is achieved by using the magnetic fields measured outside the head (the magnetoencephalogram [MEG]), which are complementary to the voltage measurements obtained from the scalp surface (electroencephalogram [EEG]). Finding electrical sources from magnetic measurements, that is, solution of the *inverse problem*, is based on the comparison of the measurements with the calculated fields. Thus, an essential part of MSI is the solution of magnetic fields outside the head for an assumed internal source distribution. This is known as the *forward problem* of MSI. In forward problem solutions an appropriate head model is used to represent the geometry and conductivity distribution of the head. The purpose of this chapter is to provide the basic properties of the forward problem and introduce different numerical approaches for its solution.

In the earliest studies, head models with simple geometries were considered that allow analytical solutions for a dipole inside the conductor model. When such models are used, the inverse problem can be solved without a need for high computational speed and computer resources. The simplest head model that has such properties is the homogeneous sphere. The magnetic fields produced by a current dipole in the homogeneous sphere have been calculated by Grynszpan and Geselowitz (1973) and Geselowitz (1973). Other homogenous head models that may represent the head shape are prolate spheroid (egg shape) and oblate spheroid (discus shape). Expressions for the magnetic fields produced by current dipoles inside such conductor models were presented by Cuffin and Cohen (1977).

To represent layers such as skull, scalp, and brain, different conductor models are proposed (Rush & Driscoll, 1968). Such models are simple in shape but have layered structures. Grynszpan and Geselowitz (1973) showed that, for MEG, a head model that consists of a set of concentric spheres is equivalent to a homogenous sphere. Another model that takes into account the effects of conductive layers is the *eccentric-spheres model*, which may also fit to the actual geometry. Use of a model of eccentric spheres to describe the head was first studied with numerical methods. It was concluded that an eccentric-spheres model should be used to interpret the EEGs, whereas a homogeneous-sphere model is a sufficiently accurate model to interpret MEGs (Meijs & Peters, 1987). The analytical solutions are then developed for the eccentric-spheres model of head (Cuffin, 1991).

The localization performance using EEG or MEG data has been investigated by a number of experimental studies and computer simulations in the literature. The localization results have shown that the use of simple head models can lead to significant errors in the source parameters. Experimental studies using EEG measurements have been carried out using a saline-filled skull (Henderson, Butler, & Glass, 1975), implanted sources in a monkey brain (Hosek, Sances, Jodat, & Larson, 1978), human head (Cohen et al., 1990; Smith, Sidman, Henke, & Labiner, 1985), and cat brain (He et al., 1987). For a single-dipole source, localization errors up to 3 cm are observed, especially when the sources are close to the inhomogeneities. Experimental studies with MEG measurements are also performed using sources in skulls filled with conductive gel and implanted sources in the human head. Significant distortion on the field maps, and localization errors up to 1 cm, have been reported (Barth, Sutherling, Broffman, & Beatty, 1986; Cohen et al., 1990, Weinberg, Brickett, Coolsma, & Baff, 1986). It should be noted that the head model alone is not the source of this error; other factors, such as measurement noise, incorrect sensor/electrode positions, and so on, are also relevant.

Simulation studies with relatively simpler head models (the concentric-spheres model for EEG and the eccentric-spheres model for MEG) are performed to add, to some degree, the effects of conductivity inhomogeneity in the head (Cuffin, 1991, 1996; Darcey, Ary, & Fender, 1980; Kavanagh, Darcey, Lehmann, & Fender, 1978; Schneider, 1974; Sidman, Giambalvo, Allison, & Bergey, 1978). Using a simple spherical volume conductor model, researchers have shown that inhomogeneities close to sources can significantly affect the calculated magnetic fields and the potential distribution (Ueno, Iramina, & Harada, 1987; Ueno, Iramina, Ozaki, & Harada, 1986). When there are simultaneously active multiple sources, the accuracy of the head shape becomes even more important. In the case of dipole pairs, a misspecified multiple-shell or single-shell sphere may produce a large amount of error in the estimation of dipole parameters (Zhang & Jewett, 1993; Zhang, Jewett, & Goodwill, 1994).

Numerical methods are used to construct head models, which have more realistic geometry and conductivity distributions. In the numerical solutions, the magnetic field distribution due to a current dipole source is obtained by first solving the potential distribution in the conductor model (Sarvas, 1987). The most common numerical methods used for this purpose are the *boundary element method* (BEM) and the *finite element method* (FEM). Once the solution for the potential is calculated, the magnetic field at a given point outside the head is obtained with Geselowitz's (1970) formula.

In the following sections, we first present the differential and integral equations governing the behavior of potentials and magnetic fields and then discuss their properties. Next, we present together formulations for the two numerical approaches—namely, BEM and FEM—with numerical results obtained in simulations.

## THEORY

For biological sources, the potentials and magnetic fields are calculated on the basis of a "quasi-static" formulation (Plonsey, 1969). In this formulation the capacitive, propagation, and inductive effects are neglected on the basis of electrical properties, the frequency of bioelectric sources, and the size of the human body. Under these assumptions, the potential and electric field expressions are exactly the same as those used in the presence of steady-state or non–time-varying currents.

In this section we present magnetic field expression due to a current source in a medium with piecewise homogeneous conductivity distribution. This is based on the formulations given by Geselowitz (1967, 1970). Excellent discussions of these formulations can be found in Gulrajani (1998); Hämäläinen, Hari, Ilmoniemi, Knuutila, and Lounasmaa (1993); and Malmivuo and Plonsey (1995).

The conductive medium is assumed to have an isotropic conductivity distribution $\sigma$ and a constant permeability $\mu = \mu_o$, where $\mu_o$ is the free space permeability. In the quasi-static limit, the Maxwell's equation reduces to:

$$\nabla \times \vec{B} = \mu_o \vec{J} , \qquad (3.1)$$

where $\vec{B}$ is the magnetic flux density and $\vec{J}$ $(= \vec{J}_i + \sigma\vec{E})$ is the total current density. Here $\vec{J}_i$ represents the impressed source current density and $\vec{E}$ is the electric field, which can be written as the negative of the gradient of an electric scalar potential $\phi$, and $\sigma\vec{E}$ is the conduction current density. Taking the curl of both sides, Equation 3.1 reduces to:

$$\nabla^2 \vec{B} = -\mu_o \left( \nabla \times \vec{J} \right) . \qquad (3.2)$$

Here the vector identity $\nabla \times \nabla \times \vec{B} = \nabla(\nabla \cdot \vec{B}) - \nabla^2 \cdot \vec{B}$ is used, and the divergence of $\vec{B}$ is assumed to be zero. Equation 3.2 is the Poisson equation along with the boundary condition that $\vec{B}$ vanishes at infinity. The solution for $\vec{B}$ at point $\vec{r}$ is

$$\vec{B}(\vec{r}) = \frac{\mu_0}{4\pi} \int_V \frac{\nabla' \times \vec{J}(\vec{r}')}{R} dV' \; , \tag{3.3}$$

where $V$ represents the volume of the conductor and $R = |\vec{r} - \vec{r}'|$. The curl operator now operates on the source coordinate $\vec{r}'$. For currents of limited extent, by using simple basic vector identities it can also be shown that

$$\vec{B}(\vec{r}) = \frac{\mu_0}{4\pi} \int_V \vec{J}(\vec{r}') \times \nabla'(1/R) dV' \; . \tag{3.4}$$

Equation 3.4 can be rewritten as

$$\vec{B}(\vec{r}) = \frac{\mu_0}{4\pi} \int_V \vec{J}(\vec{r}') dV' \times \nabla'(1/R) \; . \tag{3.5}$$

It is possible to obtain a computationally more suitable form of the magnetic field $\vec{B}$ expression when the current density is explicitly written as $\vec{J} = \vec{J}_i - \sigma \nabla \phi$ (Geselowitz, 1970),

$$\begin{aligned}
\vec{B}(\vec{r}) &= \frac{\mu_0}{4\pi} \int_V \vec{J}_i(\vec{r}') dV' \times \nabla'(1/R) \\
&\quad - \frac{\mu_0}{4\pi} \int_V \sigma \nabla \phi \times \nabla'(1/R) dV' \; .
\end{aligned} \tag{3.6}$$

If the body is divided into a number of regions in which the conductivity is uniform and isotropic, then

$$\begin{aligned}
\vec{B}(\vec{r}) &= \frac{\mu_0}{4\pi} \int_V \vec{J}_i(\vec{r}') dV' \times \nabla'(1/R) \\
&\quad - \frac{\mu_0}{4\pi} \sum_i \sigma_i \int_{V_i} \nabla \phi \times \nabla'(1/R) dV' \; .
\end{aligned} \tag{3.7}$$

Following the vector identities given by Geselowitz (1970), it is possible to obtain the following form for the magnetic field outside a body with piecewise homogeneous conductivity,

$$\vec{B}(\vec{r}) = \frac{\mu_0}{4\pi} \int_V \vec{J}_i(\vec{r}') \, dV' \times \nabla'(1/R)$$

$$+ \frac{\mu_0}{4\pi} \sum_i \int_{S_i} (\sigma_i^- - \sigma_i^+) \, \phi \, \vec{n}(\vec{r}') \times \nabla'(1/R) \, d S_i \, , \tag{3.8}$$

where $\vec{n}(\vec{r}')$ is the outward normal to the interfaces; it is directed from the region with conductivity $\sigma^-$ to the region with conductivity $\sigma^+$. The second term on the righthand side of Equation 3.8 reflects the contribution of inhomogeneities and external boundary on the magnetic field. In these terms, $S_j$ represents the $j$th interface separating regions of different conductivity $\sigma^-$ and $\sigma^+$. Equation 3.8 shows that volume currents can be replaced by an equivalent surface current distribution $- (\sigma^- - \sigma^+)\phi(\vec{r}')$ $\vec{n}(\vec{r}')$ on each interface $S_j$.

For an unbounded homogeneous conductor, the second term in the righthand side of Equation 3.8 will obviously be zero, which means that conduction current does not contribute to $\vec{B}$. Note that a similar result can be obtained from Equation 3.3. The curl operator applying on the second component of the current density at Equation 3.3 vanishes (in the quasi-static limit $\nabla' \times \vec{E} = 0$) and $\vec{B}$ is expressed only in terms of the impressed source current density:

$$\vec{B}(\vec{r}) = \frac{\mu_0}{4\pi} \int_V \frac{\nabla' \times \vec{J}_i(\vec{r}')}{R} \, dV' \tag{3.9}$$

or, similar to Equation 3.5, it can be rewritten as

$$\vec{B}(\vec{r}) = \frac{\mu_0}{4\pi} \int_V \vec{J}_i(\vec{r}') \, dV' \times \nabla'(1/R) \, . \tag{3.10}$$

In general, MEG measurements are obtained by measuring a single component of $\vec{B}$ using coils where the coil axes are normal to the surface of the conductor. For a spherically symmetric conductor this corresponds to the radial field component $B_r = \vec{B}(\vec{r}) \cdot \vec{a}_r$, where $\vec{a}_r$ represents the unit vector in the radial direction. It should be noted that for concentric shells the contribution of volume currents to $B_r$ is zero, because

$$\vec{n}(\vec{r}') \times \nabla'(1/R) \cdot \vec{a}_r = \frac{\vec{r}'}{|\vec{r}'|} \times \frac{(\vec{r} - \vec{r}')}{|\vec{r} - \vec{r}'|} \cdot \frac{\vec{r}'}{|\vec{r}'|} = 0 \, . \tag{3.11}$$

In that case, $B_r$ is obtained as

$$B_r = \frac{\mu_0}{4\pi} \int_V \vec{J}_i(\vec{r}')dV' \times \nabla'(1/R) \cdot \vec{a}_r \ . \tag{3.12}$$

Note that, if the source current is radial, then $B_r$ will be zero because of a vector property similar to Equation 3.11. Thus, for spherically symmetric conductors MEG measurements are sensitive only to the tangential components of the source. For the same conductor model, it is straightforward to show that a current dipole at the center will produce no magnetic field outside, that is, $B_r = 0$.

In the earliest studies, formulations for the solution of the forward problem are derived on the basis of Equation 3.8 for geometrically simple, homogeneous head models, such as sphere, prolate spheroid, and oblate spheroid. The magnetic fields produced by a current dipole in sphere and spheroid models have been calculated by Grynszpan and Geselowitz (1973) and Cuffin and Cohen (1977), respectively. Analytical solutions are also provided for three eccentric-spheres models (Cuffin, 1991). We conclude this section by providing the magnetic field solutions due to a current dipole in a sphere model of the head. Figure 3.1 shows the geometry for an eccentric dipole in sphere. The dipole $\vec{P} = P_x \vec{a}_x$ is placed at $z = a$. The three components of the flux density in spherical coordinates are found as (Cuffin & Cohen, 1977):

$$B_r = \frac{\mu_0 \, a \sin\theta \sin\phi \, P_x}{4\pi \, r^3 \gamma^{3/2}} \tag{3.13}$$

$$B_\theta = \frac{\mu_0 \sin\phi \, P_x}{4\pi \, r^2 \gamma^{3/2}} \left[ \frac{\gamma \cos\theta}{\sin^2\theta} \left( \cos\theta - \frac{r}{a} + \frac{r\gamma^{1/2}}{a} \right) - \frac{a}{r} \left( \cos\theta - \frac{a}{r} \right) \right]$$

$$B_\phi = \frac{\mu_0 \cos\phi \, P_x}{4\pi \, r^2 \gamma^{1/2} \sin^2\theta} \left[ \frac{r}{a} - \cos\theta - \frac{r\gamma^{1/2}}{a} \right]$$

where

$$\gamma = \left[ 1 - \frac{2a\cos\theta}{r} + \left(\frac{a}{r}\right)^2 \right]. \tag{3.14}$$

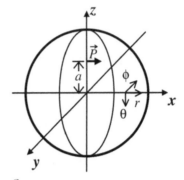

FIG. 3.1.    Current dipole $\vec{P}$ in a conductive sphere. Dipole is in x-direction and the distance
between the dipole and origin is $a$.

## FORWARD PROBLEM SOLUTION
## FOR REALISTIC HEAD MODELS

### BEM

Calculation of the electric potentials using BEM is based on the previous developments for electrocardiography (Barnard, Duck, Lynn, & Timlake,
1967; Barr, Pilkington, Boineau, & Spach, 1966; Geselowitz, 1967) and
magnetocardiography (Horacek, 1973). There are many studies in the litera-
ture that apply BEM to bioelectric and biomagnetic problems (Budiman &
Buchanan, 1993; Cuffin, 1990, 1993; de Munck, 1992; Ferguson, Zhang, &
Stroink, 1994; Fletcher, Amir, Jewett, & Fein, 1995; Fuchs, Drenckhahn,
Wisckmann, & Wagner, 1998; Gençer & Tanzer, 1999; Hämäläinen &
Sarvas, 1989; He et al., 1987; Meijs, Weier, Peters, & Van Ooesterom, 1989;
Menninghaus, Luntkenhoner, & Gonzales, 1994; Mosher, Leahy, & Lewis,
1999; Nenonen, Purcell, Horacek, Stroink, & Katila, 1991; Roth, Balish,
Gorbach, & Sato, 1993; Schimpf, Haueisen, Ramon, & Nowak, 1998;
Schlitt, Heller, Aaron, Best, & Ranken, 1995; Yvert, Bertrand, Echallier, &
Pernier, 1995, 1996). In this section, after reviewing the previous studies, we
introduce a recent BEM formulation (Gençer & Tanzer, 1999) and present
numerical results obtained from simulations.

In the BEM, the entire volume (i.e., torso or human head) is subdivided
into compartments with constant material properties. In bioelectric
studies, material property is the electrical conductivity of tissues, and it is
assumed to be isotropic in BEM formulations. To compute $\vec{B}$ from Equation 3.8, one has to solve the electric potential $\phi$ at each conductivity in-

terface. The electric potential $\phi$ due to an impressed current source $\vec{J}_i$ in a conductive body satisfies the following partial differential equation:

$$\nabla \cdot (\sigma \nabla \phi) = \nabla \cdot \vec{J}_i \quad in \ V$$

$$\sigma \frac{\partial \phi}{\partial n} = 0 \quad on \ S \ , \tag{3.15}$$

where $V$ and $S$ denote the volume and surface of the conductor body, respectively. BEM uses Green's theorem to transform the differential equation into an integral equation over the boundary surfaces, which separate regions with different conductivities. For a body with piecewise homogenous conductivity, solution of $\phi$ can be obtained using the following integral equation (Geselowitz, 1967):

$$\sigma(\vec{r})\phi(\vec{r}) = \frac{1}{4\pi} \int_V \vec{J}_i(\vec{r}')dV' \cdot \nabla'(1/R)$$

$$-\frac{1}{4\pi} \sum_i \int_{S_i} (\sigma_i^- - \sigma_i^+)\phi \vec{n}(\vec{r}') \cdot \nabla'(1/R)dS_i' \ . \tag{3.16}$$

If $\vec{r}$ approaches a point on $S_{ij}$, then it is possible to use the following form:

$$(\sigma_i^- + \sigma_i^+)\phi(\vec{r}) = \frac{1}{2\pi} \int_V \vec{J}_i(\vec{r}')dV' \cdot \nabla'(1/R)$$

$$-\frac{1}{2\pi} \sum_i \int_{S_i} (\sigma_i^- - \sigma_i^+)\phi \vec{n}(\vec{r}') \cdot \nabla'(1/R)dS_i' \ , \tag{3.17}$$

by making use of the limiting value (Vladimirov, 1971) to overcome possible singularities.

The compartment boundaries $S_{ij}$, which are surfaces in the three-dimensional space, are discretized into surface elements $\Delta_j^i$ $(j=1 \ldots n_i)$ to calculate the integrals in the second term (Barnard et al., 1967; Horacek, 1973; Lynn & Timlake, 1968). Here $n_i$ represents the number of elements on the $i$th surface. Thus integral on $S_i$ can be written as

$$\int_{S_i} (\sigma_i^- - \sigma_i^+)\phi \vec{n}(\vec{r}') \cdot \nabla'(1/R)dS_i'$$

$$= \sum_{j=1}^{n_i} (\sigma_i^- - \sigma_i^+)\int_{\Delta_j^i} \phi \vec{n}(\vec{r}') \cdot \nabla'(1/R)dS_i' \ , \tag{3.18}$$

where the effect of each compartment boundary is written as a combination of surface integrals evaluated on surface elements, which are usually planar triangles.

Different formulations in the literature are based on different approaches to the evaluation of the element surface integral. There are different assumptions about the potential function $\phi$ variation, such as regionally constant, linear, and quadratic dependencies, over the triangle area (Barnard et al., 1967, de Munck, 1992; Ferguson et al., 1994; Fletcher et al., 1995; Fuchs et al., 1998; Hämäläinen & Sarvas, 1989; Meijs et al., 1989; Schlitt et al., 1995). In the earlier calculations, the potential on each element is assumed constant and assigned the value of the potential at the centroid of the triangle (center-of-gravity method; Barnard et al., 1967). Another approach is to replace the potential term in the integral by the average of the potentials at the three vertices of the triangle (vertex method assuming average potential on each element; Schlitt et al., 1995). In both cases, the surface integral reduces to evaluation of the solid angle subtended by that triangle at point $\vec{r}$, and it can be calculated using analytical expressions (Barnard et al., 1967; Van Oosterom & Strackee, 1983).

The approximation is improved by assuming linear potential function over each triangular area (Meijs et al., 1989). The three vertices of each triangle are used to define $\phi$ as a linear function over that triangle. Note that $\phi$ will be continuous from one triangle to the next, as opposed to the case in the constant potential approach. If the potential is allowed to vary linearly on each element, then potential values at the vertices (nodes) are unknowns. This may increase the accuracy in solutions and speed of BEM calculations (de Munck, 1992; Urankar, 1990). There are $n_i$ unknowns on each surface when the potential is assumed constant on each element. However, when linear dependency is assumed the number of unknowns will drop, as there are $n_i/2 + 2$ vertices on a closed triangulated surface with $n_i$ triangles (Hämäläinen et al., 1993).

Meijs et al. (1989) made use of this linear variation assumption and expressed the integral over the triangle as a weighted sum of constant potentials on four smaller triangles. The electrical potential over the refined triangles is calculated by assuming linearity on the original triangle. The weights in the surface integral are determined by the solid-angle contributions of the four small triangles. The resultant expression is rewritten to be the weighted sum of the three potentials at the vertices of the original triangle, as opposed to the simple average.

Assuming linear potential variation on flat triangular elements, de Munck (1992) derived an analytic formula that accounts for the distribution of solid angle over the triangle. Thus, the resultant coefficient matrix elements can now be computed using analytical formulas, which may increase the accuracy and speed compared with numerical integrations. It is noted that, for field-point distances comparable to the size of the triangles, the numerical accuracy obtained using 6- and 16-point formulas is not acceptable compared with the analytical formula.

In a recent study, different approaches for the evaluation of the surface element integral were compared, including de Munck's (1992) analytical formula for linear elements (Schlitt et al., 1995). The center-of-gravity method produces smaller errors on the outermost surface and larger errors on the innermost surface compared with the either of the vertex methods. However, the analytical method is superior in terms of reliability to the center-of-gravity method and is superior in terms of accuracy to the vertex method, which replaces the potential term in the integral by the average of the potentials at the three vertices. Because both accuracy and reliability are needed, Schlitt et al. (1995) preferred the use of the vertex method with linear interpolation. Finke and Gulrajani (1999) performed a similar comparison and verified that the vertex method with linear interpolation produces less accurate solutions on the outermost surface. They proposed to double the number of triangles to recover the loss in accuracy.

Ferguson et al. (1994) noted that a possible increase in accuracy in determining the potential on the innermost surface may not necessarily produce a more accurate calculation of the magnetic field. They presented an analytic solution to the integral equation relating linearly varying surface potentials to the magnetic field, for current sources located within a tessellated surface.

De Munck (1992) also provided formulations for quadratic interpolation on flat triangles referring to a previous study (Kuwahara & Takeda, 1987) and proposed the use of the similar methods to find analytical formulas for curved (triangular) elements.

In this section we introduce a different method that again uses numerical integration to evaluate the surface integrals in Equation 3.18. However, in this study *isoparametric* elements were used (Gençer & Tanzer, 1999; Tanzer & Gençer, 1997). This means that both variation in the geometry of the element and in the potential distribution on the element are defined with the same interpolation functions.

Isoparametric elements may provide two major advantages: (a) The edges of the elements can be curved (parabolic), enabling the representation of complicated geometries with few elements (Hinton & Owen, 1983), and (b) few complex elements can be used, yielding more accurate results. Using isoparametric elements in the formulations enables one to express both the global coordinates and potentials on an element using the same interpolation (shape) functions $N_i$, $i = 1$ ... $m$, that is,

$$x = \sum_{i=1}^{m} N\hat{i}(\xi,\eta,v)x_i^e \quad z = \sum_{i=1}^{m} N\hat{i}(\xi,\eta,v)z_i^e$$

$$y = \sum_{i=1}^{m} N\hat{i}(\xi,\eta,v)y_i^e \quad \phi = \sum_{i=1}^{m} N\hat{i}(\xi,\eta,v)\phi_i^e$$

(3.19)

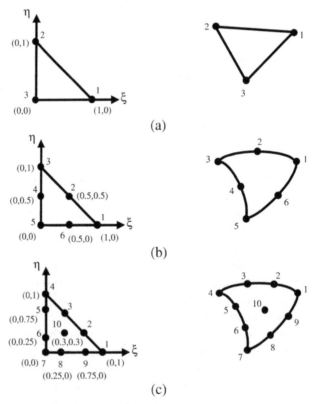

FIG. 3.2.    Isoparametric elements. Transformation from the parent element in local coordinates to the actual element in global coordinates: (a) 3-noded linear element, (b) 6-noded quadratic element, (c) 10-noded cubic element.

where $m$ is the number of nodes in an element; $x_i^e$, $y_i^e$, and $z_i^e$ are the node coordinates; and $\phi_i^e$ is the potential of the $ith$ node. The shape functions are defined on the local coordinates $(\xi, \eta, v)$ of a *parent* element. In evaluating the surface integrations defined on global coordinates, it is usually convenient to make use of a parent element. This is defined over a local coordinate system and can be mapped to the element in global coordinates (see Fig. 3.2).

In this study, linear $(m = 3)$, quadratic $(m = 6)$, and cubic $(m = 10)$ elements were used. The interpolation functions for linear elements are

$$N_1(\xi, \eta) = \xi \quad N_2(\xi, \eta) = \eta \quad N_3(\xi, \eta) = (1 - \xi - \eta) . \quad \textbf{(3.20)}$$

The interpolation functions for quadratic and cubic elements are given in Gençer and Tanzer (1999). Note that, because the parent element is planar, $v$ is a dependent variable (i.e., $v = 1 - \xi - \eta$). The element surface integrations in the right hand side of Equation 3.18 can be expressed in terms of the local coordinates $(\xi, \eta)$:

$$\int_{\Delta_j} \phi(\vec{r}')\vec{n}(\vec{r}') \cdot \nabla'(1/R) \, dS'$$

$$= \int_0^1 \int_0^{1-\eta} \phi \, \vec{n} \cdot \nabla'(1/R) G \, d\xi \, d\eta , \quad \textbf{(3.21)}$$

where the surface index is dropped for simplicity. Here $G$ is defined as

$$G = \left| \frac{\partial \vec{r}'}{\partial \xi} \times \frac{\partial \vec{r}'}{\partial \eta} \right| . \quad \textbf{(3.22)}$$

The integral on the local coordinates is approximated by using the Gauss–Legendre quadrature. That is, if $f$ is the integrand, then

$$\int_0^1 \int_0^{1-\eta} f(\xi, \eta) \, d\xi \, d\eta \approx \frac{1}{2} \sum_{j=1}^{gp} w_j \, f(\xi_j, \eta_j) , \quad \textbf{(3.23)}$$

Where $gp$ denotes the number of Gauss points and $w_j$ is the weight for each value of $f$ evaluated at a certain Gauss point. Thus the integral on the $j$th element can be evaluated as

$$\int_{\Delta_j} \phi(\vec{r}')\vec{n}(\vec{r}')\cdot\nabla'(1/R)\,dS' \tag{3.24}$$

$$= \frac{1}{2}\sum_{j=1}^{gp} w_j \left( \sum_{k=1}^{m} N_k(\xi_j,\eta_j)\phi_k \right) \frac{\vec{R}(\xi_j,\eta_j)}{R^3(\xi_j,\eta_j)} \cdot \vec{n}(\xi_j,\eta_j) G(\xi_j,\eta_j),$$

or, rearranging the terms,

$$\int_{\Delta_j} \phi(\vec{r}')\vec{n}(\vec{r}')\cdot\nabla'(1/R)\,dS' \tag{3.25}$$

$$= \sum_{k=1}^{m} \left( \frac{1}{2}\sum_{j=1}^{gp} w_j N_k(\xi_j,\eta_j) \frac{\vec{R}(\xi_j,\eta_j)}{R^3(\xi_j,\eta_j)} \cdot \vec{n}(\xi_j,\eta_j) G(\xi_j,\eta_j) \right) \phi_k.$$

In this study, the 3-point integration rule is used for linear elements and 13- and 12-point integration rules are used for quadratic and cubic elements, respectively. Recently, an alternative method was offered for the numerical integration (Frijns, de Snoo, & Schoonhoven, 2000). This is based on subdivision of the surface element into four smaller ones, over which quartic Gaussian integration can be performed more accurately. This process can be repeated recursively until the required precision is obtained.

Note that in Equation 3.25 each integration on a surface element is written as a linear combination of unknown node potentials. By including the contribution of other elements and surfaces, the second term in the right hand side of Equation 3.18 can be obtained as a linear combination of the node potentials. If $\phi$ is to be calculated at $M$ nodes, then in matrix notation, it is possible to obtain the following matrix equation:

$$\Phi = g + C\Phi , \tag{3.26}$$

where $\Phi$ is an $M \times 1$ vector of node potentials, $C$ is an $M \times M$ matrix whose elements are determined by the geometry and electrical conductivity information, and $g$ is an $M \times 1$ vector representing the contribution of the primary sources. Note that Equation 3.15 is a partial differential equation with Neumann boundary conditions, which means that all solutions are identical up to an additive constant. To find a unique solution, deflation must be applied (Barnard et al., 1967; Lynn & Timlake, 1968). This applies an additional constraint requiring that the sum of all potentials on the outer surface to be zero, thus modifying the coefficient matrix **C**. The resulting equation is solved using either iterative methods or direct inversion methods. Once $\phi$ is solved, $\vec{B}$ can be obtained from Equation 3.8 using similar integration techniques.

In the computation of $\phi$, numerical instabilities are observed when the ratio in the conductivity of skull to brain and scalp is less than 0.1, and the Richardson extrapolation technique is suggested to overcome this instability (Meijs, Peters, Van Oosterom, & Boom, 1987). In a later study, Hämäläinen and Sarvas (1989) proposed the isolated problem approach (IPA) and showed that, in a spherically symmetric conductor, this method provides accurate solutions. IPA applies a correction term, based on the solution for a homogeneous sphere, to the solution of a concentric sphere model. Recently, a modified weighted approach was proposed for IPA that reveals a parameter that can be adjusted to optimally account for the large conductivity step involved in the BEM head model (Fuchs et al., 1998).

Fletcher et al. (1995) proposed the solution of the reciprocal problem using BEM and named it the *lead field analysis algorithm*. Based on the reciprocity theorem (Rush & Driscoll, 1969), the surface potentials due to a dipole source at a given location can be obtained by computing the electric field present at the location of the dipole source due to a unit current injected at one surface point and a unit current extracted from the reference point. Fletcher et al. reported that this approach offers more accurate surface potentials, improved computational efficiency, and lower storage requirements.

It is assumed that BEM is computationally more efficient and better suited for realistically shaped homogeneous model of the head and simple nonhomogenous models with surfaces defining the cortex, CSF, skull, and scalp (Schimpf et al., 1998). Studies have been conducted, however, on developing more realistic head models using BEM, including, for example, white matter, gray matter, and the eyeballs in the model (Akalin, Acar, & Gençer, 2001).

## FEM

Compared with BEM, FEM can easily handle inhomogeneity and anisotropy. The price paid for this advantage is a need for high computational speed and computer resources. Applications of FEM to bioelectric phenomena were reviewed by Miller and Henriquez (1990), and introductions to the FEM approach have been given by Schimpf et al. (1998) and Gulrajani (1998).

In the FEM, the entire volume is discretized into volume elements on which the potential function is defined by either linear or quadratic interpolation functions. Solutions are obtained either by application of a variational principle or by the technique of weighted residuals (Gulrajani, 1998). Using the FEM approach, Sepulveda, Walker, and Heath (1983) used two-dimensional planar triangle finite elements of a midsagittal head section to compute potentials for known implanted sources. Thevenet, Bertrand, Perrin, Dumont, and Pernier (1991) applied FEM formulation to a three–concentric-sphere model of the head. They also simulated the inverse dipole solutions using the FEM model and the exact solutions. Yan, Nunez, and Hart (1991) used 20-noded hexahedral elements in their FEM formulations so that the curved geometry of the head could be well defined. In their formulations, the mathematical dipole is replaced by a number of point sources, that is, one point source for each node of the element. With this formulation the finite element model need not be altered for different dipole directions. Yan et al. computed potentials in a three–concentric-sphere region and in a head model constructed from a commercially available skull (with scalp and brain regions simulated). Le and Gevins (1993) used FEM with tetrahedral elements and developed an algorithm to reduce spatial blur distortion of scalp-recorded brain potentials due to transmission through the skull and other tissues. Van den Broek, Zhou, and Peters (1996) obtained neuromagnetic fields using the integral equation (Geselowitz, 1970) after calculating the potential distribution using a FEM model. Recently, the most detailed model of the human head was developed using FEM with 13 different tissue types (Haueisen, Ramon, Czapski, & Eiselt, 1995; Haueisen, Ramon, & Eiselt, 1997; Schimpf et al., 1998). The FEM model consists of a uniform grid of about 500,000 hexahedral elements with voxel resolution of $2 \times 2 \times 2$ mm$^3$. Solutions were obtained using a supercomputer. The magnetic fields were found sensitive to changes in the tissue resistivity in the vicinity of the source (Haueisen et al., 1997). Analytical solutions were compared to the solutions obtained from the FEM model and two BEM models (Schimpf et al., 1998). The analytical model was found to have the lowest correlation and the highest amplitude change in comparison to the FEM model for magnetic field and electric potentials. Schimpf et al. also concluded that there is a large demand for more efficient FEM al-

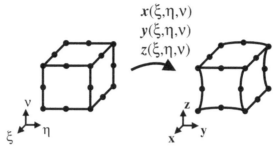

$$x(\xi,\eta,\nu)$$
$$y(\xi,\eta,\nu)$$
$$z(\xi,\eta,\nu)$$

FIG. 3.3.    20-noded basic isoparametric quadratic element in local and global coordinates.

gorithms and software in human head modeling. In a recent study, a hybrid method was introduced that use coupled FEM–BEM procedure to increase the computational efficiency and accuracy in the forward problem solutions (Bradley, Harris, & Pullan, 2001).

In this section we introduce a FEM formulation that uses isoparametric quadratic elements (Özdemir & Gençer, 1997). The fundamental element used in the FEM formulation is shown in Figure 3.3. In Galerkin's weighted residuals method, the partial differential equation (Equation 3.15) is satisfied across each element by multiplying both sides with appropriate shape functions and integrating throughout the element volume (Hinton & Owen, 1983). For each element, this yields

$$\int_{V_e} N_i \nabla \cdot (\sigma_e \nabla \phi)\, dV = \int_{V_e} N_i \nabla \cdot \vec{J}_i\, dV \quad i = 1\dots 20 , \qquad (3.27)$$

where $N_j$ is the $j$th interpolation function of the element, and subscript $e$ is used to denote the physical properties (conductivity, surface, and volume) belonging to that element. Note that a similar formulation was derived by Yan et al. (1991). In that formulation, the divergence term in the righthand side was replaced by the volume current $I$. Thereafter, $I$ was defined using Dirac delta functions to model a current dipole. Thus, dipoles can be located anywhere within an element. In this formulation, the conductivity and the impressed current density on each element are assumed to be constant. Thus, the righthand side of Equation 3.27 vanishes. After applying appropriate vector identities and Gauss's theorem to the integral term on the lefthand side, it is possible to obtain the following equation:

$$\int_{V_e} \sigma_e \nabla N_i \cdot \nabla \phi \, dV_e = \int_{S_e} N_i \sigma_e \nabla \phi \cdot d\vec{S}_e \qquad i = 1 \dots 20 , \qquad (3.28)$$

where $d\vec{S}_e$ is the differential surface element in the outward normal direction. Because $\sigma_e \partial \phi / \partial n = \vec{J}_i \cdot \vec{n}$ on every element surface, the source term reappears on the righthand side:

$$\int_{V_e} \sigma_e \nabla N_i \cdot \nabla \phi \, dV_e = \int_{S_e} N_i \vec{J}_i \cdot \vec{n} \, dS_e \qquad i = 1 \dots 20 . \qquad (3.29)$$

Because $\phi$ can be expressed as a linear combination of local node potentials $\phi_i^e$, the gradient of $\phi$ is

$$\nabla \phi = \sum_{i=1}^{20} \nabla N_i \phi_i^e . \qquad (3.30)$$

Inserting this expression into Equation 3.29, one can obtain the following equation for each element:

$$\sum_{j=1}^{20} \left( \int_{V_e} \nabla N_i \cdot \nabla N_j dV_e \right) \phi_j^e = \int_{S_e} N_i \vec{J}_i \cdot \vec{n} \, dS_e \qquad i = 1 \dots 20 . \quad (3.31)$$

In matrix form, this yields a $20 \times 20$ element matrix equation:

$$\mathbf{A}^e \, \Phi^e = \mathbf{c}^e . \qquad (3.32)$$

After an appropriate assembly process, taking into account the common nodes to the neighboring elements, the following matrix equation can be obtained:

$$\mathbf{A} \, \Phi = \mathbf{c} , \qquad (3.33)$$

where $\mathbf{A}$ is an $M \times M$ matrix that represents the geometry and conductivity information, $\Phi$ is an $M \times 1$ vector of unknown node potentials, and $\mathbf{c}$ is the $M \times 1$ source vector. Note that, just like the case for BEM, one has to modify the coefficient matrix to obtain a unique solution. This is achieved by first choosing a reference node—say, $k$—in the conductor model. Then the entries in the $k$th row and $k$th column of $\mathbf{A}$ are replaced by zero, except the entry $a_{kk}$, which is replaced by 1. The righthand side term $c_k$ is also replaced by zero to make sure that $\Phi_k$ is zero.

## Performance Assessment of BEM and FEM

The performance of the BEM formulation given is presented for a single dipole source located at different points on the z-axis in a concentric sphere model. The radii of the spheres are assumed 1.0, 0.90, and 0.80 m. The conductivity of the inner sphere (brain region) and the outer layer (scalp) are 0.2 S m$^{-1}$, whereas the conductivity of the middle layer (skull) is assumed as 0.005 S m$^{-1}$. An overall measure, the *relative difference measure* (RDM; Meijs et al., 1989), is used to test the accuracy in solutions. Three numerical models are developed using three isoparametric element types (elements that support linear, quadratic, or cubic variation). The number of nodes is kept approximately equal in different meshes (the numbers of nodes on each surface are 1026, 1026, and 1298 for meshes with linear, quadratic, and cubic elements, respectively).

Figure 3.4a shows RDM plots due to various tangential dipole (x-directed) locations on the z-axis (Gençer & Tanzer, 1999). The percentage RDM value is on the order 7% for linear elements, and this is comparable to the RDM values given by Schlitt et al. (1995), whereas RDMs for quadratic and cubic elements change between 1.2% and 1.7%. It is observed that, in general, RDMs are much smaller when the quadratic and cubic elements are used in the numerical model.

For magnetic field solutions, first a homogeneous sphere is assumed to represent the inner region of the skull. The field points are assumed to be placed on a hypothetical sphere of radius 1.1 m. Figure 3.4b shows RDMs obtained for the three models constructed using different element types (Gençer & Tanzer, 1999). RDMs are on the order of 1% for the linear-element mesh, 0.03% for the quadratic-element mesh, and 0.01% for the cubic-element mesh. When the skull layer is added in the model, RDMs in numerical solutions rise to a maximum of 0.07% when quadratic elements are used in the model.

Potential solutions using FEM are also tested for the concentric-sphere model used in the BEM studies (Acar & Gençer, 1999). There are 19,000 nodes and 4,600 quadratic elements in the FEM meshes. In FEM formulations the impressed current density is assumed constant on each element. Thus, it is possible to assign any direction to a current dipole, but it can be located at discrete positions, that is, at the centroid of an element. Because elements have an irregular shape, and no element has a center on the z-axis, it is difficult to repeat the RDM test with FEM. In this study, a group of elements were assigned appropriate values to obtain an equivalent dipole on the z-axis. If the element size is small enough, then such

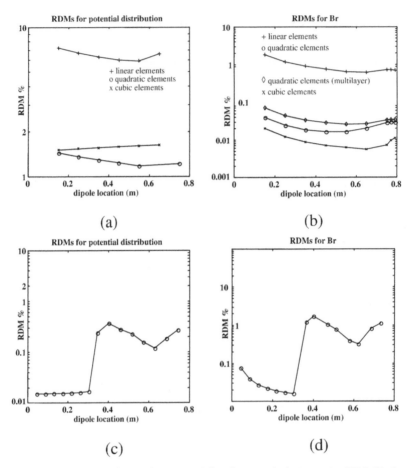

FIG. 3.4.    The RDMs for (a) the potential distribution calculations using BEM, (b) the magnetic field calculations using BEM, (c) the potential distribution calculations using FEM, (d) the magnetic field calculations using FEM.

representations can model a single dipole. As long as the distance between the source elements and field point is large, the analytical solutions for the equivalent dipole source can be used to test the accuracy in solutions. However, as the group gets closer to the field points, the equivalent dipole model is not valid, and analytical solutions must be obtained for the actual dipole distribution. Figure 3.4c shows the RDMs calculated for the potential distribution for tangential dipoles at different depths. It is found that the RDMs are less than 0.3%.

Figure 3.4d shows the RDMs for magnetic field calculations when the potential function is solved using FEM. When the source is modeled as a distributed dipole source, the RDMs are below 1.6%.

In general, both the BEM and the FEM formulations introduced in this section produce accurate potential and magnetic field solutions. All these numerical techniques, however, require state-of-the-art segmentation methods and mesh generation algorithms to develop realistic head models.

## REFERENCES

Acar, C. E., & Gençer, N. G. (1999). Forward problem solution of ESI using FEM and BEM with quadratic isoparametric elements. *Proceedings of the First Joint BMES/EMBS Conference* [CD-ROM]. Atlanta, GA: Omnipress.

Akalin, Z., Acar, C. E., & Gençer, N. G. (2001). Development of realistic head models for electromagnetic source imaging of the human brain. *Proceedings of the 23rd annual international conference of the IEEE Engineering in Medicine and Biology Society* [CD-ROM]. Istanbul, Turkey: Dört Renk Ltd.

Barnard, A. C. L., Duck, I. M., Lynn, M. S., & Timlake, W. P. (1967). The application of electromagnetic theory to electrocardiography: II. Numerical solution of the integral equations. *Biophysical Journal, 7*, 463–491.

Barr, R. C., Pilkington, T. C., Boineau, J. P., & Spach, M. S. (1966). Determining surface potentials from current dipoles with applications to electrocardiography. *IEEE Transactions on Biomedical Engineering, 13*, 88–97.

Barth, D. S., Sutherling, W., Broffman, J., & Beatty, J. (1986). Magnetic localization of a dipolar current source implanted in a sphere and a human cranium. *Electroencephalography and Clinical Neurophysiology, 63*, 260–262

Bradley, C. P., Harris, G. M., & Pullan, A. J. (2001). The computational performance of a high-order coupled FEM/BEM procedure in electropotential problems. *IEEE Transactions on Biomedical Engineering, 48*, 1238–1250.

Budiman, J., & Buchanan, D. S. (1993). An alternative to the biomagnetic forward problem in a realistically shaped head model, the "weighted vertices." *IEEE Transactions on Biomedical Engineering, 40*, 1048–1053.

Cohen, D., Cuffin, N. B., Yunokuchi, K., Maniewski, R., Purcell, C., Cosgrove, R. G., Ives, J., Kennedy, J. G., & Schomer, D. L. (1990). MEG versus EEG localization test using implanted sources in the human brain. *Annals of Neurology, 28*, 811–817.

Cuffin, N. B. (1990). Effects of head shape on EEG's and MEG's. *IEEE Transactions on Biomedical Engineering, 37*, 44–51.

Cuffin, N. B. (1991). Eccentric spheres models of the head. *IEEE Transactions on Biomedical Engineering, 38*, 871–878.

Cuffin, N. B. (1993). Effects of local variations in skull and scalp thickness on EEG's and MEG's. *IEEE Transactions on Biomedical Engineering, 40*, 42–48.

Cuffin, N. B. (1996). EEG localization accuracy improvements using realistically shaped head models. *IEEE Transactions on Biomedical Engineering, 43*, 299–303.

Cuffin, N. B., & Cohen, D. (1977). Magnetic fields of a dipole in special volume conductor shapes. *IEEE Transactions on Biomedical Engineering, 24*, 372–381.

Darcey, T. M., Ary, J. P., & Fender, D. H. (1980). Methods for the localization of electrical sources in the human brain. *Progress in Brain Research, 54*, 128–134.

de Munck, J. C. (1992). A linear discretization of the volume conductor boundary integral equation using analytically integrated elements. *IEEE Transactions on Biomedical Engineering, 39*, 986–990.

Ferguson, A. S., Zhang, X., & Stroink, G. (1994). A complete linear discretization for calculating the magnetic field using the boundary element method. *IEEE Transactions on Biomedical Engineering, 41*, 455–460.

Finke, S., & Gulrajani, R. M. (1999). Comparative accuracies of EEG forward solutions. *Proceedings of the First Joint BMES/EMBS Conference* [CD-ROM]. Atlanta, GA: Omnipress.

Fletcher, D. J., Amir, A., Jewett, D. L., & Fein, G. (1995). Improved method for computation of potentials in a realistic head shape model. *IEEE Transactions on Biomedical Engineering, 42,* 1094–1104.

Frijns, J. H. M., de Snoo, S. L., & Schoonhoven, R. (2000). Improving the Accuracy of the Boundary Element Method by the use of second-order Interpolation Functions. *IEEE Transactions on Biomedical Engineering, 47,* 1336–1346.

Fuchs, M., Drenckhahn, R., Wiscmann, H. A., & Wagner, M. (1998). An improved boundary element method for realistic volume conductor modeling. *IEEE Transactions on Biomedical Engineering, 45,* 980–997.

Gençer, N. G., & Tanzer, I. O. (1999). Forward problem solution of electromagnetic source imaging using a new BEM formulation with high-order elements. *Physics in Medicine and Biology, 44,* 2275–2287.

Geselowitz, D. B. (1967). On bioelectric potentials in an inhomogeneous volume conductor. *Biophysical Journal, 7,* 1–11.

Geselowitz, D. B. (1970). On the magnetic field generated outside an inhomogeneous volume conductor by internal sources. *IEEE Transactions on Magnetics, 6,* 346–347.

Geselowitz, D. B. (1973). Model studies of the electric and magnetic fields of the heart. *Journal of the Franklin Institute, 296,* 379–391.

Grynszpan, F., & Geselowitz, D. B. (1973). Model studies of the magnetocardiogram. *Biophysical Journal, 13,* 911–925.

Gulrajani, R. M. (1998). *Bioelectricity and Biomagnetism.* New York: Wiley.

Hämäläinen, M., Hari, R., Ilmoniemi, R. J., Knuutila, J., & Lounasmaa, O. V. (1993). Magnetoencephalography theory, instrumentation, and applications to noninvasive studies of the working human brain. *Reviews of Modern Physics, 65,* 413–497.

Hämäläinen, M. S., Sarvas, J. (1989). Realistic conductivity geometry model of the human head for interpretation of neuromagnetic data. *IEEE Transactions on Biomedical Engineering, 36,* 165–171.

Haueisen, J., Ramon, C., Czapski, P., & Eiselt, M. (1995). On the influence of volume currents and extended sources on neuromagnetic fields: A simulation study. *Annals of Biomedical Engineering, 23,* 728–739.

Haueisen, J., Ramon, C., Eiselt, M., Brauer, H., & Nowak, H. (1997). Influence of tissue resistivities on neuromagnetic fields and electric potentials studied with a finite element model of the head, *IEEE Transactions on Biomedical Engineering, 44,* 727–735.

He, B., Musha, T., Okamoto, Y., Homma, S., Nakajima, Y., & Sato, T. (1987). Electric dipole tracing in the brain by means of the boundary element method and its accuracy. *IEEE Transactions on Biomedical Engineering, 34,* 406–413.

Henderson, C. J., Butler, S. R., & Glass, A. (1975). The localization of equivalent dipoles of EEG sources by the application of electrical field theory. *Neurophysiology, 39,* 117–130.

Hinton, E., & Owen, D. R. (1983). *Finite element programming.* New York: Academic Press.

Horacek, B. M. (1973). Digital model for studies in magnetocardiography. *IEEE Transactions on Magnetics, 9,* 440–444.

Hosek, R. S., Sances, A., Jodat, R. W., & Larson, S. J. (1978). The contributions of intracerebral currents to the EEG and evoked potentials. *IEEE Transactions on Biomedical Engineering, 25,* 405–413.

Kavanagh, R. N., Darcey, T. M., Lehmann, D., & Fender, D. H. (1978). Evaluation of method for three-dimensional localization of electrical sources in the human brain. *IEEE Transactions on Biomedical Engineering, 25,* 421–429.

Kuwahara, T., & Takeda, T. (1987). An effective analysis for three dimensional boundary element method using analytically integrated higher order elements. *Transactions of IEE of Japan, 107A,* 275–281.

Le, J., & Gevins, A. (1993). Method to reduce blur distortion from EEG's using a realistic head model. *IEEE Transactions on Biomedical Engineering, 40,* 517.

Lynn, M. S., & Timlake, W. P. (1968). The use of multiple deflations in the numerical solution of singular systems of equations with applications to potential theory. *Siam Journal of Numerical Analysis, 5,* 303–322.

Malmivuo, J., & Plonsey, R. (1995). *Principles and applications of bioelectric and biomagnetic fields.* New York: Oxford University Press.

Meijs, J. W. H., Peters, M. J., Van Ooestrom, A., & Boom, H. B. K. (1987). The application of the Richardson extrapolation in simulation studies of EEGs. *Medical and Biological Engineering and Computing*, 25, 222–226.

Meijs, J. W. H., Weier, O. W., Peters, M. J., & Van Oosterom, A. (1989). On the numerical accuracy of the boundary element method. *IEEE Transactions on Biomedical Engineering*, 36, 1038–1049.

Meijs, J. W. H., & Peters, M. J. (1987). The EEG and MEG, using a model of eccentric spheres to describe the head. *IEEE Transactions on Biomedical Engineering*, 34, 913–920.

Menninghaus, E., Luntkenhoner, B., & Gonzales, S. L. (1994). Localization of a dipolar source in a skull phantom: Realistic versus spherical model. *IEEE Transactions on Biomedical Engineering*, 41, 986–989.

Miller, C. E., & Henriquez, C. S. (1990). Finite element analysis of bioelectric phenomena. *Biomedical Engineering*, 18, 207–233.

Mosher, J. C., Leahy, R. M., & Lewis, P. S. (1999). EEG and MEG: Forward solutions for inverse methods. *IEEE Transactions on Biomedical Engineering*, 46, 245–259.

Nenonen, J., Purcell, C. J., Horacek, B. M., Stroink, G., & Katila, T. (1991). Magnetocardiographic functional localization using a current dipole in realistic torso. *IEEE Transactions on Biomedical Engineering*, 38, 658–664.

Özdemir, K., & Gençer, N. G. (1997). A new finite element method formulation for the forward problem of electro-magnetic source imaging. *Proceedings of the 19th Annual International Conference of the IEEE Engineering in Medicine and Biology Society* [CD-ROM]. Netherlands: Soetekouw a/v productions.

Plonsey, R. (1969). *Bioelectric phenomena*. New York: McGraw-Hill.

Roth, B. J., Balish, M., Gorbach, A., & Sato, S. (1993). How well does a three sphere model predict positions of dipoles in a realistically shaped head? *Electroencephalography and Clinical Neurophysiology*, 87, 175–184.

Rush, S., & Driscoll, D. A. (1968). Current distribution in the brain from the surface electrodes. *Anesthesia and Analgesia: Current Research*, 47, 717–723.

Rush, S., & Driscoll, D. A. (1969). EEG electrode sensitivity—An application of reciprocity. *IEEE Transactions on Biomedical Engineering*, 16, 15–22.

Sarvas, J. (1987). Basic mathematical and electromagnetic concepts of the biomagnetic inverse problem. *Physics in Medicine and Biology*, 32, 11–22.

Schimpf, P., Haueisen, J., Ramon, C., & Nowak, H. (1998). Realistic computer modeling of electric and magnetic fields of human head and torso. *Parallel Computing*, 24, 1433–1460.

Schlitt, H. A., Heller, L., Aaron, R., Best, E., & Ranken, D. M. (1995). Evaluation of boundary element methods for the EEG forward problem: Effect of linear interpolation. *IEEE Transactions on Biomedical Engineering*, 42, 52–58.

Schneider, M. (1974). Effect of inhomogeneities on surface signals coming from a cerebral current dipole source. *IEEE Transactions on Biomedical Engineering*, 21, 52–54.

Sepulveda, N., Walker, C., & Heath, R. (1983). Finite element analysis of current pathways with implanted electrodes. *IEEE Transactions on Biomedical Engineering*, 5, 41–48.

Sidman, R. D., Giambalvo, V., Allison, T., & Bergey, P. (1978). A method for localization of sources of human cerebral potentials evoked by sensory stimuli. *Sensory Processes*, 2, 116–129.

Smith, D. B., Sidman, R. D., Henke, J., & Labiner, D. (1985). A reliable method for localizing deep cerebral sources of the EEG. *Neurology*, 35, 1702–1707.

Tanzer, I. O., & Gençer, N. G. (1997). A new boundary element formulation for the forward problem of electro-magnetic source imaging. *Proceedings of the 19th Annual International Conference of the IEEE Engineering in Medicine and Biology Society* [CD-ROM]. Netherlands: Soetekouw a/v productions.

Thevenet, M., Bertrand, O., Perrin, F., Dumont, T., & Pernier, J. (1991). The finite element method for a realistic head model of electrical brain activities: Preliminary results. *Clinical Physics and Physiological Measurement*, 12 (Suppl. A), 89–94.

Ueno, S., Iramina K., & Harada, K. (1987). Effects of inhomogeneities in cerebral modeling for magnetoencephalography. *IEEE Transactions on Magnetics*, 23, 3753–3755.

Ueno, S., Iramina, K., Ozaki, H., & Harada, K. (1986). The MEG topography and the source model of abnormal neural activities associated with brain lesions. *IEEE Transactions on Magnetics*, 22, 874–876

Urankar, L. (1990). Common compact analytical formulas for computation of geometry integrals on a basic Cartesian subdomain in boundary and volume integral methods. *Engineering Analysis with Boundary Elements, 7*, 124–129.

Van den Broek, S. P., Zhou, H., & Peters, M. J. (1996). Computation of neuromagnetic fields using finite element method and Biot–Savart Law. *Medical and Biological Engineering and Computing, 34*, 21–26.

Van Oosterom, A., & Strackee, J. (1983). The solid angle of a plane triangle. *IEEE Transactions on Biomedical Engineering, 30*, 125–126.

Vladimirov, V. S. (1971). *Equations of mathematical physics.* New York: Marcel Dekker.

Weinberg, H., Brickett, P., Coolsma, F., & Baff, M. (1986). Magnetic localization of intracranial dipoles: Simulation with a physical model. *Electroencephalography and Clinical Neurophysiology, 64*, 159–170.

Yan, Y., Nunez, P. L., & Hart, R. T. (1991). A finite element model for the human head: Scalp potentials due to dipole sources. *Medical and Biological Engineering and Computing, 29*, 475.

Yvert, B., Bertrand, O., Echallier, J. F., & Pernier, J. (1995). Improved forward EEG calculations using local mesh refinement of realistic head geometries, *Electroencephalography and Clinical. Neurophysiology, 95*, 381–392.

Yvert, B., Bertrand, O., Echallier, J. F., & Pernier, J. (1996). Improved dipole localization using local mesh refinement of realistic head geometries: An EEG simulation study. *Electroencephalography and Clinical Neurophysiology, 99*, 79–89.

Zhang, Z., & Jewett, D. (1993). Insidious errors in dipole localization parameters at a single time-point due to model misspecification of number of shells. *Electroencephalography and Clinical Neurophysiology, 88*, 1–11.

Zhang, Z., Jewett, D., & Goodwill, G. (1994). Insidious errors in dipole parameters due to shell model misspecification using multiple time points. *Brain Topography, 6*, 283–298.

# 4

## Magnetic Source Imaging: Search for Inverse Solutions

Jia-Zhu Wang
*New York Presbyterian Hospital/Cornell Medical Center*

Lloyd Kaufman
*New York University*

The ability to compute the distribution of current on the cortex that underlies observed extracranial magnetic fields will determine the ultimate usefulness of magnetic source imaging (MSI). Assuming that a current dipole is
located within a sphere filled with a uniform conducting solution, 1, and
only 1, external field pattern can be produced by that source. Thus, in principle, the so-called forward problem of computing the field has a unique solution. However, there is no unique solution to the inverse problem: that of
locating the source of a field solely on the basis of knowledge of the properties
of that field. This chapter briefly describes some efforts toward resolving the
barriers posed by the nonuniqueness of inverse solutions. It focuses on 1 approach, the *minimum norm least squares* inverse (MNLS), which explicitly incorporates knowledge of the geometry of the cortical surface and the
assumption that currents giving rise to the field are on that surface. Such
constraints make it possible to go beyond simple equivalent current dipole
sources and describe the extended patterns of current that give rise to external fields. The MNLS is then extended to account for locating on the cortical
surface the currents that give rise to regions of enhanced or depressed incoherent activity. This approach makes use of measures of field power rather
than field *per se*. In principle, it feasible to localize regions of the cortex that

are more or less active than other regions, thus mirroring modalities such as positron emission tomography and functional magnetic resource imaging, but examining altered electrical activity rather than blood flow.

Very early in the history of electroencephalography (EEG) it became apparent that many momentary spatial distributions of scalp potentials could be produced by an underlying current dipole. As described in chapter 1 of this volume, the equivalent current dipole (ECD) is a hypothetical source of observed neuromagnetic fields and electric potentials. In fact, there is no realistic way to distinguish between the effects of a point current dipole and a circumscribed population of neurons. Extraneous noise alone makes it impossible to detect statistically significant differences between the isofield or isopotential patterns produced by a point current dipole and that of a spatially confined population of neuronal sources. Despite this limitation, the positions of active neural sources were frequently found to correspond to those of current dipoles suggested by magnetoencephalography (MEG) patterns (Williamson & Kaufman, 1981, 1987). For example, some sources of interictal spikes in epileptics were found to be small tumors first identified as ECDs whose positions were confirmed during surgery. Also, current dipole sources of auditory evoked fields were located in or near the auditory cortex, and not in other arbitrary regions of the brain. In a sense, these and many other discoveries consistent with known anatomical and functional features of the brain are quite surprising. The reasons these successes surprise us stems from basic physical principles.

Gençer et al. (chap. 3, this volume) deal with predicting the extracranial fields produced by current dipole sources within the brain. In the case of a spherical head model (in which conductivity may vary only radially), it is actually quite simple to determine the strength and distribution of the external field associated with any current dipole of known strength and orientation. This is known as the *forward problem* and, since the time of Helmholtz (1853), it has been known that the forward problem has a unique solution. That is, given a known source—say, an ECD— of known position and orientation, only one extracranial field pattern will be produced. When one deals with irregularly shaped heads and multipolar sources immersed in electrically anisotropic media, the problem becomes more complicated. However, in principle this forward problem still has only one solution, although finding it entails much cleverness and enormous computational resources.

The problem unfortunately is quite different when one knows the extracranial field pattern but has no information about its source. If one starts with a simple spherical head, and has precise information regarding its external field, but has no *a priori* information regarding its source, then there is no unique solution to the problem of identifying the source of the field. The problem of determining the source of an external field from information contained in the field is known as the *inverse problem*, and it is widely accepted that there is no unique solution. The same field pattern can be produced by any number of possible sources or source configurations. This is why it is so encouraging, and surprising, that MEG data have yielded so many meaningful results.

In practice, investigators test the assumption that an observed field pattern is statistically indistinguishable from a pattern that would be produced by an ECD. Quadrupolar sources and those of yet higher orders may well be present as well, but the contributions of noise tend to mask the generally weaker contributions made by these high-order source components. Given the assumption that the actual source cannot be distinguished from an ECD, the next step may be to test a number of alternative hypotheses. That is, the investigator effectively manipulates the position orientation and strength of a hypothetical dipole until a best fit to the observed pattern is found. Prior knowledge may also play a role; for example, visual evoked fields may reasonably be presumed to originate in sources in occipital regions of the brain. Controversies can and do arise because, in some circumstances, competing hypotheses may yield equally good fits to the data. However, invasive studies using indwelling electrodes, or noninvasive studies involving both EEG and MEG, increase the probability that one of several competing hypotheses is superior. Early auditory-evoked potential (AEP) studies manifested conflicting data, with some locating the sources in or near the auditory cortex and others locating it in other areas (Vaughan & Ritter, 1970). Subsequent MEG studies were less ambiguous, because there is no need for a reference electrode, and the results of these studies placed the sources of several of AEP components in the auditory cortex. The location of the source of AEP component P300 was particularly controversial, but an early MEG study placed the source in or near the hippocampal formation (Okada, Kaufman, & Williamson, 1983). This was confirmed in studies using indwelling electrodes, but some controversy still remains. Thus, even when multiple methods converge on agreement, in principle it is not possible to be certain that some result not yet considered is better.

Our inability to find unique solutions to the inverse problem is probably the greatest barrier standing in the way of generating a form of magnetic source imaging (MSI), whose face validity is comparable to that of functional magnetic resonance imaging (fMRI). The obvious goal of MSI is to obtain time-varying images of the distributions of electric currents on the cerebral cortex. Because temporal resolutions are on the order of milliseconds, such images would beautifully complement fMRI and other measures of cerebral blood flow.

Despite the apparent difficulties facing this full development of MSI, several programs have attempted to devise methods that would make more certain solutions to the inverse problem possible. Although it is generally true that the inverse problem has no unique solution, *a priori* information may constrain the problem so that a unique solution is possible. For example, if a current dipole is placed at an arbitrary position on a planar surface, which is itself at a known location and orientation within a conducting volume (e.g., a sphere filled with saline solution), then a unique solution to the inverse problem exists. Furthermore, with the exception of weak components of auditory brain stem responses to acoustic stimuli, virtually all sources of extracranial magnetic fields are known to be located in the cerebral cortex. This thin (2-mm thick) mantle of the brain contains the dendrites that give rise to the observed fields, whereas the white matter of the brain is largely axonal and does not contribute to the MEG or the EEG. So, to a first approximation it is possible to treat the cortex as a wrinkled two-dimensional surface and the columns of cells of which it is composed as current dipoles. Sets of adjacent columns can be treated as ECDs. Furthermore, the advent of >2 Tesla magnetic resonance imaging machines make it possible to form high-resolution images of the cortex and to compute from them its precise three-dimensional geometry within an accurate representation of the skull. Some ambiguity may arise if the cortex folds back on itself, forming several active layers, but this is not commonly observed. Therefore, it is possible to go back to first principles and compute unique solutions to the inverse problem. Unfortunately, despite the existence of several programs with this as its aim, no group has yet accomplished this task. Therefore, the purpose of this chapter is to demonstrate that it is possible to find unique solutions to the inverse problem in which sources are not simple single dipoles but are areas of cortical activity.

We begin with the principles that provide the basis for this possibility. These principles are related to those involved in the forward problem, which Gençer et al. (chap. 3, this volume) discussed in detail. We begin with a more abbreviated technical discussion of the forward problem.

## LEAD FIELD ANALYSIS—THE MATHEMATICAL MODEL
## OF THE FORWARD PROBLEM IN NEUROMAGNETISM

Magnetic fields measured outside the human scalp are primarily due to the flow of ionic currents within neurons. However, the flow of extra-cellular volume currents adjacent to boundaries separating tissues of different conductivity within the skull also contributes to the field. Evaluation of the relative contributions of the primary (intracellular) currents and those of secondary sources at boundaries is possible when the skull, brain, and other tissues are modeled as piecewise homogeneous and isotropic conductors. Then field **B** can be derived from the following equations (Barr, Pikington, Boineau, & Spach, 1966; Geselowitz, 1967, 1970; Huang, Nicholson, & Okada, 1990):

$$\mathbf{B}(\mathbf{r}) = \frac{\mu_0}{4\pi} \int_\Omega \mathbf{J}(\mathbf{r}') \times \frac{(\mathbf{r}-\mathbf{r}')}{|\mathbf{r}-\mathbf{r}'|^3} d\mathbf{r}' + \frac{\mu_0 \Delta\sigma}{4\pi} \int_\Sigma \Phi(\mathbf{r}'') \frac{(\mathbf{r}-\mathbf{r}'')}{|\mathbf{r}-\mathbf{r}''|^3} \times d\mathbf{S}'' \, , \quad \textbf{(4.1)}$$

where $\mathbf{J}(\mathbf{r}')$ $(\mathbf{r}' \in \Omega)$ is the primary current density within the volume $\Omega$, and $\Phi(\mathbf{r}'')$ ($\mathbf{r}'' \in \Sigma$) the electric potential on the boundary surface $\Sigma$. The $d\mathbf{r}'$ is the differential volume element, and $d\mathbf{S}''$ is the vector surface element of size $dS$ and pointing to its normal direction $\mathbf{n}''$ at source point $\mathbf{r}''$ on the boundary ($d\mathbf{S}'' = \mathbf{n}'' \cdot dS$). (Items in boldface represent vectors.) $\Delta\sigma = \sigma_2 - \sigma_1$ is the difference in conductivity across the boundary $\Sigma$. The $\Delta\sigma \cdot \Phi(\mathbf{r}'') \cdot \mathbf{n}''$ is commonly referred to as the secondary source. Therefore, the boundary effect can be considered as the total contribution from a distribution of secondary sources: The orientation of each secondary current dipole is normal to the boundary at $\mathbf{r}''$ and generates a magnetic field element at the observation point $\mathbf{r}$ with a direction tangential to the surface at source point $\mathbf{r}''$. This result is all due to the nature of cross product in the second term of Equation 4.1.

In the special case of a semi-infinite space, where measurements are made on a plane above the conducting medium, the contributions from all secondary sources are parallel to the plane, thus making zero contribution to the normal component of the magnetic field $\mathbf{B}(\mathbf{r})$. In a spherical head model all the secondary sources are oriented along radii of the sphere. If the origin is selected at the center of the sphere, then the unit norm is given by $\mathbf{n}'' = \mathbf{r}''/|\mathbf{r}''|$. The tangential magnetic field produced by a secondary current dipole is perpendicular to the position of the source ($\mathbf{r}''$) as well as the position $\mathbf{r}$ at which the measurement is made.

This can be explained more precisely in terms of the nature of the vector cross product. As in the second term of Equation 4.1

$$(\mathbf{r} - \mathbf{r}'') \times \mathbf{n}'' = \mathbf{r} \times \mathbf{n}'' - \mathbf{r}'' \times \mathbf{n}'' = \mathbf{r} \times \frac{\mathbf{r}''}{|\mathbf{r}''|} \qquad (4.2)$$

The cross product of the two vectors $\mathbf{r}'' \times \mathbf{n}''$ with the same orientation vanishes, and the cross product of $\mathbf{r} \times \mathbf{n}''$ gives rise to a third vector that is perpendicular to both $\mathbf{r}$ and $\mathbf{n}''$. Naturally, its projection in the radial direction $\mathbf{r}$ will vanish.

$$\mathbf{r} \times \mathbf{n}'' \cdot \frac{\mathbf{r}}{|\mathbf{r}|} = 0 \quad .$$

Hence, the contribution from the secondary sources to the normal component of the magnetic field, vanishes altogether because of the nature of the dot product.

Therefore, the primary current alone determines the normal (radial) component $B(\mathbf{r})$ of the magnetic field measured at the surface of the sphere. Consequently,

$$B(\mathbf{r}) = \frac{\mu_0}{4\pi} \int_\Omega \frac{\mathbf{J}(\mathbf{r}') \times (\mathbf{r} - \mathbf{r}')}{|\mathbf{r} - \mathbf{r}'|^3} \cdot \frac{\mathbf{r}}{|\mathbf{r}|} d\mathbf{r}' \quad . \qquad (4.3)$$

Although this convolution integral appears to be complicated, the normal component of the magnetic field is linearly related to the current source density. This linearity will become clearer if the dot and the cross product in the triple scalar product are interchanged, by separating the current source density from the rest of the radial function. For a radial measurement at $\mathbf{r}$, Equation 4.3 can be rewritten

$$B(\mathbf{r}) = \int_\Omega \mathbf{L}(\mathbf{r}, \mathbf{r}') \cdot \mathbf{J}(\mathbf{r}') d\mathbf{r}' \quad , \qquad (4.4)$$

where the vector kernel $\mathbf{L}(\mathbf{r}, \mathbf{r}')$ in Equation 4.4 is known in biomagnetism as the *lead field*. It accounts for the sensitivity to the magnetic flux in the $i$th pickup coil (see chap. 1 for a description of gradiometers) at position $\mathbf{r}$ produced by unit source current density at $\mathbf{r}'$. The lead field is governed by the source geometry as well as by the geometry and orientation of the detection coil. In a spherical head model it takes the following form:

$$L(\mathbf{r}, \mathbf{r}') = \frac{\mu_0}{4\pi} \frac{\mathbf{r} \times \mathbf{r}'}{|\mathbf{r} - \mathbf{r}'|^3 \cdot |\mathbf{r}|} \quad . \tag{4.5}$$

Similar expressions of the lead field can also be derived for the case of a semi-infinite space.

It is of great interest to derive a discrete formulation of Equation 4.4, because all numeric computations involve discrete mathematics (Wang, Williamson, & Kaufman, 1992). If the source space is assumed to be a folded surface layer of uniform thickness $w$, divided into a grid of $n$ cells of area $\Delta S_j$ centered at position $\mathbf{r}'_j$, the differential volume element $d\mathbf{r}'$ can be substituted by $w \cdot \Delta S_j$. The combination of $\mathbf{J}(\mathbf{r}'_j) \cdot d\mathbf{r}'_j = \mathbf{J}(\mathbf{r}'_j) w \cdot \Delta S_j$ has the dimension of a current dipole, and the integral is reduced to a summation

$$B_i \sum_{j=1}^{n} \mathbf{L}_i(\mathbf{r}'_j) \cdot \mathbf{Q}(\mathbf{r}'_j) \quad i = 1, \ldots, m \tag{4.6}$$

where $B_i \equiv B(\mathbf{r}_i)$ is the radial component of magnetic field at observation point $\mathbf{r}_i$, $\mathbf{L}_i(\mathbf{r}'_j) \equiv \mathbf{L}(\mathbf{r}_i, \mathbf{r}'_j)$. For simplicity, the position vector $\mathbf{r}_i$ is now represented by the subscript $i$. Equation 4.6 is a matrix equation and can be explicitly expressed as follows:

$$\begin{bmatrix} B_1 \\ \vdots \\ B_m \end{bmatrix} = \begin{bmatrix} L_{11} & \cdots & L_{1n} \\ \vdots & \ddots & \vdots \\ L_{m1} & \cdots & L_{mn} \end{bmatrix} \begin{bmatrix} Q_1 \\ \vdots \\ Q_n \end{bmatrix} \quad . \tag{4.7}$$

For convenience, the matrix equation (4.7) can be rewritten in a more concise fashion:

$$\mathbf{b} = \mathbf{Lq} \quad , \tag{4.8}$$

where lowercase letters represent a column vector and uppercase a matrix.

## CURRENT SOURCE GENERATOR: THE EQUIVALENT CURRENT DIPOLE AND OTHER APPROACHES

It is of some interest to review the electrostatics. The description of a localized distribution of charges requires an infinite number of terms. The first term is the simple static point charge, which, incidentally, is not associated with any magnetic field. The next order involved in the description consists, for example, of an opposed pair of static charges, or a dipole. Other terms of higher order include the quadrupole; the octopole; and, in general, multipoles. Similarly, in magnetostatics for a general current distribution that occupies a small region of space, a complete treatment of this problem is possible by using the multipole expansion, with the magnetic dipole being the lowest and also the dominant component (Jackson, 1974). If a charge should move, it is accompanied by a magnetic field. In this case the fundamental term describing moving charges is the current dipole. By analogy with electrostatics, a multipole expansion is needed to describe more complicated current distributions.

Searching for cortical sources that generate neuromagnetic fields is of major importance in many MEG studies. Although the cortical source of a neuromagnetic field may be extended and convoluted, it may well occupy a region of space that is small relative to the distance at which its field is measured. In many cases neuronal sources producing the dominant extracranial magnetic fields are confined to specific regions of the brain. Thus, the ECD is a valuable concept (chap. 1, this volume). The concept of multipole expansion can also be applied to the electric potential and the neuromagnetic field produced by the neural current distribution. One may be content here with only the lowest order of approximation, as it is the dominant component in the expansion as well and is often the only component to emerge from both environmental and instrumental noise. In many cases, especially those involving event-related fields, the task is therefore reduced to determining the first order of the expansion, ECD (Cuffin & Cohen, 1977; chap. 2, this volume).

It is obvious that two concurrently active sources at widely separated places in the brain will produce their own, possibly independent neuromagnetic field patterns. Successful examples include the bilateral sources of fields evoked by acoustic stimuli (Curtis, Kaufman, & Williamson, 1988). A major question, however, concerns the ability to describe extended current patterns on the cortex. This requires rather sophisticated approaches to solving the inverse problem. Examples of efforts in this direction are those of Ioannides (1990); Sarvas (1987); Smith, Dallas, Kullman, & Schlitt (1990); Okada and Huang (1990); and Mosher, Lewis, and Leahy (1992). Some of these approaches entailed the *so-called least-squares minimization* or *minimum norm technique*, which minimizes a certain cost function to fit the inverse solution. Hämäläinen and Ilmoniemi (1984) used Bayesian parameter estimation in making inferences about extended sources of neuromagnetic fields.

Spatial filtering approaches have been applied to determine how well various sensing coil configurations could resolve two dipoles separated by various distances (Tan, Roth, & Wikswo, 1990; Wikswo, Roth, & Sepulveda, 1989). This may be extended to deal with describing extended sources. The operation defined in Equation 4.4 is actually a convolution of two functions: the lead field **L** and the current density **J** over the source space $\Omega$. By virtue of the Fourier transform, convolution in the spatial domain will become simple multiplication in the frequency domain. One can solve the inverse problem using the Fourier components in the frequency domain and then perform the inverse Fourier transform to derive the extended (spatial) source distribution.

Readers are referred to the foregoing sources for various approaches of overcoming the obstacle of the nonuniqueness of solutions to the inverse problem. Our purpose in this chapter is to present one more or a less coherent approach, based largely on the work of Wang, Williamson, and Kaufman (1992–1995).

## UNDERSTANDING NONUNIQUENESS OF THE INVERSE PROBLEM: AN ILL-CONDITIONED SYSTEM

In biomagnetism, inverse approaches frequently use the least-squares method to fit one or more current dipoles, by iteratively minimizing the difference between observed and theoretical field patterns, where this difference is expressed as a cost function. In practice, however, searching for a minimum least squares difference may well lead to a false result; that is, it may be merely local and not a global minimum.

It is well known that knowledge of a field outside the human scalp is not sufficient to determine uniquely the sources of neuronal activity within the brain (Helmholtz, 1853). The inverse solution of Equation 4.4 can never be mathematically unique, for there may exist a family of functions $\mathbf{J}^*$, that are the solutions of the homogeneous equations corresponding to Equation 4.4:

$$\int_{\Omega} \mathbf{L}(\mathbf{r}, \mathbf{r}') \cdot \mathbf{J}^*(\mathbf{r}') d\mathbf{r}' = 0 \tag{4.9}$$

Numerically, it is an underconditioned problem. This is implicit in the lead field analysis in Equation 4.4, where one wishes to determine the source current distribution based on a set of measurements. In effect, one is seeking an infinite number of parameters from a finite number of measurements.

A more detailed explanation can be seen in the matrix form of Equation 4.7. The lead-field matrix is in general a rectangular matrix, where the number of measurements is less than the number of unknowns ($m < n$). One may think that a unique solution can be found if the number of dipole parameters (dipole moments and orientations) is equal to the number of measurements, such that there are $m$ equations to solve for the same number of unknowns ($m = n$). This intuitive concept is wrong. The exact solution does not exist because the ill-conditioned nature of the inverse solutions is not reduced by artificially restricting it into a square matrix, for this square matrix may well be a singular matrix. In other words, these $m$ measurements may not be independent, and errors in the measurements contribute further indeterminacy to the inverse solutions. Apart from additive noise in the observations, there are also nonadditive errors in determining the positions of measurements. The mathematical model representing the physical problem itself introduces error into the inverse problem. Selecting a number of discrete sources to represent a continuous source distribution is one such example. Furthermore, because almost all computation is now carried out on digital computers, errors are introduced into the solution of all problems. Round-off errors and their accumulation and propagation are inevitable when floating-point arithmetic is used in the fundamental computer operations.

Statistics generally deals with cases where the number of measurements (i.e., the number of equations) is greater than the number of unknowns ($m > n$), and the unknowns are always linearly independent. In such conditions, and only in such conditions, can one form a nonsingular square matrix by multiplying the transpose $\mathbf{L}^T$ to its left and compute the inverse $(\mathbf{L}^T\mathbf{L})^{-1}$. This way, one can obtain a unique inverse estimation in a least-squares sense.

$$\mathbf{q} = (\mathbf{L}^T\mathbf{L})^{-1}\mathbf{L}^T \quad . \tag{4.10}$$

In inverse problems, the number of unknowns often exceeds the number of measurements, such as in the extended source imaging ($m < n$). The least-square approach is no longer valid, because the matrix of $\mathbf{L}^T\mathbf{L}$ is singular. Instead, one shall construct a square matrix by multiplying its transpose to the right side: $\mathbf{L}\,\mathbf{L}^T$. If this square matrix is nonsingular, then one can then form a *minimum-norm inverse:*

$$\mathbf{q} = \mathbf{L}^T(\mathbf{L}\,\mathbf{L}^T)^{-1} \quad . \tag{4.11}$$

It is noteworthy that Equation 4.10 implies a situation in which the number of equations exceeds the number of unknowns. This approach implies a classic least-squares fit. Whereas in Equation 4.11 the number of unknowns exceeds the number of equations. Only under the condition of being a nonsingular square matrix, may it directly lead to a minimum norm solution of the inverse problem.

## THE MINIMUM-NORM AND LEAST-SQUARE INVERSE: WHY AND HOW?

It is possible, at least in theory, to find a unique estimate of the unknown elements of the current image by imposing proper constraints on the problem, such as *a priori* knowledge of anatomy, as may be provided by magnetic resonance images. Equipped with such knowledge, one may assume that the *image space,* where the inverse solution is sought, coincides with the *source space,* where the actual primary currents are located. Thus, the detailed elements of the lead field matrix in the forward model can be constructed.

First, however, one must still contend with the *ill-conditioned* problem encountered in all inverse problems. As we have discussed, the number of unknowns ($n$) is greater than the number of equations ($m$ measurements), and the measurements themselves may not be independent. Therefore, the lead field matrix **L** is in general an $m \times n$ rectangular matrix with $m < n$. The least-square inverse can apply to a system only with $m > n$. As explained earlier, the minimum-norm inverse does not exist either, because the square matrix $\mathbf{L}\,\mathbf{L}^T$ may be singular, if its rank $r < min\,(m, n)$. In this case, one has to use the generalized inverse (Moore, 1920; Penrose, 1955) of the lead-field matrix **L**, which provides an estimation $\hat{\mathbf{q}}$ of the current dipoles **q**.

$$\hat{\mathbf{q}} = \mathbf{L}^+ \mathbf{b} \quad . \tag{4.12}$$

The generalized inverse of a matrix **L** is defined mathematically as

$$\mathbf{L}^+ = \mathbf{D}^T (\mathbf{D}\,\mathbf{D}^T)^{-1} (\mathbf{C}^T \mathbf{C})^{-1} \mathbf{C}^T \tag{4.13}$$

where **C** and **D** are two full rank matrices (rank $= r$); (for any $m \times n$ matrix of rank $r$, **L** can be factored into the product of two matrices $\mathbf{L} = \mathbf{C} \cdot \mathbf{D}$, with dimension $(m \times r)$ and $(r \times n)$ (Ben-Israel & Greville, 1974).

Numerically, the generalized inverse can be directly computed using the well-known *singular value decomposition* (SVD) method given in many textbooks on numerical analysis (Golub et al., 1983). Its application to neuromagnetism has been discussed in detail by Wang et al. (1992) and Wang (1993).

This generalized inverse estimation, or pseudo-inverse, is better known as the *Moore–Penrose inverse*. It is also called the *minimum-norm least-squares* (MNLS) inverse, for the following important reason: It has the least residual error as well as the minimum power among all least-squares solutions, as indicated in Equation 4.14:

$$\left\| \mathbf{L}\hat{\mathbf{q}} - \mathbf{b} \right\|^2 = \sum_{i=1}^{m} \left( \frac{\hat{B}_i - B_i}{\sigma_i} \right)^2 = minimum \qquad (4.14a)$$

$$\left\| \hat{\mathbf{q}} \right\| = \sqrt{\sum_{j=1}^{n} Q_i^2} = minimum \qquad (4.14b)$$

where $\left\| \cdot \right\|$ is the Euclidean norm of a vector, and $\hat{\ }$ indicates the estimated values. In the presence of noise, the radial components of magnetic field $B_i$ are weighted by the standard error $\sigma_i$ in the measurements, so does each element of the lead field matrix: $L_{ij}/\sigma_i$. More important, Penrose (1955) proved that the solution set of the MNLS inverse contains only one element; that is, the MNLS inverse is *mathematically unique*.

## SIMULATION OF MNLS INVERSE OF EXTENDED SOURCE DISTRIBUTION IN A SEMI-INFINITE SPACE

A small portion of a simulated sulcus is configured as a vertical *L*-shaped wall of the cortex extending below a horizontal surface representing the scalp, as shown in Fig. 4.1. Each plane of the *L*-shaped wall of the cortex is $5 \times 5$ cm. This is called the *source space*. One also assumes that the prior knowledge of anatomy provides enough information of the source space so that one can assume that the *image space*, where inverse solutions will be sought, coincides with the source space. The "measurements" are taken across a horizontal plane of $12 \times 12$ cm (*observation space*) and located 1 cm above the top edge of the image surface.

In one example, two current dipoles of equal strength 3 cm apart and at the same depth are located on the left side of the *L*-shaped cortex. Three simulations on dipole depths of 2, 3, and 4.5 cm were carried out, and the magnetic fields on the observation space produced by those cur-

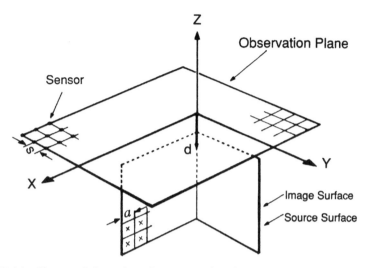

FIG. 4.1. Horizontal plane where observations of the field are made by point sensors at nodes of a square array of side $s$. The source space consists of two vertical walls meeting at right angles at 2 cm from the center of the observation plane. The top edge of the image surface is located 1 cm below the observation plane. The image surface coincides with the source surface, and inverse computations are carried out to deduce the image density on nodes of a square array of side $a$.

rent dipoles were computed. These furnished the data of our so-called measurements. Because opposing fields from the two parallel dipole sources are partially self-canceling, the magnetic field pattern closely resembles that of a single current dipole (see Fig. 4.2). The MNLS inverse solution clearly locates the two dipoles even without introducing an explicit source model, as shown in Fig. 4.3, where dipole images are well resolved even at the greatest depth. However, the peaks of the image in the deepest case lie at a slightly shallower depth (4.2 cm) than the actual source depth (4.5 cm). The image density in the right plane is very low (less than 0.1 μA/m), so it is not shown here.

A particularly interesting example of the versatility of the MNLS inverse is the computation of the image of an extended source, that is, one having activity distributed over a finite area of the source plane. A configuration shaped like a crescent moon is illustrated in the lefthand panels of Fig. 4.4. Two cases are considered: a continuous current distribution (a) whose top is at a depth of $d = 2.5$ cm and bottom at $d = 4.5$ cm and (b) that defines a source of the same shape but with source strength increasing at depth to better emphasize the lower region in the field pattern. The inverse dipole distributions in the middle panels generally mimic the

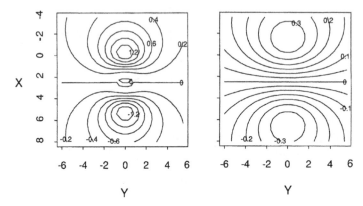

FIG. 4.2. Isocontours of a magnetic field across the observation plane produced by two dipoles 3 cm apart horizontally and at shallow depth $z = -2$ cm (left panel) and at deep depth $z = -4.5$ cm (right panel).

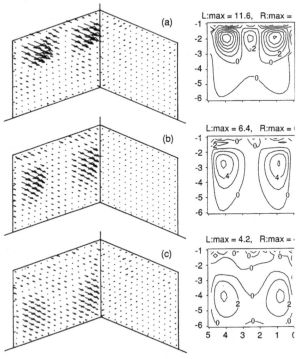

FIG. 4.3. Magnetic source images of two dipoles, each of a dipole moment q = 1 nAm, separated by 3 cm horizontally and at $z = -2$ cm (Panel a), $z = -3$ cm (Panel b), and $z = -4.5$ cm (Panel c) for a field sampling interval of $s = 1$ cm. The values ($\mu$A/m) for the left (L) and right (R) extrema are indicated above each panel where images of the dipoles are represented by contours of constant current dipole moment density. max = maximum.

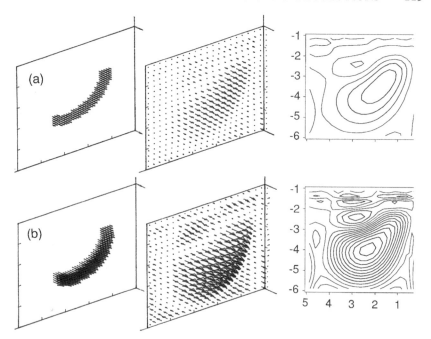

FIG. 4.4.    Panel a: extended source of uniform source density with the upper edge at $z$ = –2.5 cm and the lower edge at –4.5 cm. Panel b: source of the same outline but with the source density at the bottom quadruple that of the top. With a field sampling interval of $s$ = 0.5 cm, and measurements across an observation plane of boundaries 14 × 14 cm, the corresponding magnetic source images are shown in the middle panel and their isocontour representations in the right panel.

overall shape but exhibit some distortion as more strength is pushed toward the region near the center of gravity. Isocontour representation of the inverse distributions is illustrated in the righthand panel.

The practical limit to the quality of a magnetic source image in neuromagnetic measurements is generally determined by noise. To discuss the influence of noise, both sides of the forward equation of Equation 4.8 are normalized with the standard error of each measurement, so that the noisy measurements would play less of a role in the inverse approach. For a detailed discussion of methods and results, see the article by Wang et al. (1992).

## CONSERVATION OF DIPOLAR STRENGTH:
## AN EVALUATION OF CONVERGENCE
## IN THE INVERSE APPROACH

An important property of these images is that their total strength, expressed as the total current dipole moment, is essentially independent of the depth of the maximum and matches the total source strength. Integrating over the whole image surface provides values that are consistently within 0.1% of the deviation of the source's dipole moments. Such a conservation law may be expected to hold if the field pattern across the observation plane is properly sampled and the computation of the SVD is accurate.

This observation reveals an important feature and may be explained by the conservation of energy. Assume the cortex is immersed in a fictitious uniform external magnetic field $\mathbf{B}_{ext}$ with a uniform strength $B_{ext}$ and a fixed angle between the direction of the external field and the dipole orientation. The potential energy of the current dipoles in an external field $\mathbf{B}_{ext}$ can be written:

$$U_{int} = \sum_j -\mathbf{Q} \cdot \mathbf{B}_{ext} = \sum_j Q_j \cdot \cos\alpha \cdot B_{ext} = const \qquad (4.15)$$

Here Equation 4.15 is given as a helpful service for our understanding. It indeed has the dimension of energy. We may, therefore, interpret the conservation of total dipole strength as the consequence of the energy conservation.

$$\sum_j Q_j = const \qquad (4.16)$$

It should be noted that although Penrose's proof guarantees a unique solution to the MNLS inverse problem it does not guarantee the convergence of the numeric computations. As we explained earlier, because of the intrinsic features of floating-point form used in all computers, that is, the arithmetic performed in a computer involves numbers with only a finite number of digits. Round-off errors could accumulate and propagate, causing a divergence of solutions. The integral of dipole strength can serve as a powerful tool to evaluate the convergence of inverse solutions. For example, if the threshold chosen to truncate the near-zero eigenvalues in the SVD process is not appropriate, then conservation of inverse dipole source strength would be violated, and the corresponding resulting "MNLS inverse" could be a spiky chaos.

## SIMULATION OF MNLS INVERSE OF EXTENDED SOURCE DISTRIBUTION IN A SPHERICAL HEAD MODEL

The typical spherical head model consists of a set of three concentric spherical layers of different conductivity, representing the scalp, skull, and cerebrospinal fluid. Their features have no effect on the radial component of the magnetic field. As explained before, an $L$-shaped wall is adopted to represent a part of the folded cortex, the source space. Each plane is 5 cm wide. The height of each plane falls off from 5 cm along the $z$-axis to 3.48 cm on the ends, as shown in Fig. 4.5. The image surface is assumed to coincide with the source surface for the ideal case, as the prior knowledge provided enough information. The nonideal case, in which the image surface had a few-millimeter displacement error as the prior knowledge rendered nonperfect information, was also discussed (Wang, 1993). A total of 127 hypothetical sensors, an entirely realistic number by today's standards, were spaced on the observation surface with axial symmetry, and the spacing between neighboring sensors was about 1.75 cm. A grid of size 0.357 cm was set up across the image surface with a total of 356 nodes representing the magnetic source image.

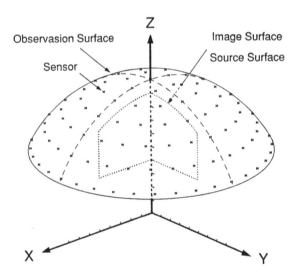

FIG. 4.5. Spherical surface on which observations of the normal components of the magnetic field are made by point sensors placed with axial symmetry about the $z$-axis. The source space is an $L$-shaped wall formed by two vertical planes. The top boundary of each plane is about 1 cm below the observation surface, and the two planes intersect at the $z$-axis. The image surface, if correctly placed, coincides with the source surface.

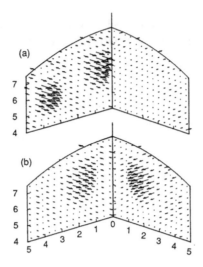

FIG. 4.6.   Magnetic source images for two current dipoles on the same wall, Panel a: $(x, z) = (1, 7)$ and $(4, 6)$ cm, and on different walls, Panel b: $(x, z) = (2, 7)$ and $(y, z) = (2, 7)$ cm.

Two dipoles of equal strength were located at $(x, z) = (4, 6)$ and $(1, 7)$ cm. The magnetic field map of two such parallel dipoles closely resembles that of a dipolar distribution. Conventional methods may not be able to distinguish this source from a single dipole source; however, the MNLS inverse automatically resolves two dipoles in the magnetic source image (see Fig. 4.6a). In Fig. 4.6b, the magnetic source image from the MNLS inverse indicates two dipoles on different walls, located at $(x, z) = (2, 7)$ and $(y, z) = (2, 7)$ cm and oriented at a right angle to each other.

Figure 4.7a represents an extended source configuration in which the cerebral cortex is populated by a large number of primary current elements. The strength of the activity in this example was assumed to be normally distributed, centered at $(x, z) = (2.5, 7)$ cm, with a standard deviation $\sigma = 0.5$ cm. The active area of the circular region extends to $3\sigma = 1.5$ cm in radius. The magnetic source image from the MNLS inverse is shown in Fig. 4.7b. The center of the image describes the peak of the source distribution, and the spread of the image is about 1 cm, comparable to $2\sigma$.

Some two thirds of cerebral cortex lie within fissures and sulci, where neuronal activity occurs on opposite walls. One wants to assess how well the MNLS inverse can distinguish between these walls when they are separated by only a few millimeters. As shown in Fig. 4.8, the skull cap is

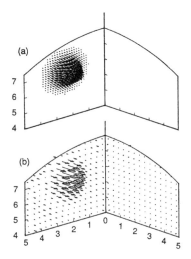

FIG. 4.7. Panel a: extended source of normal distributed density with the center at $(x, z) = (2.5, 7)$ cm and a standard deviation of 0.5 cm. Panel b: magnetic source image obtained from the minimum norm least squares inverse.

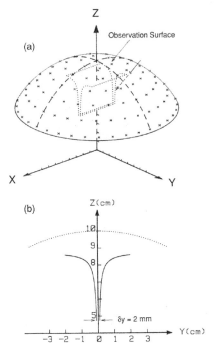

FIG. 4.8. Panel a: spherical surface on which observations of the normal component of the magnetic field are made by an array of point sensors. The source space consists of two walls of a sulcus, modeled as a two-sheeted hyperbolic cylinder. Panel b: The projection of these two surfaces onto the $y$–$z$ plane. Each surface is 5 cm wide and about 5 cm deep.

119

simulated by a partial sphere (basically the same spherical model of the skull used previously), and the cortex is folded to resemble a real sulcus by adopting the shape of a two-sheeted hyperbolic cylinder (Wang, Kaufman, & Williamson, 1995a; Wang, 1994).

In Fig. 4.9, two dipolar sources of equal strength are located on the opposing walls at the same height. They are oriented normally to the walls of the cortex and point toward each other. These sources are at an elevation angle of 32° above the horizontal (Fig. 4.9a). The magnetic source image from the MNLS inverse is shown in both dipolar (Fig. 4.9b) and isocontour representation (Fig. 4.9c). In (Fig. 4.9b) the two sheets are pulled apart from each other by 4 cm in order to present a better view of the image. The wide separation of two surfaces is added only for display purposes.

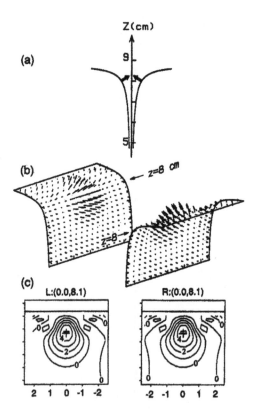

FIG. 4.9.   Panel a: the front view of the sulcus with two current dipoles of the same strength located on the opposite walls: $(x, z) = (0, 8)$ cm, pointing toward each other. Panel b: minimum norm least squares (MNLS) inverse solution represented by a dipole distribution. Panel c: isocontour representation of the MNLS inverse.

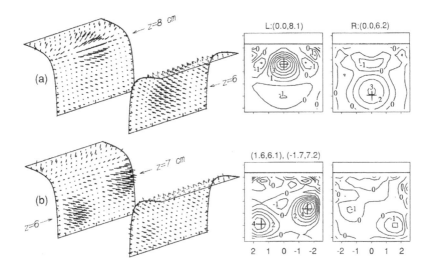

FIG. 4.10.    Panel a: magnetic source image (MSI) of two dipoles on different walls: left: $(x, z) = (0, 8)$, right: $(0, 6)$ cm. Panel b: the MSI for two dipoles on the left wall at positions $(x, z) = (-1.5, 7)$ and $(1.5, 6)$ cm.

In another two dipole simulation (Fig. 4.10), two dipoles are located at different heights, either on different walls (Fig. 4.10a) or on the same wall (Fig. 4.10b) of the sulcus. Three-dimensional display and isocontour representation of the MNLS inverses are shown side by side. The horizontal and the vertical position $(x, z)$ of the peaks in the inverse solution are printed on top of the isocontour plot. The location of each source dipole is marked by a cross for purposes of visual comparison.

## INVERSE OF MAGNETIC FIELD POWER: HOW IS THAT POSSIBLE?

All the other inverse approaches, as well as the MNLS solutions discussed earlier, apply only to coherent (synchronous) patterns of primary current. Synchronized current elements, where current flows normally to the surface of the cortex, provide a reasonable source model for spatially coherent event-related fields (Kaufman, Kaufman, & Wang, 1991).

Many experiments have shown that incoherent activity revealed by power patterns of extracranial fields are differentially affected by the performance of cognitive tasks. Evidence suggests (Kaufman, Schwartz, Salustri, & Williamson, 1990; Kaufman, Curtis, Wang, & Williamson,

1992) that power of the spontaneous alpha-band activity originating in the right temporal lobe is suppressed while a participant scans his or her memory for previously heard musical tones. It is clear that early sensory–perceptual and some cognitive processes are reflected in the coherent event-related responses. It is also clear that local changes in incoherent activity reflect other cognitive processes as well.

In this section we describe a method for discerning the patterns of incoherent cortical activity, for example, relative increases or decreases in activity, regardless of the direction of current flow. As we pointed out earlier, adjacent dipoles of opposed orientation tend to generate self-canceling fields. Therefore, simple averaging could not reveal an increase or decrease in such asynchronous activity of many concurrently active units, despite the fact that regions of the cortex may be either more or less active than neighboring regions. We now consider a process for identifying such regions, in which average field power is the basic measure. The MNLS method is extended to make it possible to delineate the cortical areas exhibiting changes in incoherent activity (Wang, Kaufman, & Williamson, 1993).

In practice, to study variations in field power one needs simply to compute the variance of the average field, because the variance is of the same order as the field power. A novel mathematical development for solving the inverse problem for such measures is derived as follows. First, an autocorrelation matrix $\mathbf{B}_p$ is introduced in terms of the magnetic field vector $\mathbf{b}$:

$$\mathbf{B}_p = \mathbf{b}\,\mathbf{b}^T \qquad (4.17)$$

with elements $(B_p)_{ij} = B_i \cdot B_j$, where $i, j = 1, 2, \ldots, m$. Therefore, the diagonal elements of $\mathbf{B}_p$ are the field power $B_i^2$ ($i = 1, 2, \ldots, m$). Recall Equation 4.8, which is the forward model of the magnetic field. By substituting Equation 4.8 into Equation 4.17, one obtains

$$\mathbf{B}_p = \mathbf{L}\,\mathbf{Q}_p\,\mathbf{L}^T \qquad (4.18)$$

where $\mathbf{Q}_p = \mathbf{q}\,\mathbf{q}^T$ is the autocorrelation matrix of the source dipoles with elements $(Q_p)_{kl} = Q_k \cdot Q_l$, where $k, l = 1, 2, \ldots, n$. The diagonals of $\mathbf{Q}_p$ are the power of each source dipole element. Note that Equation 4.18 is an all-matrix equation.

Relying on the theory and properties of the MNLS inverse (Ben-Israel & Greville, 1974; Penrose, 1955), we are able to derive an extended MNLS inverse of the field power distribution given by Equation 4.18 ( Wang et al., 1995b):

$$\hat{Q}_p = L^+ B_p (L^+)^T \tag{4.19}$$

where $(L^+)^T$ is the transpose of the MNLS inverse matrix, and $\hat{Q}_p$ represents the MNLS estimate of the source dipole power matrix. Equation 4.18 makes it possible to delineate regions of cortex whose levels of incoherent activity deviate from a baseline because of, for example, some ongoing cognitive process or pathological state.

$$<\hat{Q}_p> = L^+ <B_p> (L^+)^T \tag{4.20}$$

where $<>$ denotes the time average. Note that the lead field matrix $L$ is time invariant and so is its MNLS matrix $L^+$, provided that the measures made at different times are taken at the same positions. Equation 4.20 forms the basis for the extended MNLS inverse. Again, because of the minimum-norm and least-square nature of the inverse, the extended MNLS approach guarantees that the result is the best estimate. An iterative search process in which residual errors are compared at each step to find a minimum, as in the typical nonlinear least-square approach, is unnecessary.

In various simulations, the geometry of the cortex and the skull is the same as that in Fig. 4.1. However, here surfaces representing the cerebral cortex are populated by a large number of perpendicular primary current dipoles of random orientation and magnitudes to reflect their incoherence. Subsets of these elements are either increased or decreased in magnitude, and the net fields of all the elements are summed at the observation surface, then averaged. The background activity is spread over the entire source surface. The randomized magnitudes and directions of current flow, which simulates background noise, are given values that range from −1 to 1. A smooth attenuation of the magnitudes of random dipoles at the top and side edges of the L-shaped wall is added to simulate the rounded contours of the actual cortex.

A small circular region of radius 0.6 cm on one wall is enhanced by a factor of 10 as compared with the surrounding region. Figure 4.11a shows one sample of 100 such source distributions. Note that the arrows signify current elements where the directions of current flow are randomly related to each other, unlike the sources of evoked responses. The extended MNLS inverse is shown in Fig. 4.11b. The inverse power at each point is a scalar. Arrowheads are included to better illustrate their length. Figure 4.11c is an isocontour plot representing the same inverse.

In Fig. 4.12, two incremented circular subsets are located on the source surface. Although the current elements vary at random over time inside

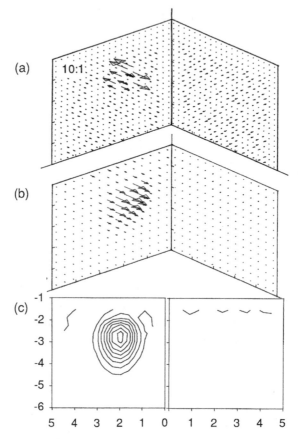

FIG. 4.11.   Panel a: the source surface is populated with a large number of current dipoles of randomly selected orientations and strengths, but those within a small (0.6-cm radius) region are, on average, 10 times stronger than those in the surrounding region. The current power image distribution (Panel b) and isopower density contours (Panel c) are shown on the image surface. Arrows in Panel b do not represent current. The arrowhead is added to better illustrate its length, which is proportional to the average power at each location.

as well as outside the incremented regions, the ratio of the averaged amplitude of the two incremented regions relative to their surroundings is 10:1. One of the 100 source samples is shown in Fig. 4.12b. Figure 4.12a is the plot of the magnetic field power averaged over all 100 samples; Fig. 4.12c is the inverse solution computed using the extended MNLS.

In the next simulation, a crescent-shaped portion of the source surface contains current elements, which on average are 10 times stronger than those in the surrounding region. Figure 4.13a shows 2 of the 100 samples

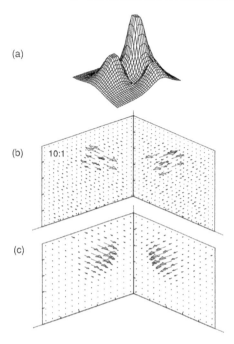

FIG. 4.12.    This figure is similar to Fig. 4.11, except that two 0.6-cm radius regions—one on each wall of the source surface—have current dipole moments increased by an average factor of 10. The average power distribution is computed for 100 random arrays of dipole moments. The bottom of the figure shows the current power image distribution determined from the average field power pattern and the known shape of the source surface.

of the random distributions used in computing the average field power at the observation plane. The extended MNLS inverse provided the current power image, as shown in Fig. 4.13b, which gives a reasonable rendition of the crescent shape. This is made clearer by the isocontours display (Fig. 4.13c) of the current power image.

Thus far we have dealt only with target areas whose activity is at a somewhat higher level than that of the surroundings. We must also consider patterns in which the activity of the target is less than that of its surroundings, simulating selective suppression of the activity of a region of cortex, as presumably occurs when participants scan short-term memory for previously heard tones and seen images (Kaufman, Curtis, Wang, & Williamson, 1992). Therefore, it would be of considerable value to be able to locate and delineate such areas.

One of the difficulties associated with detecting small target areas of suppressed activity is that the extracranial field is dominated by the background activity, which originates in a relatively much larger area of

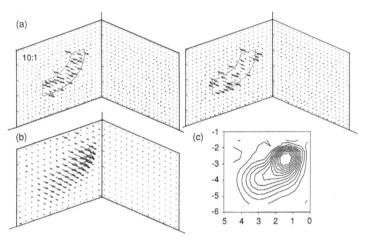

FIG. 4.13. Panel a: two of the 100 samples used in computing average field power for a crescent-shaped area of incoherent activity. Panel b: the inverse solution representing the spatial distribution of current power. Panel c: the corresponding isodensity current power plot.

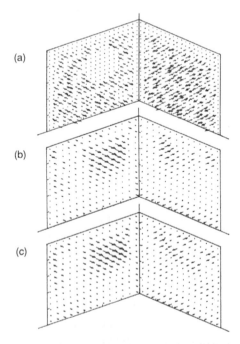

FIG. 4.14. Panel a: sample of a source distribution with a circular region that is decremented. Panels b and c: image power distributions obtained by subtracting the average of 100 such samples from the baseline inverse of 100 different samples of uniform but incoherent activity, beginning with different seeds in the random number generator.

cortex. As a simulation, a circular target area with a radius of 1 cm is selected. The strength of activity within this target is 1:10 that of its surroundings on average. A single sample of a source distribution is shown in Fig. 4.14a. One hundred such samples with different initial seeds of random number generator were used in the simulation. The current power image when the source is decremented is subtracted from the current power image of the baseline when no power depression is present. Figures 4.14b and 4.14c display these power image difference plots.

The above procedures are used to detect a crescent-shaped region of suppressed activity, as shown in Fig. 4.15a. The power image difference pattern extends over a wide range in depth, and the lower part of the current power image is buried in the noise (see Fig. 4.15b). If the surrounding activity is more stable over time, it is possible to obtain an image of higher quality. For example, the image in Fig. 4.15c is one where the baseline of background activity and the distributions containing the target shapes are created by applying the same initial seed to the random number gen-

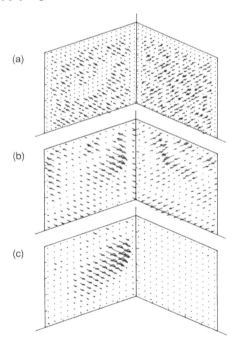

FIG. 4.15.    Panel a: a crescent-shaped source region of suppressed activity. Panel b: the image power distribution difference obtained by subtracting the current power image of 100 samples of Panel a from the current power image of 100 samples of uniform activity obtained from different initial seeds. Panel c the image power distribution difference obtained as in Panel b but starting from the same initial seeds.

erator. The resulting power image difference plot shows a well-defined crescent, because there is a better cancellation of the background activity. The poorer image of Fig. 4.15b is what results when there is no correlation of baseline and target.

## SPATIOTEMPORAL INVERSE—REMEMBER RELATIVITY: TIME IS JUST ONE ADDITIONAL DIMENSION IN A SPACETIME MANIFOLD

The developments in the MNLS approach in forming images of extended distributions of neuronal currents or power that we have discussed is based on the static characterization of the inverse problem. However, brain activity is time dependent, and it results in an ever-changing pattern of extracranial magnetic field. Because the spatial distribution of brain activity continuously evolves with time, the inverse solution that describes this time evolution is of great potential value. Oster and Rudy (1992) took temporal information into account in an attempt to stabilize the inverse solution for epicardial potential distribution from ECG data. Also, Mosher et al. (1992) proposed a multiple-dipole approach based on spatiotemporal MEG data, with the inverse solution limited to a set of dipoles. However, difficulties in numerical calculations when simultaneously fitting many dipoles have, so far, restricted its usefulness in practice.

Wang et al. (1995b) proposed an alternative approach to integrating temporal information with the spatial distribution in which the MNLS approach for the static case is extended to deal with the inverse of time-dependent problems. Large arrays of sensors now make it possible to obtain a large sample of measurements at a given instance. The time dependence in the sampling can be considered as an explicit variable; the forward model in Equation 4.8 can be extended to incorporate the time dependence as well:

$$\mathbf{b}(t) = \mathbf{L}\mathbf{q}(t) + \mathbf{n}(t) \ . \tag{4.21}$$

The noise vector $\mathbf{n}(t)$, which is associated with the measurements, is explicitly included in the forward model for the benefit of later discussions. Note that the lead field matrix is time invariant as long as all the sensors are kept at the same positions during the sampling. For the noise-free case, the MNLS inverse assumes a simple expression:

$$\hat{\mathbf{q}}(t) = \mathbf{L}^+ \mathbf{b}(t) \ . \tag{4.22}$$

Samples of field measurements taken at different time are then combined into a matrix form to include the temporal information:

$$\mathbf{B} = \begin{bmatrix} \mathbf{b}(t_1), & \mathbf{b}(t_2), & ..., & \mathbf{b}(t_l) \end{bmatrix} = \begin{bmatrix} B_1(t_1) & \cdots & B_1(t_l) \\ \vdots & \ddots & \vdots \\ B_m(t_1) & \cdots & B_m(t_l) \end{bmatrix} \quad \textbf{(4.23)}$$

The explicit time dependence of each variable in Equation 4.23 can be further absorbed into the subscript of the column index, ranging from 1, ..., $l$. In the same manner, the noise matrix $\mathbf{N}$ and source matrix $\mathbf{Q}$ can also be constructed with elements $N_{ij} = n_i(t_j)$ and $Q_{ij} = q_i(t_j)$, respectively. From Equations 4.21 and 4.23 one is able to form an all-matrix equation that provides the framework of the spatiotemporal source model. Capital letters in boldface type denote the matrices,

$$\mathbf{B} = \mathbf{L}\,\mathbf{Q} + \mathbf{N} \quad\quad\quad (4.24)$$

Note that $\mathbf{B}$ and $\mathbf{N}$ are $m \times l$ matrices, $\mathbf{L}$ is an $m \times n$ matrix, and $\mathbf{Q}$ is an $n \times l$ matrix. In terms the indices, one can write:

$$B_{ik} = \sum_{j=1}^{n} L_{ij}\, Q_{jk} + N_{ik} \quad\quad i = 1, ..., m; \quad k = 1, ..., l \;. \quad \textbf{(4.25)}$$

Although Equation 4.24 resembles Equation 4.21, they differ from each other not only in their physical meanings but also in their mathematical structures. Equation 4.21 represents the forward model for the static case, where $\mathbf{b}$, $\mathbf{q}$, and $\mathbf{n}$ are column vectors; whereas Equation 4.24 describes the time evolution and the spatial distribution of the source currents, as well as their accompanying magnetic field patterns, in which all quantities are matrices. Despite the matrix nature of Equation 4.24, the field matrix $\mathbf{B}$ is still linearly related to the source matrix $\mathbf{Q}$. Moreover, for the noise-free case, the solution can also be given by the MNLS inverse as follows:

$$\hat{\mathbf{Q}} = \mathbf{L}^+\mathbf{B} \;. \quad\quad\quad (4.26)$$

It is worth noting that the time and the space dimensions play equal roles in this model in the following sense: Both the temporal and the spatial components are linearly related to the field measurements in the forward model, so they can be treated as a single entity. It is these equal roles of time and space in this model that make the inverse procedure much simpler than other spatiotemporal models and entails no ad hoc assumptions regarding which dipole parameters are to be fixed.

Because of the time dependence of the noise level, one is no longer able to use a single weight to normalize each row of the matrices **B** and **L**, as was proposed earlier; neither can one use a different weight to normalize individual elements in the same row of the matrices. Therefore, a novel noise-deduction technique was derived by Wang et al. (1995b) and implemented in the following simulations.

The same source geometry described in Fig. 4.5 is chosen to demonstrate the method and result. Three dipolar sources are chosen for this simulation. Two dipoles, denoted S1 and S2, are fixed in positions on the left wall but have time-dependent magnitudes; the third dipolar source, S3, lies on the right wall and moves from the upper left toward the right along a curved line. The instantaneous moments and phases of these time-varying dipoles can be best illustrated by the functions in Fig. 4.16. The moments of S1 and S2 vary sinusoidally with a phase difference of 90°. Meanwhile, the moment of the moving dipole, S3, abruptly reverses in square wave fashion with a shorter period.

To compute the inverse, a grid was set up across the image surface of a grid size of 0.357 cm, with a total of 356 nodes representing the image. As

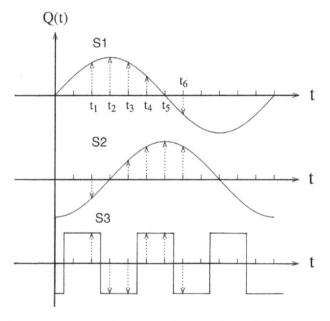

FIG. 4.16.   Time evolution of the strength of activity of three dipolar sources.

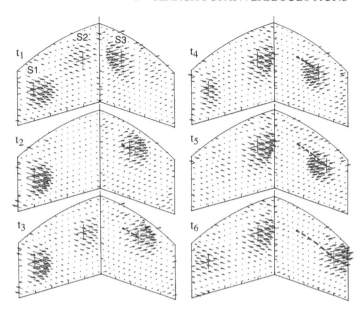

FIG. 4.17. Kinetic magnetic source image computed from the minimum norm least squares inverse for two stationary sources (S) and one moving source is shown as six time slices. Three cross marks indicate the actual source dipole positions at different time instances in the simulation. The trajectory of the third moving dipole is represented by the broken line.

we explained earlier, the MNLS inverse does not entail any assumption about the number of dipoles in the image. Six time slices $t_1, ..., t_6$ of simulation results are displayed in Fig. 4.17. At the first instance, $t_1$, the image shows three dipoles with different strengths and positions. For the next time instance, $t_2$, the image of dipole S1 grows stronger, but the image of S2 vanishes, and the image of S3 changes its orientation and moves toward the right. If one compares the rest of the image slices in Fig. 4.17 with the evolution of the sources in Fig. 4.16, one can see that at each time instance the strength of an image and the location of its strongest element match the strength and location of the respective source. For purposes of comparison, the positions of actual sources are marked on the image surface, and the trajectory of source S3 is indicated by the broken line on the right wall. This simulation was repeated in the presence of noise (10% noise level) or in the position errors of the image surface (Wang et al., 1995b). Noise or position errors cause blur in the resulting images. However, the kinetic MNLS image still provides useful information on the spatial distribution and the time evolution of the source current.

## CONCLUSION

This chapter represents a very early attempt to develop a practical means for forming magnetic source images. These images of distributions of currents and of altered levels of incoherent brain activity will depend on the ways in which investigators come to grips with solving the inverse problem. Our only contribution here is to show that it is possible in principle to solve this problem. This is especially true today with the availability of large arrays of sensors and of high resolution magnetic resonance imaging machines. It is also clear that in some cases it may not be possible to form magnetic source images based solely on MEG data. Data obtained using EEG, which is well suited for deep sources within the brain, may be integrated with MEG data and enable some MNLS solutions (cf. Gençer & Williamson, 1998). Also, Bayesian approaches, with which we have not dealt, may well permit *a posteriori* source identification, or least localization of centers of gravity of extended but deep-lying sources.

We hope that future investigators will take the results reported here and attempt to extend them (as well as related results obtained by other investigators) and develop a form of MSI that will truly complement other functional imaging modalities.

## REFERENCES

Barr, R. C., Pikington, R. C., Boineau, J. P., & Spach, M. S. (1966). Determining surface potentials from current dipole, with application to electrocardiography. *IEEE Transactions on Biomedical Engineering, 113,* 88–92,

Ben-Israel, A., & Greville, T. N. E. (1974). *Generalized inverses: Theory and applications.* New York: Wiley.

Cuffin, B. N., & Cohen, D. (1977). Magnetic fields produced by models of biological current sources. *Journal of Applied Physics, 48,* 3971–3980

Curtis, S., Kaufman, L., & Williamson, S. J. (1988). Divided attention revisited: Selection based on location or pitch. In K. Atsumi, M. Kotani, S. Ueno, T. Katila, & S. J. Williamson (Eds.), *Biomagnetism, 87* (pp. 138–141). Tokyo: Tokyo Denki University Press.

Gençer, N. G., & Williamson, S. J. (1998). Differential characterization of neural sources with the bimodal truncated SVD pseudo-inverse for EEG and MEG measurements. *IEEE Transactions on Biomedical Engineering, 45,* 827–838.

Geselowitz, D. B. (1967). On bioelectric potentials in an inhomogeneous volume conductor. *Biophysics Journal, 7,* 1–11.

Geselowitz, D. B. (1970). On the magnetic field generated outside an inhomogeneous volume conductor by internal current sources. *IEEE Transactions on Magnetism, 6,* 346–347.

Golub, G. H., & Van Loan, C. F. (1983). *Matrix computations.* Baltimore: Johns Hopkins University Press.

Hämäläinen, M. S., & Ilmoniemi, R. J. (1984). Interpreting measured magnetic fields of the brain: Estimates of current distributions. Report TKK-F-A559. Helsinki University of Technology.

Helmholtz, H. (1853). Über einige Gesetze der Vertheilung elektrischer Ströme in körperlichen Leitern, mit Anhwendung auf die thierischelektrischen Versuche. *Annelen der Physik und Chemie, 89,* 211–233, 353–377.

Huang, J. C., Nicholson, C., & Okada, Y. C. (1990). Distortion of magnetic evoked fields and surface potentials by conductivity differences at boundaries in brain tissue. *Biophysics Journal, 57,* 1155–1166.

Ioannides, A. A., Bolton, J. P. R., Hasson, R., & Clarke, C J. S. (1990). Continuous probabilistic solutions to the biomagnetic inverse problem. *Inverse Problems, 6,* 1–20.

Jackson, J. D. (1974). *Classical Electrodynamics* (2nd ed.). New York: Wiley.

Kaufman, L., Curtis, S., Wang, J.-Z., & Williamson, S. J. (1992). Changes in cortical activity when subjects scan memory for tones. *Electroencephalography and Clinical Neurophysiology, 82,* 266–284.

Kaufman, L., Kaufman, J. H., & Wang, J.-Z. (1991). On cortical folds and neuromagnetic fields. *Electroencephalography and Clinical Neurophysiology, 79,* 211–226.

Kaufman, L., Schwartz, B., Salustri, C., & Williamson, S. J. (1990). Modulation of spontaneous brain activity during mental imagery. *Journal of Cognitive Neuroscience, 2,* 124–132.

Moore, E. H. (1920). On the reciprocal of the general algebraic matrix. *Bulletin of the American Mathematical Society, 26,* 394–495.

Mosher, J., Lewis, P., & Leahy, R. (1992). Multiple dipole modeling and localization from spatio-temporal MEG data. *IEEE Transactions on Biomedical Engineering, 39,* 541–557.

Okada, Y. C., & Huang, J. C. (1990). "Current-density imaging as method of visualizing neuronal activities of the brain," in proc. Annual Meeting of the Society of Neuroscience, St. Louis, MO.

Okada, Y. C., Kaufman, L., & Williamson, S. J. (1983). The hippocampal formation as a source of the slow endogenous potentials. *Electroencephalography and Clinical Neurophysiology, 55,* 417–426.

Oster, H. S., & Rudy, Y. (1992). The use of temporal information in the regularization of the inverse problem of electrocardiography. *IEEE Transactions on Biomedical Engineering, 39,* 65–75.

Penrose, R. (1955). A generalized inverse for matrices. *Mathematical Proceedings of the Cambridge Philosophical Society, 51,* 406–413.

Sarvas, J. (1987). Basic mathematical and electromagnetic concepts of the biomagnetic inverse problem. *Physics in Medicine and Biology, 32,* 11–22.

Smith, W. E., Dallas, W. J., Kullmann, W. H., & Schlitt, H. A. (1990). Linear estimation theory applied to the reconstruction of a 3-D vector current distribution. *Applied Optics, 29,* 658–667.

Tan, S., Roth, B. J., & Wikswo, J. P., Jr. (1990). The magnetic field of cortical current sources: The application of a spatial filtering model to the forward and inverse problem. *Electroencephalography and Clinical Neurophysiology, 76,* 73–85.

Vaughan, H. G., Jr., & Ritter, W. (1970). The sources of auditory evoked responses recorded from the human scalp. *Electroencephalography and Clinical Neurophysiology, 28*(4), 360–367.

Wang, J.-Z. (1993). Minimum-norm least-squares estimation: Magnetic source images for a spherical model head. *IEEE Transactions on Biomedical Engineering, 40,* 387–396.

Wang, J.-Z. (1994). MNLS inverse discriminates between neuronal activity on opposite walls of a sulcus of the brain. *IEEE Transactions on Biomedical Engineering, 40,* 387–396.

Wang, J.-Z., Kaufman, L., & Williamson, S. J. (1993). Imaging regional changes in the spontaneous activity of the brain: An extension of the minimum-norm least-squares estimate. *Electroencephalography and Clinical Neurophysiology, 86,* 36–50.

Wang, J.-Z., Kaufman, L., & Williamson, S J. (1995a). MNLS inverse applied to complex source geometric. In C. Baumgartner, L. Deecke, G. Stroink, & S. J. Williamson (Eds.), *Biomagnetism: Fundamental Research and Clinical Applications* (pp. 394–397). Amsterdam: Elsevier Science, IOS Press.

Wang, J.-Z., Williamson, S. J., & Kaufman, L. (1992). Magnetic source images determined by a lead-field analysis: The unique minimum-norm least-squares estimation. *IEEE Transactions on Biomedical Engineering, 39,* 665–675.

Wang, J.-Z., Williamson, S. J., & Kaufman, L. (1995b). Kinetic images of neuronal activity of the human brain based on the spatio-temporal MNLS inverse: A theoretical study. *Brain Topography, 7,* 193–200.

Wikswo, J. P., Jr., Roth, B. J., & Sepulveda, N. G. (1989). Using a magnetometer to image a two-dimensional current distribution. *Journal of Applied Physics, 65,* 361–372.

Williamson, S. J., &. Kaufman, L. (1981). Magnetic fields of the cerebral cortex. In S. N. Erné, H.-D. Hahlbohm, & H. Lubbig (Eds.), *Biomagnetism* (pp. 353–402). Berlin: de Gruyter.

Williamson, S. J., & Kaufman, L. (1987). Analysis of neuromagnetic signals. In A. S. Gevins & A. Remond (Eds.), *Handbook of Electroencephalography and Clinical Neurophysiology:* Vol. 1. Methods of analysis of brain electrical and magnetic signals (pp. 405–444). Amsterdam: Elsevier.

# 5

## Techniques for Investigating and Exploiting Nonlinearities in Brain Processes by Recording Responses Evoked by Sensory Stimuli

M. P. Regan
D. Regan
*York University*

As W. Reichardt and T. Poggio (1981) noted, every nontrivial neural computation must be essentially nonlinear. If this is so, then linear systems analysis is not even an approximately valid approach to any nontrivial neural computation. Although there is only 1 kind of linear behavior, the number of kinds of nonlinear behavior is indefinitely large, and the nonlinear analytic method chosen must be tailored to the particular nonlinearity. Furthermore, nonlinear systems analysis is considerably more demanding than linear systems analysis. On the other hand, the application of methods of nonlinear systems analysis to sensory systems offers insights that are hidden to linear systems analysis.

A hybrid frequency domain–time domain technique has been developed that allows time-varying processes (such as adaptation) to be tracked and is the basis of the sweep-averaging technique. Turning to steady-state (frequency domain) analysis, when the input to a system that consists of 1 or more nonlinear stages is the sum of 2 sinusoids of different frequencies, $F_1$ and $F_2$, the output may contain multiple crossmodulation terms of frequency $nF_1 \pm mF_2$ (where $n$ and $m$ are integers.) A mathematical method has been developed to model a sensory pathway and predict the pattern of harmonic and crossmodulation terms; the model consists of multiple nonlinear rectifier-like elements, each representing a neuron. By using nondestructive zoom-FFT (Fast Fourier transform) to analyze brain responses so as to give a spectrum at the physical limit of resolution, the harmonic and cross-modulation terms can be recorded even when they are very weak. In principle, this technique gives an advantage to nonlinear analysis in the frequency domain as compared with the time-domain white noise (Wiener kernel) method, because terms of considerably higher order can be recorded, thus allowing sharper testing of models. Further illustrations of the exploitation of nonlinearities include the use of "frequency tagging" to (a) identify and locate an audiovisual convergence area in the human brain, (b) estimate neural tuning bandwidths for orientation and spatial frequency, (c) demonstrate the presence of functioning binocular neurons in people with low visual acuity, and (d) test a theoretical model of distortion at the level of auditory hair cells.

## LINEAR SYSTEMS AND THE WIDE AND WILD WORLD OF NONLINEAR SYSTEMS

A system or part of a system is said to behave *linearly* if the relation between its output and its input obeys the following requirement:

1. If input $I_a(t)$ produces output $O_a(t)$, and input $I_b(t)$ produces output $O_b(t)$, then input $[I_a(t) + I_b(t)]$ produces output $[O_a(t) + O_b(t)]$. (This requirement is sometimes called the *superimposition requirement*.)

Any system that does not obey this requirement is said to be *nonlinear*. Although all linear systems are similar in that they obey Requirement 1, the number of kinds of nonlinear behavior is indefinitely large. A smoothly curved input–output characteristic is a *nonessential nonlinearity* that behaves more and more linearly as the amplitude of the input is progressively reduced. An *essential nonlinearity* does not approximate linear behavior even when the input signal is small. A threshold, multiplication, and rectification are examples of essential nonlinearities that are commonly encountered in magnetoencephalography (MEG), evoked-potential (EP) studies, and neurophysiology in general.

*Time invariance* means that the system's output $O(t)$ does not depend on the time at which the input $I(t)$ is applied; that is, the response to $I(t - T)$ is $O(t - T)$ for all $T$ and $I(t)$. A consequence of linearity plus time invariance is as follows:

2. A pure sinusoidal input produces a pure sinusoidal output of the same frequency as the input (Bracewell, 1965, pp. 185–186).

A system whose output does not depend on the previous history of inputs is called a *zero-memory system*. The hysteresis curve of an iron transformer's core is a familiar example of memory. As D. Regan (1975a) discussed and illustrated, when using the sweep method with MEG or EP recording it is essential to check for hysteresis. A perhaps less familiar manifestation of memory is the phenomenon of *nonlinear resonance,* in which the output of a system fed with a sinusoidal input depends on whether the frequency of the input is increasing or decreasing so that there is a region of instability within which the output produced by a particular input may have two possible values (the *jump effect*.) Formal discussions of nonlinear oscillations and the jump effect are available (Blaquière, 1966; Hagedorn, 1982; Hayashi, 1964; Stoker, 1950). A dramatic illustration of complex nonlinear oscillations in EP recording was given by D. Regan, Schellart, Spekreijse, and van den Berg (1975).

A very convenient feature of linear system behavior is that if a sinusoidal input is applied to a linear system and the amplitude and phase of the steady-state output are recorded over the range of input frequencies that produce an output, then the time-domain output produced by a single input pulse *or any other transient waveform* can be computed by means of the inverse Fourier transform. Furthermore, the minimum possible phase shift produced by any linear system can be calculated if the effect of input frequency on output amplitude is known (Aseltine, 1958; Bracewell, 1965).

In a certain sense, however, linear systems are tame and somewhat boring: Both the static and dynamic behavior of a linear system are severely restricted, and their range of possible behaviors is narrow (Hirsch & Smale, 1974). As Reichardt and Poggio (1981, p. 187), writing on the topic of neural information processing, noted: "Every nontrivial computation has to be essentially nonlinear, that is, not representable (even approximately), by linear operations."

Although any linear system can be analyzed by the same method of linear systems analysis there is, unfortunately, no single method of analysis that can be applied to all nonlinear systems: For nonlinear systems the method of analysis depends on the type of nonlinear behavior. Also, as mentioned earlier, the number of different kinds of possible nonlinear behavior is indefinitely large. For the engineer, this offers an indefinitely large range of nonlinear behaviors to be exploited while at the same time challenging him or her with mathematical and conceptual problems that are seldom straightforward and may even exceed the competence of any living mathematician. On the other hand, although considerably more demanding than linear systems analysis, the application of methods of nonlinear systems analysis to sensory systems offers insights that are hidden to linear systems analysis. For example, although the sequence and characterization of processing stages within a linear system cannot be obtained by comparing the system's output and input, this analysis is possible for some systems that contain a nonlinear stage (Jenkins & Watts, 1968, p. 45).

## TECHNIQUES FOR INVESTIGATING ADAPTATION AND OTHER NONSTATIONARY PROCESSES

Adaptation, an often-encountered characteristic of sensory systems, violates the requirement for a zero-memory system. A simple procedure, first developed for recording evoked electrical responses, can be used to investigate either electrical or magnetic correlates of sensory adaptation.

Strictly speaking, a transient waveform is one that is repeated once only. The *averaged* "transient" evoked brain response can be regarded as a true transient response only to the extent that the relevant brain mechanisms are in their resting states before each successive stimulus and return to their resting state before the next stimulus. This requirement implies that the response to any given trial does not depend on any previous trial.

In coining the term *steady-state evoked potential,* D. Regan (1964, 1966) defined the idealized response as a repetitive evoked potential whose constituent discrete frequency components remain constant in amplitude and phase over an infinitely long time period. Although this definition does imply that the idealized steady-state EP is an infinitely long train of identical waveforms, it is more helpful to think of the steady-state EP in terms of its constituent frequency components rather than in terms of a complex waveform, endlessly repeated.

Note that, in principle, neither the repetition rate of the EP waveform nor the repetition rate of the stimulus is germane to this definition of steady-state EP. The significance of repetition rate is merely that the higher the repetition rate, the wider the spacing of the steady-state EP's constituent frequency components. Consequently, at high repetition rates only a few harmonic components fall within the brain's passband so that the steady-state EP waveform is simpler than at low repetition rates.

D. Regan (1964, 1966) recorded steady-state brain responses by multiplying the electroencephalogram by the sine and cosine of the stimulus repetition frequency and combining the low-pass filtered outputs of the multipliers in such a way as to obtain the amplitude and phase of the brain response (D. Regan, 1989, pp. 81–90). The use of low-pass filters rather than integrators means that the recorded signal could be used to verify that the response was indeed steady state before integrating the multiplier's outputs over 0.5–2 min so as to give a frequency-domain analysis.

Further to this point, the use of low-pass filters allows the signal to follow progressive changes in the brain response that are caused by sensory adaptation, for example, adaptation caused by exposure to very bright lights (D. Regan, 1964). This technique is a hybrid frequency domain–time domain analysis and is the basis of the single-sweep method that allows the effect of any given variable to be explored within a recording period as short as 10 sec, up to 100 times faster than a comparable time-domain averaging procedure (D. Regan, 1973, 1974, 1975a). Figure 5.1 illustrates Nelson, Seiple, Kupersmith, and Carr's (1984) use of the single-sweep method to demonstrate rapid adaptation to spatial contrast.

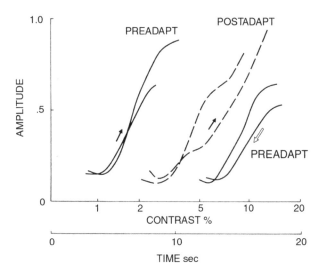

FIG. 5.1. *Visual adaptation to contrast: rapid measurement of contrast threshold by the sweep visual evoked potential method.* The continuous lines are upward sweeps starting at 0.1% contrast before adapting for 60 sec to a 75% contrast grating. The dashed lines are upward sweeps recorded immediately after adaptation, showing a roughly threefold increase of threshold. Note, however, that this threshold was lower than the preadaptation (preadapt) threshold for 20% to 0.1% downward sweeps of contrast. Postadapt = postadaptation. From "A Rapid Evoked Potential Index of Cortical Adaptation" by J. I. Nelson, W. H. Seiple, M. J. Kupersmith, and R. E. Carr, 1984, *Electroencephalography and Clinical Electrophysiology, 59*, p. 460. Copyright 1984 by Elsevier Science. Adapted with permission.

In the sweep-averaging technique, multiple sweeps are averaged (D. Regan, 1974, 1975a). Rather than laboriously constructing a graph (e.g., of response amplitude vs. stimulus intensity) point by point, the graph is quickly sampled (swept) many times, and the sweeps are averaged. This technique reduces the effect of slow variations of visual sensitivity and is particularly useful when investigating labile visual or auditory characteristics. For example, a problem in using a monochromatic test light to measure the spectral sensitivities of parallel color channels is that the test light progressively desensitizes one or more channels. This problem can be reduced by using the sweep-averaging method (D. Regan, 1974, 1975a).

The running average feature can also be exploited to place the brain within a feedback loop such that the brain exerts direct moment-to-moment control over some feature of the stimulus so as to maintain the amplitude of the brain response constant. (This feedback loop operates below the level of consciousness.) For example, this brain-feedback technique has been used to control the luminance of a desensitizing light superimposed on a monochromatic checkerboard stimulus so as to keep constant the brain response evoked by the checkerboard while the wavelength of the desensitizing light was progressively swept (D. Regan, 1975a, 1979).

The steady-state technique allows different submodalities or stimulus features to be "tagged" by slightly different frequencies (also called the *method of multiple stimuli*). The different frequencies can be sufficiently close that they are identical to the brain yet easily separated by a sine–cosine analyzer (e.g., 10.0 Hz and 10.1 Hz.) This technique was originally used to tag the two retinal half-fields (later four retinal quadrants ) so as to allow responses evoked from two (or four) retinal locations to be recorded simultaneously from any given recording location, a procedure that allows the responses from different sites in the visual field to be compared much more rapidly and accurately when the different sites are stimulated one at a time rather than simultaneously (Cartwright & Regan, 1974; D. Regan & Cartwright, 1970; D. Regan & Heron, 1969). This feature showed to advantage in an investigation in which D. Regan and Heron (1970) measured how the balance of visual excitability in the left and right hemispheres varied during the course of migraine attacks by recording responses evoked simultaneously by left and right half-field stimulation. The frequency tagging technique has also been used to record simultaneous responses to three stimulus frequencies so as to track progressive changes of visual response latency in patients with multiple sclerosis whose body temperature was being progressively changed (Regan, 1976; Regan, Murray, & Silver, 1977) and, as we discuss later, to identify an audiovisual convergence area in the human brain, to estimate the tuning bandwidths of neurons sensitive to orientation and spatial frequency, to isolate the responses of binocular neurons, and to distinguish between brain responses evoked by signals from the left and right eyes. This last application was recently used to study retinal rivalry (Tonini, Srinivasan, Russell, & Edelman, 1998).

## LOCATING A FREQUENCY-DOUBLING NONLINEARITY

The brain response evoked by flickering a light at about 5 Hz or at about 40 Hz contains a strong component at twice the input frequency (Spekreijse & van der Tweel, 1965; van der Tweel, 1961; van der Tweel & Verduyn Lunel, 1965). Thus, the visual processing of flicker violates Requirement 2, presented earlier, for linear processing. The frequency-doubled response component can be abolished by superimposing noise-modulated light on the sinusoidal stimulus and viewing the combination with one eye (which is an example of the linearizing phenomenon, well known in engineering). On the other hand, presenting the sinusoidal stimulus to one eye and the noise to the other eye does not abolish the frequency-doubled response component. This demonstrates that the nonlinearity that causes the frequency doubling is located before convergence of signals from the left and right eyes (Spekreijse, 1966).

Spekreijse (1966) modeled the early processing of flicker in terms of a "sandwich system" in which the first and last stages are linear frequency filters and the middle stage is a frequency-independent rectifier (a static nonlinearity.) Suppose that the input to the first stage is a light flickering sinusoidally at $F$ Hz. Realizing that the second harmonic distortion (frequency doubling) cannot occur until the input signal reaches the rectifier, Spekreijse proceeded as follows. He kept the $F$ Hz input constant and measured the amplitude of the $2F$-Hz component in the brain response. When a second sinusoidal input flicker (the *auxiliary signal*) was added, the amplitude of the $2F$-Hz component was reduced because of the linearizing effect caused by the auxiliary signal. Reasoning that a constant linearizing effect means that the amplitude of the auxiliary signal *on its arrival at the rectifier* is constant, Spekreijse adjusted the amplitude of the auxiliary signal while varying its frequency so as to maintain a constant linearizing effect. The reciprocal of the amplitude of the auxiliary signal gave the attenuation characteristic of the filter that preceded the rectifier. The attenuation characteristic of the entire sandwich system was then obtained by comparing the amplitude of the output and input over a range of input signal frequencies (in the absence of an auxiliary signal.) The attenuation characteristic of the second filter could be derived straightforwardly from the two characteristics already obtained (see also Spekreijse & Oosting, 1970; Spekreijse & Reits, 1982; van der Tweel & Spekreijse, 1969).

Flicker excites the following three parallel subsystems in the human brain: (a) the low-frequency subsystem, whose peak response is at 9 to 11 Hz (Spekreijse, 1966; van der Tweel & Verduyn Lunel, 1965); (b) the medium-frequency subsystem, whose peak response is at 14 to 20 Hz (D. Regan, 1968a, 1970a); and (c) the high-frequency subsystem, whose peak response is near 40 Hz (D. Regan, 1968b; Spekreijse, 1966; van der Tweel & Verduyn Lunel, 1965). The properties of the low-frequency (Spekreijse, 1966) and 40-Hz (D. Regan, 1968a, 1968b, 1970b) responses are similar regardless of whether they are generated as fundamental or second harmonic responses. The finding that multiple sclerosis (a demyelinating disease) increases the delay of the medium-frequency flicker response while not affecting the delay of the 40-Hz response implies that these two subsystems are separate from retinal level (D. Regan, 1975b). (This topic was reviewed by D. Regan, 1975b, and D. Regan, 1989, pp. 380–386.)

The color and saturation characteristics of the 40-Hz subsystem closely match those of macaque monkeys' magnocellular retinal ganglion cells, whereas the quite different characteristics of the medium-frequency subsystem match those of parvocellular retinal ganglion cells (D. Regan & Lee, 1993). On this basis Regan and Lee proposed that the 40-Hz flicker response and the medium-frequency flicker response allow one to isolate and study noninvasively the magnocellular and parvocellular streams in humans.

## RESPONSE SPECTRUM RECORDED AT ULTRA-HIGH FREQUENCY RESOLUTION

Before going on to the next section we should discuss a signal-to-noise issue. The theoretical limit of resolution in the spectrum of a time series, the Gabor–Heisenberg limit, is given by $\Delta F = 1/\Delta T$, where $\Delta T$ is the length of the time series in seconds, and $\Delta F$ Hz is the frequency resolution.[1] Although the simple analog technique described earlier can deliver

---

[1]The relation involves a scaling constant that depends on how one chooses to describe frequency bandwidth $\Delta F$ and how one chooses to define the duration of the signal. Gabor (1946) chose the root mean square (RMS) definition of bandwidth and duration, giving $\Delta F = 1/2\Delta T$. The $\Delta F = 1/\Delta T$ version implies a different definition of bandwidth in which $\Delta F$ is measured between the first two zero crossings in the amplitude spectrum.

this theoretical limit of resolution for harmonic and even crossmodulation frequency components, it is inconvenient. The FFT algorithm is convenient, but the best possible frequency resolution provided by the approach is determined by the number of samples used to describe the time series and is far below the Gabor–Heisenberg limit for long recording durations. We adapted the zoom-FFT technique to nondestructive form (nondestructive zoom-FFT; M. P. Regan & Regan, 1988, 1989) so as to attain the theoretical limit of frequency resolution over an indefinitely wide bandwidth (see also D. Regan, 1989, pp. 98–108). Provided that the variability of the frequency components in the brain response is not too great, the bandwidth of these components is set by the recording duration rather than by signal variability. For example, after recording brain responses for 520 sec while the observer viewed a counterphase-modulated grating, a harmonic component of the EP fell within a bandwidth of 0.002 Hz (D. Regan, 1989, Fig. 1.70B). A bandwidth of 0.004 Hz or 0.008 Hz can be used on an everyday basis, as illustrated in Fig. 5.2. The point of this high resolution is that all the signal power is concentrated into a few very narrow regions along the frequency axis while the noise is distributed continuously along the frequency axis. This allows very weak signals to be recorded at high signal-to-noise levels. This topic was discussed more fully by D. Regan (1989, pp. 103–111). A device for delivering spectra at the theoretical limit of resolution over bandwidths suitable for MEG recording is now available commercially (Bruel and Kjaer signal analyzer, Model 2035).

## TWO-SINEWAVE METHOD USED TO MEASURE THE SPATIAL–FREQUENCY TUNING, TEMPORAL–FREQUENCY TUNING, AND ORIENTATION TUNING OF A BRAIN MECHANISM

The method we describe next can, in principle, be used to measure the tuning characteristics of neural mechanisms within any sensory modality. To illustrate the general idea, we choose the particular example of a neural mechanism sensitive to spatial contrast.

The rationale in this particular case is as follows. When the eye is stimulated by two superimposed gratings, nonlinear grating–grating interactions in the brain response can be produced only if the neural mechanism that generates the brain response "sees" both gratings simultaneously. In other words, nonlinear interaction terms cannot be generated if only one grating is within the spatial frequency, temporal frequency, and orienta-

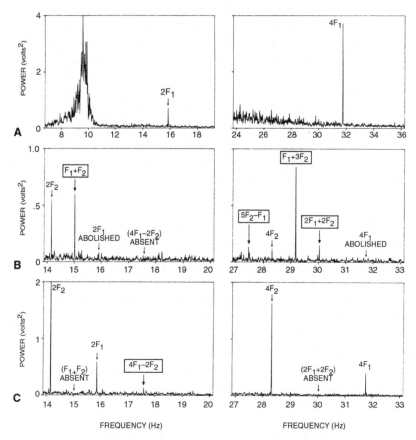

FIG. 5.2. *Nonlinear interaction between two gratings.* Two sections of the DC–100-Hz power spectrum are shown at ultranarrowband 0.0078-Hz resolution, giving 801 frequency bins in each section and a total of 12,800 real frequency bins from DC to 100 Hz. Panel A: The stimulus was a single grating that was counterphase modulated at a nominal 8 Hz (actually 7.938 Hz.) For comparison purposes. the alpha region is included in the spectrum. Panel B: The grating in A was exactly superimposed on a second grating that was counterphase modulated at a nominal 7 Hz (actually 7.080 Hz.) Panel C: The grating in A was superimposed on an unpatterned field flickering at 7.080 Hz. For any small retinal area, the superimposed $F_2$ Hz grating in B was identical to the superimposed flicker in C. The terms boxed in B index nonlinear interactions. Ordinates are in arbitrary units with the dimensions of $V^2$. The gratings were both 5 cycles/degree, oriented vertically and subtended 10°. Viewing was binocular. Recording between the inion and an electrode midway between inion and vertex with vertex grounded. Recording duration was 320 sec using a Bruel and Kjaer Model 2032 analyzer. From "Objective Evidence for Phase-Independent Spatial Frequency Mechanisms in the Human Visual Pathway" by D. Regan and M. P. Regan, 1988, *Vision Research, 28,* p. 188. Copyright 1988 by Elsevier Science. Reprinted with permission.

tion bandwidth of the generator mechanism. Given this rationale, the tuning bandwidths of the mechanism that responds to any given grating can be estimated in the following way (D. Regan, 1983).

1. *Spatial frequency bandwidth:* Superimpose on the reference grating a grating of closely similar orientation and closely similar counterphase-modulation frequency and then vary the spatial frequency of this second grating.
2. *Orientation bandwidth:* Superimpose on the reference grating a second grating of closely similar spatial frequency and closely similar counterphase-modulation frequency and then vary the orientation of this second grating.
3. *Temporal bandwidth:* Superimpose on the reference grating a second grating of closely similar spatial frequency and orientation and then vary its counterphase-modulation frequency.

The nonlinear grating–grating interactions between a grating that exchanges bright and dim bars $2F_1$ times/sec and a grating that exchanges bars $2F_2$ times/sec comprise (a) suppression of the $2F_1$ Hz, $2F_2$ Hz, and other harmonic components of the response and (b) generation of crossmodulation components of frequency $(nF_1 \pm mF_2)$ Hz (where $n$ and $m$ are integers.) Figures 5.2A–5.2C show the following. Figure 5.2A shows the $2F_1$ and $4F_1$ responses to a single grating that was counterphase-modulated at $F_1$ Hz (so that it exchanged bright and dim bars $2F_1$ times/sec.) Figure 5.2B shows the suppression of these components and generation of crossmodulation components when a grating that was counterphase-modulated at $F_2$ Hz was superimposed on the first grating. Figure 5.2C shows the very different effect of superimposing a blank field whose luminance was modulated at $F_2$ Hz (D. Regan & M. P. Regan, 1988a).

Figure 5.3B shows how suppression of the $2F_1$ component in Fig. 5.2A was used to show that the broad spatial frequency tuning bandwidth observed when only one grating was used (Fig. 5.3A) was composed of multiple narrow-bandwidth submechanisms even at contrast levels that were well above threshold (D. Regan, 1983).

The temporal-frequency tuning of any one of these submechanisms fell into one of only two classes: lowpass or bandpass (D. Regan, 1983).

Figure 5.4 shows that suppression of the $2F_1$ Hz component was greatest and the $(2F_1 + 2F_2)$ Hz component was largest when the two gratings were parallel. These nonlinear interactions were much weaker

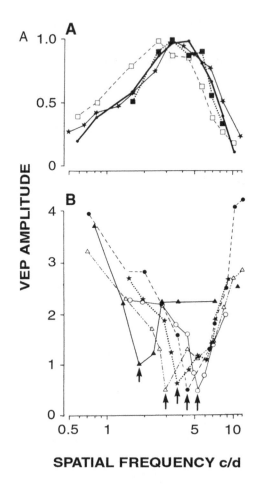

FIG. 5.3. *Spatially selective subunits.* Panel A: normalized evoked potential amplitudes for a single grating of fixed temporal frequency (20 reversals/sec) plotted versus the spatial frequency of the grating for contrasts of 15% (large solid squares, dotted line), 30% (open squares, broken line), 60% (solid circles, heavy continuous line), and 100% (stars, fine continuous line.) Panel B: evoked potential amplitude (in microvolts) for a reference grating in the presence of a superimposed variable grating. The temporal frequencies of both gratings were fixed: No. 1 at 20 and No. 2 at 18 reversals/sec. The spatial frequency of Grating 1 was constant, while the spatial frequency of Grating 2 was varied. The five plots show data for five experiments in which, as indicated by vertical arrows, the spatial frequency of Reference Grating 1 was fixed at 1.6, 3.0, 3.7, 4.4, and 5.2 cycles/degrees in different experiments. Amplitudes shown are for the visual evoked potential frequency component at the reversal rate of Grating 1. c/d = cycles/degrees. From "Spatial Frequency Mechanisms in Human Vision Investigated by Evoked Potential Recording" by D. Regan, 1983, *Vision Research, 23,* p. 1402. Copyright 1983 by Elsevier Science. Reprinted with permission.

when the gratings differed in orientation by about 40 degrees. This finding is consistent with a full half-sensitivity bandwidth of about 25 degrees for orientation-tuned cortical neurons. However, nonlinear interactions were again strong when the two gratings were at right angles. This finding could not have been predicted from data obtained with a single grating. It can be understood if there is a strong nonlinear interactions between orthogonal orientation-tuned neural mechanisms (D. Regan & Regan, 1987).

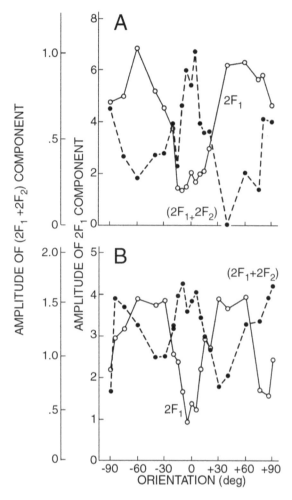

FIG. 5.4. *Visual response to a two-dimensional pattern that cannot be explained in one-dimensional Fourier terms.* A vertical grating was counterphase modulated at $F_1$ Hz. A second grating was optically superimposed and counterphase modulated at $F_2$ Hz. The orientation of the second grating was varied. Filled symbols plot the amplitudes of the $(2F_1 + 2F_2)$ Hz nonlinear interaction term versus the second grating's orientation. Open symbols plot the amplitude of the $2F_1$ terms produced by the fixed grating. There was a strong nonlinear interaction when the gratings were parallel (zero on abscissa) and also ($\pm$ 90 degrees [deg] on abscissa) when the gratings were orthogonal. From "Nonlinearity in Human Visual Responses to Two-Dimensional Patterns and a Limitation of Fourier Methods" by D. Regan and M. P. Regan, 1987, *Vision Research, 27,* p. 2182. Copyright 1987 by Elsevier Science. Reprinted with permission.

## TWO-SINEWAVE METHOD USED TO REVEAL
## AND TO LOCATE A MULTISENSORY CONVERGENCE
## AREA IN THE HUMAN BRAIN

A variant of the frequency-tagging method just described can be used to investigate and localize brain regions where information about two (or even three) sensory modalities converge. An illustration follows.

Subjects viewed a light flickering at $F_V$ Hz while listening to an auditory tone that was amplitude modulated at $F_A$ Hz. The auditory pathway of the brain could generate responses at harmonic frequencies of $F_A$ (i.e., $F_A$, $2F_A$, $3F_A$, etc.), and the visual pathway of the brain could generate response at harmonic frequencies of $F_V$ (i.e., $F_V$, $2F_V$, $3F_V$, etc.), but crossmodulation frequencies $[(F_A+F_V), (2F_A+2F_V), (3F_A-2F_V), $ etc.$]$ could be generated only after auditory and visual signals had converged. Cross-modality crossmodulation components were, therefore, a signature of audiovisual convergence areas of the brain (M. P. Regan, He, & Regan, 1995).

The magnetic field of the brain was analyzed in the frequency domain at 0.008 Hz resolution at recording sites that are marked + or − in Figs. 5.5A to 5.5C according to the phase of the response. The lines are isofield contour maps for the $2F_V$ (Fig. 5.5A), the $2F_A$ (Fig. 5.5B) and the $(2F_A + F_V)$ (Fig. 5.5C) components of the brain's magnetic field. Magnetic source location placed the intracranial source of the $(2F_A + F_V)$ field component approximately 2 cm inferior to the source of the $2F_A$ component, in fair agreement with the relative locations of the primary auditory cortex and an audiovisual convergence area in monkey brains (Tigges & Tigges, 1985).

## TWO-SINEWAVE METHOD USED TO TEST MODELS
## OF VISUAL AND AUDITORY PROCESSING

Response asymmetry (e.g., to light on vs. off), a frequently encountered property of neurons at both peripheral and central levels in sensory pathways, can be modeled as rectification. A series of neurons can be modeled as a series of rectifiers, and the rectifier arms can be of differing kinds (e.g., linear, compressive, accelerating, or mixed accelerating–compressive). A double Fourier series method has been described that allows the output of such a multistage model to be calculated when the input is a sum of sinewaves (M. P. Regan & Regan, 1988). If one of the inputs is held constant while the other's amplitude is varied, one can calculate a family

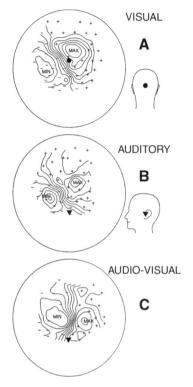

VISUAL

**A**

AUDITORY

**B**

AUDIO-VISUAL

**C**

FIG. 5.5. *Audiovisual convergence area in the human brain.* Isofield contour maps of magnetic response amplitude recorded from the human brain during simultaneous visual and auditory stimulation. Panel A: responses generated in the visual system. Panel B: responses generated in the auditory system. Panel C: responses generated in an audiovisual convergence area. The circle around the map is a best fit to the curvature of the skull over the region of the head from which recordings were made. Recording sites are marked + and – according to the phase of the response. The viewpoint was from the left side of the head in Panels B and C and from directly behind the head in Panel A. The inion is marked with a filled circle in Panel A. The left periauricular point is marked with a filled triangle in Panels B and C. max = maximum; min = minimum. From "An Audio-Visual Convergence Area in Human Brain" by M. P. Regan, P. He, & D. Regan, 1995, *Experimental Brain Research, 106*, p. 486. Copyright 1996 by Springer-Verlag. Reprinted with permission.

of curves: a curve for each harmonic and a curve for each $(nF_1 \pm mF_2)$ component. *The family of curves seems to be characteristic of the particular nonlinear model.*

Figure 5.6 illustrates this point for the case of three cascaded square-root rectifiers. This family of curves is changed very greatly when the number of cascaded rectifiers or the shape of their arms is varied.

By recording magnetic or electrical brain responses at ultrahigh resolution in the frequency domain, up to 30 response components may be recorded at high signal-to-noise levels, even up to the 10th order. (In principle, this technique gives an advantage to nonlinear analysis in the frequency domain as compared with the time–domain white noise [Wiener kernel] method [Marmarelis & Marmarelis, 1978], in that high-order terms allow sharper testing of models.)

For example, Fig. 5.7 shows the following three simultaneous recorded responses: (a) a $2F_1$-Hz response produced by stimulating one eye with $F_1$ Hz flicker, (b) a $2F_2$-Hz response produced by stimulating the other eye

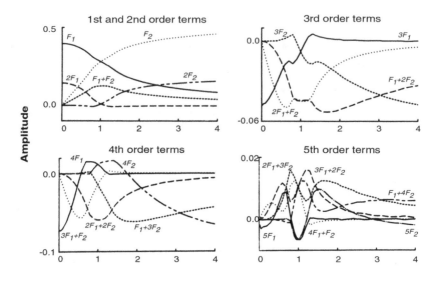

**Ratio of input amplitudes: k**

FIG. 5.6.    *Mathematical basis for testing multi-neuron nonlinear models.* Ordinates plot the amplitudes of frequency terms in the output of three cascaded square-root rectifiers whose input is the sum of two sinusoids, one of frequency $F_1$ and the other of frequency $F_2$. The amplitude ($A_1$) of the $F_1$ input is held constant while the amplitude ($A_2$) of the $F_2$ input is varied. Values of $k$ are plotted along the abscissa, where $k = A_2/A_1$. From "A Frequency Domain Technique for Characterizing Nonlinearities in Biological Systems" by M. P. Regan and D. Regan, 1988, *Journal of Theoretical Biology, 133*, p. 303. Copyright 1988 by Academic Press. Reprinted with permission.

with $F_2$-Hz flicker, and (c) a nonlinear response component generated by binocular neurons. This last response can be used to demonstrate the presence of binocular neurons even in patients with very low acuity in both eyes. Figure 5.8 shows how the theoretical approach described earlier can be used to test models of such binocular processing (e.g., to test whether a patient's binocular neurons function normally.) The data shown in Fig. 5.8 rejected many plausible models and were most compatible with two monocular linear rectifiers that fed a binocular compressive (square root) rectifier (M. P. Regan & Regan, 1989).

### TWO-SINEWAVE METHOD FOR AMPLITUDE-MODULATED AND FREQUENCY-MODULATED STIMULI

A mathematical method is available for calculating the output of a rectifier whose input is a single amplitude-modulated (AM) sinusoid or the

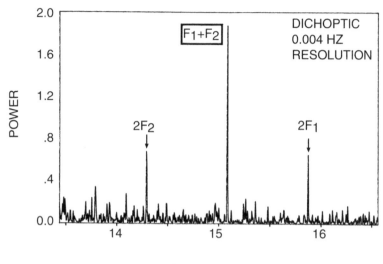

FIG. 5.7.    *Demonstration of binocular neurons.* One eye viewed homogeneous field flickering at of $F_1$ = 8Hz while the other eye viewed a similar homogeneous field flickering at $F_2$ = 7 Hz. The electroencephalogram spectrum was recorded at a resolution of 0.004 Hz by zoom-FFT. The ($F_1$ + $F_2$) component is due to a nonlinear interaction between signals from the left and right eyes, demonstrating the presence of binocular neurons. From "Objective Investigation of Visual Function Using a Nondestructive Zoom-FFT Technique for Evoked Potential Analysis" by M. P. Regan and D. Regan, 1989, *Canadian Journal of Neurological Science, 16*, pp. 168–179. Reprinted with permission.

sum of two AM sinusoids (M. P. Regan, 1994). Although this method has not yet been exploited in MEG or EEG studies of visual or somatosensory processing, an example of its use in the auditory modality is available (D. Regan & Regan, 1988b, M. P. Regan & Regan, 1993). The mathematical method was used to derive the output of the hair cell transducer function (a rectifier-like function) in the following cases: (a) the input is a single carrier whose amplitude is modulated by the sum of two sinusoids and (b) the input is the sum of two carriers, each of which is amplitude modulated by a single sinusoid. The theoretical results were similar to the results of an experiment in which EPs were recorded from the scalp while one ear was stimulated with either Waveform 1 or Waveform 2.

In particular, the rather complex behavior illustrated in Fig. 5.9 was predicted by the theory. This means that the "signature" imposed on neural signals by rectification at the first stage of auditory processing was clearly present in slow-wave signals generated at a much later stage of processing.

## EVOKED POTENTIAL DATA

### DICHOPTIC VIEW OF FLICKER

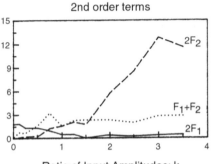
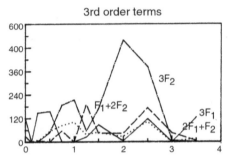

5.8.   Investigation of binocular neurons. Ordinates plot the powers of some of the frequency components in the evoked potential recorded while a subject viewed a homogeneous field flickering at 9 Hz with 20% modulation depth in the left eye while a second homogeneous field flickering at 7 Hz in the right eye was varied in modulation depth from 0% to 70%. From "Objective Investigation of Visual Function Using a Nondestructive Zoom-FFT Technique for Evoked Potential Analysis" by M .P. Regan and D. Regan, 1989, *Canadian Journal of Neurological Science, 16*. Reprinted with permission.

An interesting result of mathematical analysis of the effect of rectification on a frequency-modulated (FM) tone is as follows. It is well known that the power spectrum of a quasi-FM tone is exactly the same as the power spectrum of an AM tone, namely, a carrier plus two sidebands. The difference between quasi-FM and AM lies entirely in the phase spectrum. However, after rectification, the two signals differ in their power spectra (M. P. Regan, 1996). Furthermore, many frequency components are present that do not exist in the sound waveforms. This finding implies that studies on the processing of complex auditory waveforms such as speech might more profitably regard the stimulus as being the output of the hair cells rather than the auditory waveform that

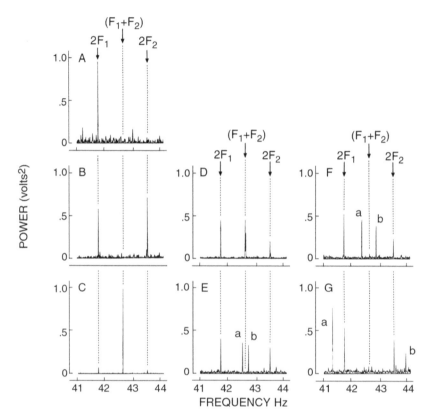

FIG. 5.9.   *The two-sinewave approach in audition: splitting of the ($F_1 + F_2$) Hz component.* The traces are short sections of ultrahigh-resolution response spectra recorded between the vertex and right earlobe. Three auditory waveforms were used: (a) S1, an $f_1$ Hz audio carrier amplitude modulated at $F_1$ Hz; (b) S2, an $f_1$ Hz carrier modulated at $F_2$ Hz; and (c) S3, an $f_2$ Hz carrier modulated at $F_2$ Hz. Panel A: S1 to left ear, Panel B: S1 to left ear and S2 to right, Panel C: S1 plus S2 to left ear. Panels D–G: S1 plus S3 to left ear. Panel E: $f_2 - f_1 = 0.01$ Hz, Panel E: $f_2 - f_1 = 0.1$ Hz, Panel F: $f_2 - f_1 = 0.25$ Hz, Panel G: $f_2 - f_1 = 1.3$ Hz. Ordinates are power with the dimensions of volts squared. Signals were analyzed over a DC–200-Hz bandwidth using zoom-FFT by a Bruel and Kjaer Model 2032 analyzer controlled by a digital computer giving 0.0078-Hz frequency resolution (approximately 25,000 real frequency bins). From "The Transducer Characteristic of Hair Cells in the Human Ear: A Possible Objective Measure" by D. Regan and M. P. Regan, 1988, *Brain Research, 438*, p. 364. Copyright 1988 by Elsevier Science. Reprinted with permission.

reaches the hair cells. These two waveforms are very different. At the time this is being written, however, the mathematical method has not yet been exploited in MEG studies.

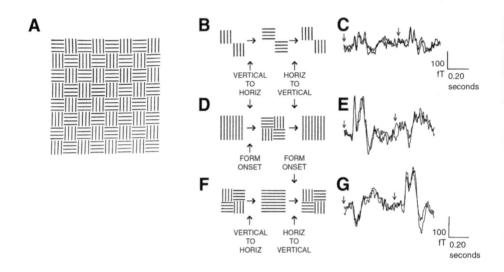

FIG. 5.10.    *Magnetic brain responses to texture-defined form.* Panel A: The stimulus was an 8 × 8 checkerboard pattern of checks. Panels B and C: Abrupt changes in the orientation of lines within alternate checks produced little magnetic response. Panels D–G: When the blank checks were filled with stationary vertical (D and E) or horizontal (horiz; F and G) lines, the abrupt changes of orientation produced strong magnetic responses that correlated with the onset and offset of spatial form rather than by the sense of line orientation change. After "Magnetic and Electrical Responses of the Human Brain to Texture-Defined Form and to Textons" by D. Regan and P. He, 1995, *Journal of Neurophysiology, 74,* pp. 1168–1171. Copyright 1995 by the American Physiological Society. Reprinted with permission.

## THE AVERAGED TRANSIENT EVOKED RESPONSE IN THE EXPLOITATION OF NONLINEARITY: AN EXAMPLE

Magnetic and electrical averaged evoked responses were recorded while observers viewed a pattern of 8 × 8 texture-defined checks that subtended 4° × 4° (see Fig. 5.10A). Each stimulus consisted of an abrupt change in the orientation of the lines within alternate checks, as depicted in Figs. 5.10B, 5.10D, and 5.10F (D. Regan & He, 1995).

At the recording location used to obtain the data shown in Fig. 5.10, the abrupt changes in line location produced little magnetic response (see Figs. 5.10B and 5.10C). In Fig. 5.10D, the blank checks were filled with stationary vertical lines. (These stationary lines would not, of course, evoke any averaged magnetic response.) However, the abrupt changes in line orientation that produced little response in Fig. 5.10C now gave a clear magnetic response (see Fig. 5.10E). Furthermore, the response to an abrupt vertical to horizontal change of orientation was quite different from the response to an abrupt horizontal to vertical change of orientation. In Fig. 5.10F the blank checks of Fig. 5.10B were filled with stationary horizontal (rather than vertical) lines. Figure 5.10G shows that an abrupt vertical to horizontal change of orientation now evoked a response similar to that evoked by an abrupt horizontal to vertical change of orientation in Fig. 5.10E, and vice versa.

The magnetic responses shown in Figs. 5.10E and 5.10G are clearly not the sum of responses to the time-varying checks (Figs. 5.10B and 5.10C) and to the stationary checks. Therefore they violate the superimposition requirement for linearity.

Although, as already stated, the two response waveforms in Figs. 5.10E and 5.10G are dissociated from the sense of line orientation change, they correlate with the appearance/disappearance of a texture-defined checkerboard pattern. In particular, the onset of form produced a double-peaked response, whereas form offset produced a single peak that was directed oppositely to the double peak.

## ACKNOWLEDGMENTS

We thank Derek Harnanansingh for assistance in the preparation of this chapter. D. Regan holds the National Science and Engineering Research Council/Canadian Aviation Electronics (NSERC/CAE) Industrial Research Chair in Vision and Aviation at York University. Work for this chapter was sponsored by the U.S. Air Force Office of Science Research, Air Force Material Command, under Grant F40620-00-1-0053. The U.S. Government is authorized to reproduce and distribute reprints of this chapter for governmental purposes notwithstanding any copyright violation thereon. The views and conclusions contained herein are ours and should not be interpreted as necessarily representing the official policies or endorsements, either expressed or implied, of the U.S. Air Force Office of Scientific Research or the U.S. government.

## REFERENCES

Aseltine, J. A. (1958). *Transform methods in linear systems analysis*. New York: McGraw-Hill.

Blaquière, A. (1966). *Nonlinear Systems Analysis*. New York: Academic Press.

Bracewell, R. (1965). *The Fourier transform and its application*. New York: McGraw-Hill.

Cartwright, R. F., & Regan, D. (1974). Semi-automatic multi-channel Fourier analyzer for evoked potential analysis. *Electroencephalography and Clinical Neurophysiology, 36*, 547–550.

Gabor, D. (1946). Theory of communication. *Journal of the Institute of Electric Engineers (London), 93*, 429–456.

Hagedorn, P. (1982). *Nonlinear oscillations*. Oxford, England: Oxford University Press

Hayashi, C. (1964). *Nonlinear oscillations in physical systems*. New York: McGraw-Hill.

Hirsch, M., & Smale, S. (1974). *Differential equations, dynamical systems and linear algebra*. New York: Academic.

Jenkins, G. M., & Watts, D. G. (1968). *Spectral analysis*. Oakland, CA: Holden-Day.

Marmarelis, P. A., & Marmarelis, V. Z. (1978). *Analysis of physiological systems: The white noise approach*. New York: Plenum.

Nelson, J. I., Seiple, W. H., Kupersmith, M. J., & Carr, R. E. (1984). A rapid evoked potential index of cortical adaptation. *Investigative Ophthalmology and Visual Science, 59*, 454–464.

Regan, D. (1964). *A study of the visual system by the correlation of light stimuli and evoked electrical responses*. Unpublished PhD thesis, Imperial College, London.

Regan, D. (1966). Some characteristics of average steady-state and transient responses evoked by modulated light. *Electroencephalography and Clinical Neurophysiology, 20*, 238–248.

Regan, D. (1968a). Chromatic adaptation and steady-state evoked potentials. *Vision Research, 8*, 149–158.

Regan, D. (1968b). A high frequency mechanism which underlies visual evoked potentials. *Electroencephalography and Clinical Neurophysiology, 25*, 231–237.

Regan, D. (1970a). Evoked potentials and psychophysical correlates of changes in stimulus colour and intensity. *Vision Research, 10*, 163–178.

Regan, D. (1970b). Objective method of measuring the relative spectral luminosity curve in man. *Journal of the Optical Society of America, 60*, 859–859.

Regan, D. (1973). Rapid objective refraction using evoked brain potentials. *Investigative Ophthalmology, 12*, 669–679.

Regan, D. (1974). Electrophysiological evidence for colour channels in human pattern vision. *Nature, 250*, 437–449.

Regan, D. (1975a). Colour coding of pattern responses in man investigated by evoked potential feedback and direct plot techniques. *Vision Research, 15*, 175–183.

Regan, D. (1975b). Review: Recent advances in electrical recording from the human brain. *Nature, 250*, 437–449.

Regan, D. (1976). Latencies of evoked potentials to flicker and to pattern speedily estimated by simultaneous stimulation method. *Electroencephalography and Clinical Neurophysiology, 40*, 654–600.

Regan, D. (1979). Electrical responses evoked from the human brain. *Scientific American, 241*, 134–146.

Regan, D. (1983). Spatial frequency mechanisms in human vision investigated by evoked potential recording. *Vision Research, 23*, 1401–1408.

Regan, D. (1989). *Human brain electrophysiology*. New York: Elsevier.

Regan, D., & Cartwright, R. F. (1970). A method of measuring the potentials evoked by simultaneous stimulation of different retinal regions. *Electroencephalography and Clinical Neurophysiology, 28*, 314–319.

Regan, D., & He, P. (1995). Magnetic and electrical responses of the human brain to texture-defined form and to textons. *Journal of Neurophysiology, 74*, 1167–1178.

Regan, D., & Heron, J. R. (1969). Clinical investigation of lesions of the visual pathway: A new objective technique. *Journal of Neurology, Neurosurgery and Psychiatry, 32*, 479–483.

Regan, D., & Heron, J. R. (1970). Simultaneous recording of visual evoked potentials from the left and right hemispheres in migraine. In A. L. Cochrane (Ed.), *Background to migraine*. (pp. 66–77. London: Heinemann.

Regan, D., & Lee, B. B. (1993). A comparison of the human 40Hz response with the properties of macaque ganglion cells. *Visual Neuroscience, 10*, 439–445.

Regan, D., Murray, T. K., & Silver, R. (1977). Effect of body temperature on visual evoked potential delay and visual perception in multiple sclerosis. *Journal of Neurology, Neurosurgery and Psychiatry, 40*, 1083–1091.

Regan, D., & Regan, M. P. (1987). Nonlinearity in human visual responses to two-dimensional patterns and a limitation of Fourier methods. *Vision Research, 27,* 2181–2183.

Regan, D., & Regan, M. P. (1988a). Objective evidence for phase-independent spatial frequency mechanisms in the human visual pathway. *Vision Research, 28,* 187–191.

Regan, D., & Regan, M. P. (1988b). The transducer characteristic of hair cells in the human ear: A possible objective measure. *Brain Research, 438,* 363–365.

Regan, D., Schellart, N. A. M., Spekreijse, H., & van den Berg, T. J. T. P. (1975). Photometry in goldfish by electrophysiological recording: Comparison of criterion response method with heterochromatic flicker photometry. *Vision Research, 15,* 799–807.

Regan, M. P. (1994). Linear half-wave rectification of modulated sinusoids. *Applied Mathematics and Computation, 62,* 61–79.

Regan, M. P. (1996). Half-wave linear rectification of a frequency modulated sinusoid. *Applied Mathematics and Computation, 79,* 137–162.

Regan, M. P., He, P., & Regan, D. (1995). An audio-visual convergence area in human brain. *Experimental Brain Research, 106,* 485–487.

Regan, M. P., & Regan, D. (1988). A frequency domain technique for characterizing nonlinearities in biological systems. *Journal of Theoretical Biology, 133,* 293–317.

Regan, M. P., & Regan, D. (1989). Objective investigation of visual function using a nondestructive zoom–FFT technique for evoked potential analysis. *Canadian Journal of Neurological Science, 16,* 168–179.

Regan, M. P., & Regan, D. (1993). Nonlinear terms produced by passing amplitude-modulated sinusoids through a hair cell transducer function. *Biological Cybernetics, 69,* 439–446.

Reichardt, W., & Poggio, T. (1981). (Eds.). *Theoretical approaches in neurobiology.* Cambridge, MA: MIT Press.

Spekreijse, H. (1966). *Analysis of EEG responses in man.* The Hague, The Netherlands: Dr. Junk.

Spekreijse, H., & Oosting, H. (1970). Linearizing, a method for analyzing and synthesizing nonlinear systems. *Kybernetik, 7,* 23–31.

Spekreijse, H., & Reits, D. (1982). Sequential analysis of the visual system in man: Nonlinear analysis of a sandwich system. *Annals of the New York Academy of Sciences, 388,* 72–97.

Spekreijse, H., & van der Tweel, L. H. (1965). Linearization of evoked responses to sine wave modulated light by noise. *Nature, 205,* 913.

Stoker, J. J. (1950). *Nonlinear vibrations.* New York: Wiley Interscience.

Tigges, J., & Tigges, M. (1985). Subcortical sources of direct projections to visual cortex. In H. Peters & E. G. Jones (Eds.), *Cerebral cortex* (Vol. 3, pp. 351–378). New York: Plenum.

Tonini, G., Srinivasan, R., Russell, D. P., & Edelman, G. M. (1998). Investigating neural correlates of conscious perception by frequency-tagged neuromagnetic responses. *Proceedings of the National Academy of Sciences of the USA, 95,* 3198–3203.

van der Tweel, L. H. (1961). Some problems in vision regarded with respect to linearity and frequency response. *Annals of the New York Academy of Sciences, 89,* 829–856.

van der Tweel, L. H., & Spekreijse, H. (1969). Signal transport and rectification in the human evoked response system. *Annals of the New York Academy of Sciences, 156,* 678–695.

van der Tweel, L. H., & Verduyn Lunel, H. F. E. (1965). Human visual responses to sinusoidally modulated light. *Electroencephalography and Clinical Neurophysiology, 18,* 587–598.

# 6

## Independent Components of Magnetoencephalography: Localization and Single-Trial Response Onset Detection

Akaysha C. Tang
Barak A. Pearlmutter
*University of New Mexico*

Independent component analysis (ICA) is a class of decomposition methods that separate sources from mixtures of signals. In this chapter, we used second order blind identification (SOBI), one of the ICA methods, to demonstrate its advantages in identifying magnetic signals associated with neural information processing. Using 122-channel magnetoencephalography data collected during both simple sensory activation and complex cognitive tasks, we explored SOBI's ability to help isolate and localize underlying neuronal sources, particularly under relatively poor signal-to-noise conditions. For these identified and localized neuronal sources, we used a simple threshold-crossing method, with which single-trial response onset times could be measured with a detection rate as high as 96%. These results demonstrated that, with the aid of ICA, it is possible to noninvasively measure human single-trial response onset times with millisecond resolution for specific neuronal populations from multiple sensory modalities. This capability makes it possible to study a wide range of perceptual and memory functions that critically depend on the timing of discrete neuronal events.

The goal of this chapter is to introduce the basic concept of independent component analysis (ICA), a class of algorithms that decompose a multidimensional time series into a set of components, each with a one-dimensional time course and a fixed spatial distribution. For magnetoencephalography (MEG) as well as electroencephalography (EEG), the multidimensional time series corresponds to the multichannel MEG or EEG recordings, the component time series to simultaneously separated and temporally overlapping signals from various neuronal populations, and the spatial distributions to the set of attenuations from the neuronal sources to the sensors. Whereas the component time series provides temporal information about the evoked neuronal responses and ongoing activity, the sensor projection vectors give information about the spatial locations of the neuronal sources.

We use one particular ICA algorithm, second-order blind identification (SOBI; Belouchrani, Meraim, Cardoso, & Moulines, 1993; Cardoso, 1994), as an example to illustrate the procedures for separating the mixture of noise and neuromagnetic signals into neurophysiological and neuroanaotmically meaningful components, for localizing their corresponding source generators, and for measuring single-trial response onset times from the localized neuronal populations. Systematic comparisons between SOBI and alternative ICA algorithms (e.g., InfoMax [Bell & Sejnowski, 1995] and Fast ICA [fICA; Hyvriänen & Oja, 1997]) using the same data set, remain to be conducted.

The chapter is organized into six parts.

- In Part 1 we define the ICA problem and offer the reader considerations in selecting a specific ICA algorithm. Second-order blind identification (SOBI) will be introduced as our algorithm of choice for separation of MEG data. The relation between ICA and other decomposition and source localization methods is briefly discussed.
- In Part 2 we discuss the task conditions under which ICA is most likely to be beneficial, specifically, low signal-to-noise ratio (S/N) conditions resulting from large trial-to-trial variability and small number of trials in behavioral tasks. The behavioral tasks used in this chapter are described.
- In Part 3 we describe the process of SOBI application to neuromagnetic signals. SOBI components are characterized in both time and space using *MEG images* and *field maps,* respectively. We identify a variety of common neuronal and nonneuronal SOBI components using both temporal and spatial information as constraints.

- In Part 4 we describe the process of finding equivalent current dipole models for SOBI neuronal components. The time invariance of a SOBI component's field map and the resulting reduction in the subjectivity of localization process are discussed. Cross-task and cross-subject reliability will be examined. Systematic comparisons between source localizations with and without the aid of SOBI will be made.
- In Part 5 we describe the process of detecting single-trial response onset times in SOBI-separated neuronal components. An iterative threshold-crossing method is used to measure single-trial response onset times. We provide examples of onset time detection for three major sensory modalities. Cross-subject reliability is demonstrated for each of three major sensory modalities.
- In Part 6 we summarize the capabilities and advantages that SOBI offers to the analysis of MEG data, and we discuss assumptions and future directions.

We assume that readers have a basic knowledge of MEG and the standard analysis tools offered by commercially available Neuromag software. We avoid comprehensive reviews on ICA algorithms because of space limitation. For reviews of ICA see Amari and Cichocki (1998); Cardoso (1998); Hyvärinen (1999); Vigário, Särelä, Jousmäki, Hämäläinen, and Oja (2000) and Stone (2002).

## INTRODUCTION

### ICA: Definition

Let x($t$) be an $n$-dimensional vector of sensor signals, which we assume to be an instantaneous linear mixture of $n$ unknown independent underlying components $s_i(t)$, *via* the unknown $n \times n$ mixing matrix **A**,

$$\mathbf{x}(t) = \mathbf{A} \, \mathbf{s}(t) \tag{6.1}$$

The ICA problem is to recover **s**($t$), given the measurement **x**($t$) and nothing else. This is accomplished by finding a matrix **W** that approximates $\mathbf{A}^{-1}$.

For MEG, $x_i(t)$ corresponds to either continuous or averaged sensor readings from a magnotometer or gradiometer, and $s_i(t)$ corresponds to a recovered neuronal or noise source; $n$ is the number of sensors available. ICA decomposes the mixed-sensor signals **x**($t$) into $n$ components.

The output of the algorithm is an $n \times n$ matrix, $\mathbf{W}$, which maps from the vector of sensor values $\mathbf{x}(t)$ to the vector of recovered component values $\hat{s}(t) = \mathbf{W}\,\mathbf{x}(t)$ (Fig. 6.1), up to a scaling and permutation of the components.

The types of true sources that affect MEG sensor readings are summarized on the lefthand side of Fig. 6.1. When ICA does a good job, the recovered components $(t)$ correspond to the true sources.

### ICA Components in Time

The recovered components $\hat{s}_i(t)$ can be displayed as a plot of signal strength as a function of time or in an *MEG image* (e.g., Fig. 6.4 righthand side), a pseudocolored bitmap in which the responses of a given component during an entire experiment can be parsimoniously displayed. Typically, each row represents one discrete trial of stimulation, and multiple trials are ordered vertically from top to bottom. MEG images can be very informative in providing not only averaged but trial-to-trial temporal information about the source activation, such as the single-trial re-

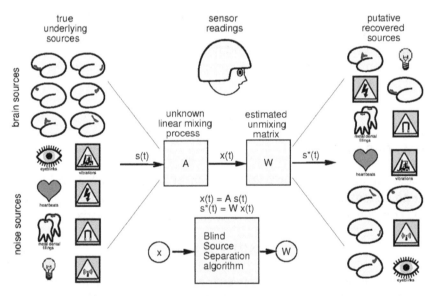

FIG. 6.1.    The independent-components analysis (ICA) process. Signals from the brain and other noise sources $\mathbf{s}(t)$ are mixed through an unknown linear mixing process $\mathbf{A}$, resulting in the sensor readings $\mathbf{x}(t) = \mathbf{A}\,\mathbf{s}(t)$. ICA finds an unmixing matrix $\mathbf{W}$ that maps from the sensor signals to recovered components $\hat{s}(t) = \mathbf{W}\,\mathbf{x}(t)$. The entries of the attenuation matrix $\mathbf{A} = \mathbf{W}^{-1}$ describe how strongly each sensor responds to each component. From "Independent components of magnetoencephalography: Single-trial onset times," by A. C. Tang et al., 2002b, *NeuroImage, 17*(4). Copyright © 2002 by Elsevier. Reprinted with permission.

sponse-onset times of a given separated component. For examples of MEG images of noise sources see Fig. 6.4 and for examples of neuronal sources, see Figs. 6.12b, 6.13c,d, and 6.14b.

### ICA Components in Space

Although ICA does not assume any physical model of the neuronal source generators, spatial information concerning a separated component is given by the *field map* of the component, which represents the measured *sensor* response to the activation of the component $\hat{s}_i(t)$. In other words, the field map of a neuronal component gives the sensor readings when the corresponding neuronal *source* alone is activated. Examples of field maps for a visual, somatosensory, and auditory components are shown in Fig. 6.5b. The field map of the $i$th component $\hat{s}_i(t)$ is the $i$th column of the estimated attenuation matrix $\hat{\mathbf{A}}$, where $\hat{\mathbf{A}} = \mathbf{W}^{-1}$. In combination with structural magnetic resonance image (MRI), the field maps can be used as input to any localization tools for localizing the separated components within the brain. For example, after calculating its sensor projection, we can repackage a component for localization by Neuromag dipole modeling tools.

### Selection of ICA Algorithms

ICA algorithms (for review, see Amari & Cichocki [1998], Cardoso [1998], Hyäarinen, [1999], and Vigário et al. [2000]) fall between two extremes: instantaneous and summary algorithms, which differ in whether each point in time is considered in isolation. Instantaneous algorithms (such as Bell-Sejnowski Infomax and fICA) make repeated passes through the dataset to update the unmixing matrix in response to the data at each time-point. Signals are assumed to have no temporal correlation, and the results are meant to be invariant to shuffling of the data. In contrast, summary algorithms, such as SOBI (Belouchrani et al., 1993; Cardoso, 1994), first make a pass through the data whereas summary statistics are accumulated by averaging; they then operate solely on the summary statistics to find the separation matrix.

In selection of ICA algorithms for MEG applications, one important consideration is the robustness of the algorithm to noise. In general, summary algorithms are more likely to be less sensitive to noise because their summary statistics are averages over time. The relatively poor signal-to-noise ratio in MEG data suggests the choice of a summary algorithm, such as SOBI, over an instantaneous algorithm. When it can be assumed that each source has a broad autocorrelation function, as is the case with brain signals, SOBI can give high quality separation while imposing rather modest computational requirements.

SOBI extracts a large set of statistics from the dataset, which it uses for the separation. Each of these statistics is calculated by averaging across the dataset, which makes the algorithm robust against noise. The particular statistics calculated are the correlations between pairs of sensors at a fixed delay, $\tau \langle (x_i(t) x_i(t + \tau) \rangle$. This makes good use of abundant but noisy data, and most important, SOBI can be tuned by modifying its set of delays, allowing its users to gently integrate a very weak form of prior knowledge.

## Second Order Blind Identification (SOBI)

SOBI is considered blind because it makes no assumptions about the form of the mixing process. In other words, *SOBI does not attempt to solve the inverse problem* or use the physics of the situation in any way. It does not try to estimate currents or to know about Maxwell's equation or any of its consequences. The only physical assumption made about the mixing process is that it is instantaneous and linear.

As stated before, the ICA problem is to recover $s(t)$, given the measurement $x(t)$ and nothing else. This is accomplished by finding a matrix $W$ that approximates $A^{-1}$, up to permutation and scaling of its rows. SOBI assumes that the components are statistically independent in time and not necessarily orthogonal in space. It finds $W$ by minimizing the total correlations between one component at time $t$ and another at time $t + \tau$, computed with a set of time delays $(\tau s)$.[1]

The particular set of delays $\tau$ can be chosen to cover a reasonably wide interval without extending beyond the support of the auto-correlation function. Measured in units of samples at a 300-Hz sampling rate, a reasonable set of delays is:

$$\tau \in \{1, 2, 3, 4, 5, 6, 7, 8, 9,$$
$$10, 12, 14, 16, 18,$$
$$20, 25, 30, 35, 40, 45, 50, 55,$$
$$60, 65, 70, 75, 80, 85, 90, 95, 100\}.$$

---

[1]For justification for this minimization, see pp. 196–197.

It is important to point out that the choice of delays can affect the results of separation. Depending on the types of sources activated by the behavioral task, the selection of delays can have complex interactions with the latency of evoked responses. Prior knowledge about the sources can be incorporated by setting these parameters.

## ICA Versus Other Decomposition Methods

Both PCA (principal-components analysis (PCA; Hotelling, 1933) and ICA (Comon, 1994) can be thought of as decomposing the matrix whose rows are the sensor values at various points in time into a sum of rank-one matrices. Each of these rank-one matrices is an outer product of two vectors: one representing a time course, the other a set of spatial attenuations. The question is: What is the best decomposition? PCA assumes that the data are Gaussian and requires the vectors that form the outer products to be *orthogonal*, whereas ICA models the data as generated by *statistically independent* but *non-Gaussian* processes.

Jung et al. (1999) applied both PCA and ICA to electroencephalogram (EEG) data and assessed their ability to segregate various known sources of noise. They found that ICA was superior in this regard. Vigário, Särelä, Jousmäki, and Oja (1999) applied both methods to MEG data and found that the auditory and somatosensory ICA components were physiologically more reasonable than the PCA components. These results are not surprising, given the poor match between PCA's assumptions (Gaussian, orthogonal) and the actual processes generating the data (highly non-Gaussian, highly correlated spatial attenuations).

## ICA and Other Source Modeling Methods

Beside ICA, a variety of algorithms have been developed (Aine, Huang, Stephen, & Christner, 2000; Ermer, Mosher, Huang, & Leahy, 2000; Gavit et al., 2001; Huang et al., 2000; Ioannides et al., 1995; Kinouchi et al., 1996; Mosher & Leahy, 1998, 1999; Mosher, Lewis, & Leahy, 1992; Nagano et al., 1998; Schmidt, George, & Wood, 1999; Schwartz, Badier, Bihoue, & Bouliou, 1999; Sekihara et al., 2000; Sekihara, Peoppel, Marantz, Koizumi, & Miyashita, 1997; Uutela, Hämäläinen, & Salmelin, 1998) to localize neuronal sources or to simultaneously localize and recover the time course of these neuronal sources from a mixture of source signals recorded at multiple sensors. Because ICA can generate sensor projections of functionally independent components, ICA can be viewed not as an alternative to an existing source modeling method but as a preprocessing tool that generates "cleaner" sensor readings from functionally unique neuronal populations. Given their ability to separate the noise from neuronal signals, ICA algorithms are expected to benefit all source-localization methods by providing them with input signals that are more likely to be associated with functionally independent neuronal sources.

## ICA and MEG

Since the initial application of ICA to EEG (Makeig, Bell, Jung, & Sejnowski, 1996) ICA algorithms, such as SOBI (Belouchrani et al., 1993; Cardoso, 1994), Infomax (Bell & Sejnowsk, 1995), and fast independent component analysis (fICA; Hyvärinen & Oja, 1997), have been applied to EEG data (Jung, Humphries, et al., 2000; Makeig, Jung, Bell, Ghahremani, & Sejnowski, 1997; Makeig et al., 1999) and MEG data (Cao et al., 2000; Tang et al., 2002ab; Tang, Pearlmutter, Zibulevsky, 2000a; Tang, Pearlmutter, Zibulevsky, Hely, & Weisand, 2000b; Vigário, Jousmäki, Hämäläinen, Hari, & Oja, 1998; Vigário et al., 2000; Vigário, Särelä, Jousmäki, & Oja, 1999; Wübbeler et al., 2000; Ziehe, Müller, Nolte, Mackert, & Curio, 2000). In both applications, ICA methods have been proven useful for artifact removal (Jung, Humphries, et al., 2000; Jung, Makeig, et al., 2000; Tang, Pearlmutter, Zibulevsky, 2000a; Vigário et al., 1998; Ziehe et al., 2000). Neurophysiologically meaningful components have been separated (Makeig et al., 1997, 1999; Vigário et al., 1999; Tang et al., 2000abc, 2002ab; Wübbeler et al., 2000). For MEG, these neurophysiologically meaningful ICA components have been further localized using equivalent current dipole models (Tang et al., 2002a; Tang, Phung, Pearlmutter, & Christner, 2000; Vigário et al., 1999). Most recently, single-trial response onset times have been estimated with a success rate of over 90% from these functional components (Tang et al., 2002b).

## WHEN TO USE ICA?

Typical magnetic signals associated with neuronal activity are on the order of 100 fT, whereas the noise signals within a shielded room tend to be much larger (Lewine & Orrison, 1995). Furthermore, the intrinsic sensor noise is comparable in magnitude to some small neuronal signals. Therefore, what the sensors record during an experiment is always a mixture of small neuromagnetic and large noise signals. This poor signal-to-noise ratio[2] can affect the estimation of temporal profile and localization of neuronal activity.

Because one strength of ICA is its ability to separate various noise sources from the signals of interest, ICA is most likely to be useful when the experimental conditions necessitate relatively poor $S/N$. For example, the somatosensory responses associated with thumb mouse-button presses without any constrains on the resting position of the hand and on how the hands hold the mouse would have a relatively poor $S/N$, whereas somatosensory responses associated with well-controlled median nerve stimulation would have a much higher $S/N$. If more or few trials of stimulation are conducted, the $S/N$ in the average responses can be higher or lower accordingly. ICA is expected to be particularly useful when a small number of trial data are collected; when the behavioral tasks involve large variability in stimulus presentation or in the behavioral-responses required; when neuronal sources of interests lie beyond the early sensory processing areas; and when the tasks are highly cognitive in contrast to sensory activation tasks. Therefore, ICA may support experimental designs that more closely approximate perceptual, motor, and cognitive processing taking place in the real world.

Because the details of the behavioral tasks are critical in assessing the utility of ICA, we briefly describe the tasks used in generating the data for the following ICA application. We collected MEG data from 4 subjects during four visual reaction time tasks, originally designed for studying temporal lobe memory. In each task, a pair of colored patterns was presented on the left and right halves of the display screen. The subject was instructed to press either the left or right button when the target appeared on the left or right side of the screen, respectively. In all tasks, the target was not described to the subject prior to the experiment. The subject was to discover the target by trial and error using auditory feedback (low and high tones that corresponded to correct and incorrect responses, respectively). All subjects were able to discover the rule within a few trials.

The tasks differed in the memory load required for determining which of the pair is the target. Task 1 served to familiarize the subjects with all visual patterns. The subjects simply viewed the stimuli and were asked to press either the left or right button at their own choice while making

---

[2]Unless otherwise indicated, we use the term *signal-to-noise ratio* in the sense defined in signal detection theory. *Signals* refer to the neuromagnetic signal of interest; noise refers to all other signals, including environmental and sensor noise and other background brain signals.

sure approximately equal numbers of left and right button presses were performed. As such, Task 1 placed little memory demand on the subject. Task 2 involved remembering a single target pattern that appeared on each trial paired with other patterns. Subjects were to press the corresponding button to indicate the side of the screen on which the target pattern was displayed. Task 3 involved remembering multiple targets, each always paired with the same nontargets. Task 4, in which whether a pattern was a target was context sensitive, as in the game of rock–paper–scissors, was the most complex. The amount of cognitive processing beyond the initial sensory processing increased from Task 1 to Task 4.

We used data from these complex cognitive tasks to evaluate the capability of SOBI because of the relatively poor signal-to-noise ratios involved in comparison to simple sensory activation tasks. Specifically, these tasks involved (a) large visual field stimulation without the use of fixation points, (b) incidental somatosensory stimulation as a result of button presses during reaction time tasks, and (c) highly variable button press responses because precisely what form of the thumb movement should be made, how the mouse was held, and where the hands rest were not specified. These sources of variability in visual and somatosensory activation can lead to poor signal-to-noise ratios in the average responses, making it particularly difficult to localize the neuronal sources from unprocessed averaged sensor data. In addition, the involvement of higher level cognitive functions, memory demand, and the small number of trials collected under each task condition—90 trials in most cases—could further decrease the signal-to-noise ratio in the average sensor data. As such, these tasks offer challenging cases in which the unique advantages of ICA methods may be revealed.

To include data from high signal-to-noise experimental conditions, data from a separate *auditory sensory activation task* (binaural 500-Hz tone, of 200-ms duration, $3.25 \pm 0.125$ msec stimulus onset asynchrony, 150 trials) will also be used. Together, these tasks offer data collected under both poor and good signal-to-noise conditions (cognitive tasks: poor; sensory activation task: good) and data involving activation of neuronal sources from three major sensory modalities.

## IDENTIFICATION OF SOBI NEURONAL COMPONENTS

Using SOBI, continuous MEG signals from 122 channels were separated into 122 components. Each of the components has a time course, which can be averaged across multiple trials using either the visual stimulus onset or the button press as a trigger. As shown in the overlay plots of the visual stimulus and button press triggered averages for *all* 122 SOBI components (Fig. 6.2c and d), only a subset of the components showed task-related responses, shown separately in Fig. 6.2a and b.

The SOBI components can be displayed in the sensor domain by using the Neuromag software xfit (fullview). The sensor projections for two SOBI components are shown: one for a visual component (Fig. 6.3a) and the other for a right sensory–motor component Fig. 6.3c. It is clear that the two SOBI components are projected selectively to sensors over the visual and right sensory–motor cortices. In contrast, the full-view plots of the sensor projections from the corresponding raw data (mixture of all components) have much wider distributions of sensor activation (Fig. 6.3b and d).

In the following example, 122 SOBI components were separated from continuous 122-channel, unaveraged, unepoched data collected during cognitive and simple sensory-activation tasks (300-Hz and 600-Hz sampling rates respectively, and band-pass filtered at 0.03–100 Hz).

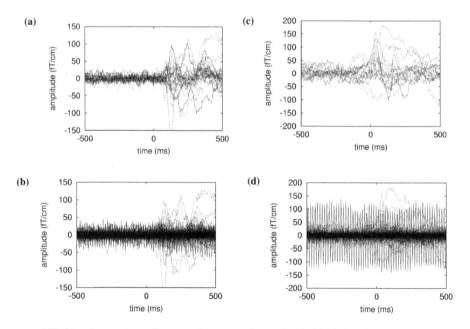

FIG. 6.2. Event-triggered averages for groups of second-order blind identification (SOBI) components ($N$ = 90 trials). Panel a: components showing visual-stimulus-triggered responses, triggered on visual stimulus onset. Panel b: components showing button-press-triggered responses triggered on button presses. Panel c: all components, triggered on visual-stimulus onset. Panel d: all components, triggered on button presses. From "Independent components of magnetoencephalography: Localization," by A. C. Tang et al., 2002a, *Neural Computation, 14*(8). Copyright © 2002 by MIT Press. Reprinted with permission.

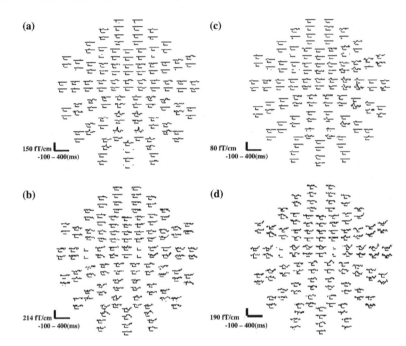

FIG. 6.3.   Sensor projections of second-order blind interaction (SOBI) components and the mixed raw magnetoencephalography (MEG) data. $N = 90$ trials, Panels a and c: visual-stimulus-triggered; Panels b and d: button-press-triggered averages. Panel a: SOBI component showing selective sensor activation over the occipito-parietal cortex. Panel c: A SOBI component showing selective activation over the right fronto–parietal cortex. Panel b: all components (unseparated data), triggered on visual stimulation. Panel d: all components (unseparated data), triggered on button presses. Aberrant sensors are shaded. From "Independent components of magnetoencephalography: Localization," by A. C. Tang et al., 2002a, *Neural Computation, 14*(8). Copyright © 2002 by MIT Press. Reprinted with permission.

## SOBI Nonneuronal Components

As illustrated in Fig. 6.1, MEG records magnetic signals associated with both noise and neuronal signals. These nonneuronal noise sources include ambient noises, such as 60 Hz or slow DC drift, ocular artifact-related signals, signals associated with large amplitude quantum state changes, and other unknown noise sources. Ocular artifacts were identified by the component's characteristic activation patterns in the field map and large-amplitude responses in the MEG image (Fig. 6.4a), which match responses in separately recorded electrooculographic data (not shown). In these particular experimenters, a motor response typically triggered an eyeblink response. The 60-Hz source was identified by the component's clearly visible cyclic activity in the MEG images in Fig. 6.4b (right). Components corresponding to large amplitude sensor noise were easily identified by the single-sensor activation in the field maps and sometimes by high-contrast lines or dots in the MEG images (Fig. 6.4c). DC drift can be identified in the MEG image by a change of color from one block of trials to another, and sources associated with such drift tend to have a broad activation pattern in the scalp projection (data are not shown, but see Tang, Pearlmutter, & Zibulevsky (2000a).

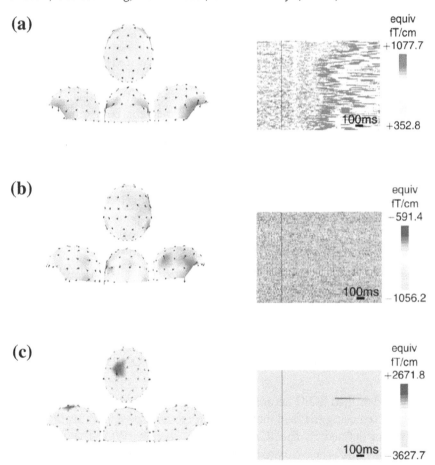

FIG. 6.4.   Field maps and unfiltered magnetoencephalography (MEG) images for **(a)** an ocular artifact component, **(b)** a 60-Hz component, and **(c)** a sensor noise component. equiv = equivalent. Left: field maps or sensor projections of SOBI components. Right: time course of SOBI components shown in MEG images. From "Independent components of magnetoencephalography: Localization," by A. C. Tang et al., 2002a, *Neural Computation, 14*(8). Copyright © 2002 by MIT Press. Reprinted with permission. See Color Panel A.

## SOBI Neuronal Components

Before one can localize a neuronal source or estimate its single-trial response onset times, neuronal sources must first be identified among all $n$ separated components ($n$ = number of sensors). The first step in identification is to compute various event-triggered averages for each of the $n$ components, (e.g., visual, auditory, or somatosensory stimulus-locked, or motor-response-locked averages). If a component unambiguously shows an event-triggered response in the average, it becomes a candidate for being a neuronal source.

To identify neuronal sources that are directly task-related, both temporal and spatial constraints are used. For a task related component, if its field map and time course were consistent with known neurophysiological and neuroanatomical facts, we considered it a neuronal component reflecting the activity of a neuronal generator. For example, if the field map of a component shows activation over the occipital cortex, and the visual stimulus triggered average for this component contains an evoked response that peaks between 50 msec and 100 msec, then it is considered to reflect the activity of a visual source in the occipital lobe.

Figure 6.5a shows the stimulus or response triggered averages for the evoked visual, somatosensory, and auditory responses in three SOBI components. The field maps of these SOBI components (Fig. 6.5b) have activations over the occipital–parietal, parietal, and temporal lobes that correspond to the expected visual, somatosensory, and auditory activation. For more details on the interpretation of these components in relation to the cognitive tasks, see Tang et al. (2002a). For identification of SOBI components within the same modality see Tang et al. (2000a).

## LOCALIZATION OF SOBI COMPONENTS

For the identified SOBI neuronal components, equivalent current dipoles can be fitted using the field maps as inputs to any source-localization algorithm. As defined in the ICA Definition section, $\mathbf{W}$ is the estimated unmixing matrix, the estimated time courses for the sources are $\hat{s}(t) = \mathbf{W}\mathbf{x}(t)$, and the corresponding estimated mixing matrix is $\hat{\mathbf{A}} = \mathbf{W}^{-1}$. Using these, the sensor signals resulting from just one of the components can be computed as $\hat{\mathbf{x}}(t) = \hat{\mathbf{A}}\mathbf{D}\mathbf{W}\mathbf{x}(t) = \hat{\mathbf{A}}\mathbf{D}\hat{s}(t)$, where $\mathbf{D}$ is a matrix of zeros except for those on the diagonal entries corresponding to each component that is to be retained. To localize a single SOBI component, one computes

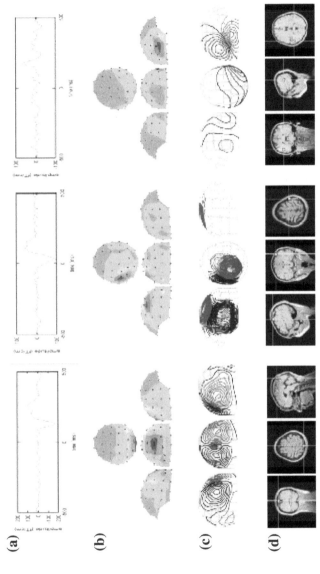

FIG. 6.5.  Examples of second-order blind identification (SOBI) separated visual **(left)**, somatosensory **(middle)**, and auditory **(right)** components, shown in (Panel a) event triggered averages ($N = 90$ trials), (Panel b) field maps, (Panel c) contour plot, and (Panel d) the fitted dipole superimposed on the subject's own magnetic resonance image (MRI). All sensors (channels) were used in generating the contour plots and fitting the dipoles. From "Independent components of magnetoencephalography: Localization," by A. C. Tang et al., 2002a, *Neural Computation, 14*(8). Copyright © 2002 by MIT Press. Reprinted with permission. See Color Panel B.

$$\hat{\mathbf{x}}^{(i)}(t) = \hat{s}_i(t)\hat{a}^{(i)} \qquad\qquad (6.2)$$

where $\hat{a}^{(i)}$ is the $i$th column of $\hat{\mathbf{A}}$ and $\hat{\mathbf{x}}^{(i)}(t)$ is the sensor-space image of source $i$. Because $\hat{\mathbf{x}}^{(i)}(t)$ is at each point in time equal to the unchanging vector $\hat{a}^{(i)}$, scaled by the time course $\hat{s}_i(t)$, dipole fitting algorithms will localize $\hat{\mathbf{x}}^{(i)}(t)$ to the same location no matter what window in time is chosen.

Theoretically, one sampling point in time across all sensors contains all information about the source. In practice, Neuromag software needs a time series of at least several samples. Therefore, we calculated the event-locked average for the component of interest and made a .fif file containing such averages for the dipole fitting algorithm.

## Localization Across Multiple Modalities

The process of localizing SOBI components is simple. For each component of interest, one computes its sensor projections described earlier, and we repackage a .fif file for the Neuromag dipole fitting software. One can select any time during the average time window to fit the dipole because the dipole solution is invariant to time. In contrast, when localizing sources directly from the mixed sensor data, the resulting dipole solution is sensitive to the dipole-fitting time. The independence of SOBI localization from time selection can significantly simplify the dipole-localization process by reducing the subjective input needed during time selection.

The contour plots of the visual, somatosensory, and auditory components and their corresponding dipole locations are shown in Fig. 6.5c and d. These SOBI components have naturally dipolar contour plots without channel selection or reduction. Without SOBI preprocessing, manual selection of a subset of channels (20–30) or exclusion of channels is often needed in order to obtain dipolar field patterns when modeling dipole sources from the mixed-sensor data. Using SOBI preprocessing, one can remove this subjective step from the localization process.

Localization results shown in Fig. 6.5c and d can be obtained directly from fitting dipoles to the field maps by a naive user who simply follows instructions without selecting dipole-fitting time and without selecting channels.

## Cross-Task and Cross-Subject Reproducibility

To show how reproducible the localization of SOBI components can be *across the four cognitive tasks,* we examined SOBI-separated visual components from 1 subject. Across four tasks, the two occipito–parietal visual sources (Fig. 6.6c and d) can be reliably localized within the same subjects for two SOBI-separated components . For both visual sources, the time course of the response is highly repeatable across multiple tasks, as shown in the overlay plot (Fig. 6.6a and b). The earlier visual responses were almost identical in both amplitude and response latency (Fig. 6.6a) while the later responses varied only in amplitude across tasks (Fig. 6.6b). These visual SOBI components were localized to similar locations within the occipital and parietal lobes, as shown in Fig. 6.6c and d, in which fitted dipoles from multiple experiments are superimposed on the subject's own structural MRI. Notice that in the field map the right side of the head is shown on the right, whereas in the MRI image, following radiological convention, the right is shown on the left.

To show how reproducible the localization of SOBI components can be *across subjects,* we examined SOBI-separated somatosensory components from 3 subjects.[3] In all 3, we reliably identified two components (left and right) with button press locked responses in the somatosensory areas. Figure 6.7 shows the time course, field map, contour plot, and fitted dipole for the SOBI somatosensory components in the right hemisphere of the 3 subjects. Notice the cross-subject similarity in the field maps, contour plots, and dipole locations (somatosensory cortex in the anterior parietal lobe, postcentral sulcus).

**Localization With and Without SOBI**

To offer quantitative comparison in the relative performance of source localization with and without SOBI, we attempted to identify and localize the most reliable occipito–parietal visual source, and both the left and right somatosensory sources, in 4 subjects and four cognitive tasks[4] from SOBI components and from the unprocessed data. As all four tasks involved bilateral presentation of visual stimuli, we expected that at least one visual source would be found active in the occipito–parietal cortex. Similarly, because separate left and right button presses were required by all the tasks, we also expected that at least one left and one right somatosensory source would be active. For these *expected sources* we attempted to localize the source with dipole fitting from SOBI components and from the raw sensor data (without SOBI). The percentage of the ex-

---

[3]The fourth subject did right-hand index-mid finger button presses that differed from the rest of the subjects.

[4]For detailed description of the tasks, see Tang et al. (2002a).

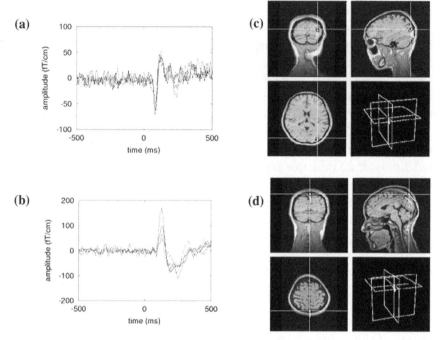

FIG. 6.6. Cross-task consistency in the temporal profile (Panels a and b) and dipole location (Panels c and d) of two second-order blind interaction (SOBI) visual components. Occipital (Panels a and c) and occipito–parietal (Panels b and d) sources can be identified and localized consistently across multiple tasks (overlay). Panels a and b: visual stimulus-locked averages from four visual tasks, overlaid ($N = 90$ trials per task). Panels c and d: corresponding single equivalent current dipoles (ECDs) for visual sources in Panels a and b. Notice the consistency of the dipole locations across tasks. Notice also that the temporal profile of the earlier visual source (Panel a) did not differ across tasks, but the amplitude of the later visual source (Panel d) was modulated by the task conditions. From "Independent components of magnetoencephalography: Localization," by A. C. Tang et al., 2002a, *Neural Computation, 14*(8). Copyright © 2002 by MIT Press. Reprinted with permission.

pected sources for which dipole solutions can be found are compared for localization with and without the aid of SOBI.

For a SOBI component to be considered a detectable neuronal source, there must be an evoked response that clearly deviates from the baseline in the averaged component data. We rejected all SOBI components with any ambiguity on this criterion. Second, the SOBI components must have a field map showing focal activation of sensors over the relevant brain regions (occipito–parietal cortex and anterior parietal cortex in this study). Third, the contour plot for the SOBI component must be dipolar.

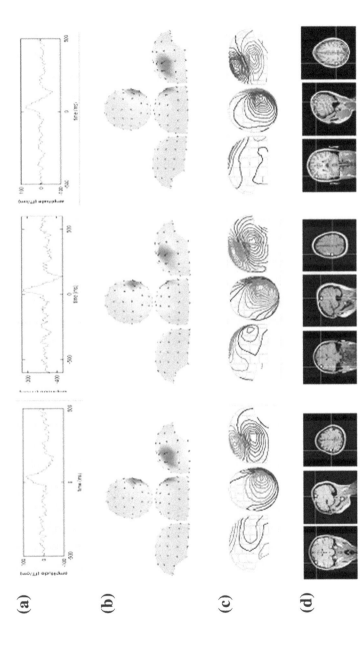

FIG. 6.7. Somatosensory sources can be identified and localized consistently across multiple subjects (shown for the left source). The figure is similar to Fig. 6.5 except the responses were locked onto the button press. From "Independent components of magnetoencephalography: Localization," by A. C. Tang et al., 2002a, *Neural Computation, 14*(8). Copyright © 2002 by MIT Press. Reprinted with permission.

Finally, the fitted dipole must be in the relevant cortical areas. For a source to be considered detectable using the conventional method of localization from raw sensor data one must first identify a sensor at which the largest evoked response is found. Second, the contour plot must be dipolar at the peak time. Finally, in a few cases when multiple-dipole solutions are needed, at least one of the dipoles is localized to the expected brain region. By allowing multiple-dipole solutions for localization without SOBI preprocessing, our comparison was biased against the SOBI method.

### Visual Sources

Among all SOBI components, for each subject and each task, we were able to identify and localize an occipito–parietal visual source with a single dipole (100% detectability). These occipito–parietal components invariantly had very focal sensor projections, and the contour plots were invariantly dipolar even without channel selection (e.g., see field map and contour plot in Fig. 6.5b and c, left). A subset of channels (20–30) over the occipito–parietal lobe were used for the purpose of fair comparison with the conventional analysis method without the aid of SOBI. The peak response latencies of these SOBI components ($N = 16$) were 139.0 ± 7.6, and the dipole coordinates (X, Y, Z) were 7.5 ± 2.6, -49.4 ± 3.2, and 68.6 ± 3.4 mm.

Using the conventional method of source localization directly from the unseparated sensor data, we fitted dipoles using the same or similar subset of channels selected over the occipito–parietal cortex. In all subjects and all tasks, the conventional method identified and localized at least one visual source in the occipitoparietal lobe (100% detectability). Of a total of 16 expected sources (4 tasks by 4 subjects), 10 could be fitted with a single dipole, 4 were fitted with two-dipole solutions, 1 was fitted with a three-dipole solution, and 1 was fitted with a four-dipole solution. When multiple-dipole solutions were needed, at least one of them was localized to the occipito–pariental cortex. This variation in dipole solutions may reflect some individual differences in visual processing occurring outside of the occipito–parietal cortex. The peak response latencies of these occipito–parietal visual sources ($N = 16$) were 143.6 ± 5.5, and the dipole coordinates (X, Y, Z) were 4.21 ± 4.8, -55.89 ± 2.68, and 59.42 ± 3.83 mm.

### Somatosensory Sources

For each subject and each task, with only 2 failures we were able to identify and localize 22 out of the 24 expected left and right somatosensory sources with a single dipole from SOBI components (3 subjects × 4 tasks ×

2 hemispheres). All 22 somatosensory components invariantly had very focal sensor projections, and the contour plots were invariantly dipolar even without channel selection (e.g., see field map and contour plot in Fig. 6.7 b & c). Single dipoles were fitted for these components, with a subset of channels (20–30) over the somatosensory cortex selected for the purpose of fair comparison with the conventional analysis method. The peak response latencies were $3.3 \pm 4.2$ and $0.8 \pm 3.4$ msec for the left ($N = 11$) and right ($N = 11$) somatosensory sources. The dipole coordinates (X, Y, Z) were $-39.4 \pm 2.4$, $7.8 \pm 2.7$, and $84.6 \pm 1.7$ for the left somatosensory sources and $45.69 \pm 2.1$, $5.6 \pm 2.2$, and $84.1 \pm 3.1$ for the right somatosensory sources.

Using the conventional method of source localization directly from the unseparated sensor data, we fitted dipoles using the same or similar subset of channels selected over the somatosensory cortex. Of 24 sources expected, in 7 cases no visible peak response could be identified in any of the sensors. Of the remaining 17 cases in which peak responses could be found in at least one sensor over the somatosensory cortex, 4 did not have dipolar fields, and 4 resulted in dipole locations outside of the head or in the auditory cortex. Single-dipole solutions were found in only 9 cases. The peak response latencies of these somatosensory sources were $-5.2 \pm 2.5$ for the left hemisphere ($N = 5$) and $1.6 \pm 1.8$ for the right hemisphere ($N = 4$). The dipole coordinates (X, Y, Z) were $-43.3 \pm 3.9$, $12.1 \pm 5.6$, and $82.8 \pm 3.8$ for the left sources and $42.3 \pm 5.5$, $15.9 \pm 2.7$, and $89.9 \pm 1.4$ for the right sources.

### *Statistical Comparisons*

There were no significant differences in the detectability for the occipito-parietal source measured with and without SOBI. In both cases, 100% detectability (16 out of 16 expected sources) was achieved. In contrast, SOBI resulted in an increase in the detectability of the expected somatosensory sources (22 out of 24 for SOBI and 9 out of 24 for unprocessed data; $\chi^2$ test, $p < .0001$; Fig. 6.8). The peak response latencies for the visual and somatosensory sources did not differ significantly when measured using SOBI and without using SOBI. For the visual sources, the precise dipole locations estimated with and without SOBI did not differ in the X and Y dimensions but nearly differed significantly in the Z dimension ($p = .05$). For the somatosensory sources, the precise dipole locations differed significantly in the Y dimension ($p < .05$) for the left source and in the Y and Z dimensions for the right source ($p < .05$). Because the

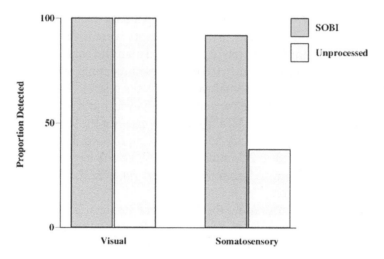

FIG. 6.8.    Second-order blind identification (SOBI) increased the detectability of expected neuronal sources for the more variable somatosensory activation. From "Independent components of magnetoencephalography: Localization," by A. C. Tang et al., 2002a, *Neural Computation, 14*(8). Copyright © 2002 by MIT Press. Reprinted with permission.

true accuracy of source locations cannot be determined from these experiments without a depth electrode, no quantitative comparisons can be made concerning accuracy.

## SOBI Reduced Subjectivity and Labor

Because each component has a fixed field map, the dipole fitting solutions for SOBI components were sensitive to neither the time at which the dipoles were fitted nor the sensor used for determining the time of fit. Within this map, each sensor reading reflects only activation due to a single source generator, or several temporally coherent generators, as opposed to activation due to a combination of multiple generators, each with a different time course. Therefore, using SOBI, there is no need to subjectively select a time from a sensor for dipole fitting. One way to view the difference between dipole localization with and without SOBI processing is to view SOBI as an automatic and a more objective tool that allows the isolation of sensor activation due to an already isolated functionally independent generator. Second, simple SOBI components, which have field activation over early sensory processing areas, were almost always dipolar

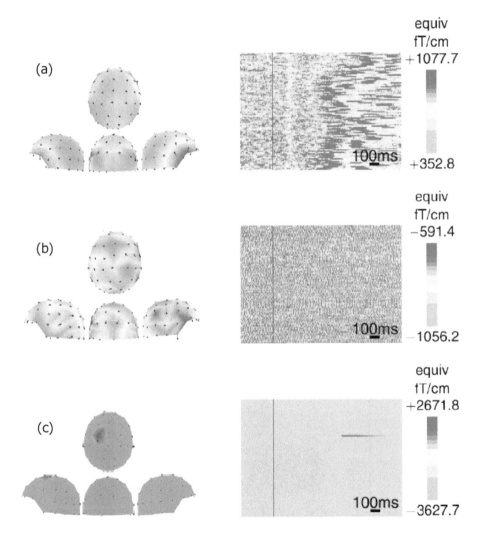

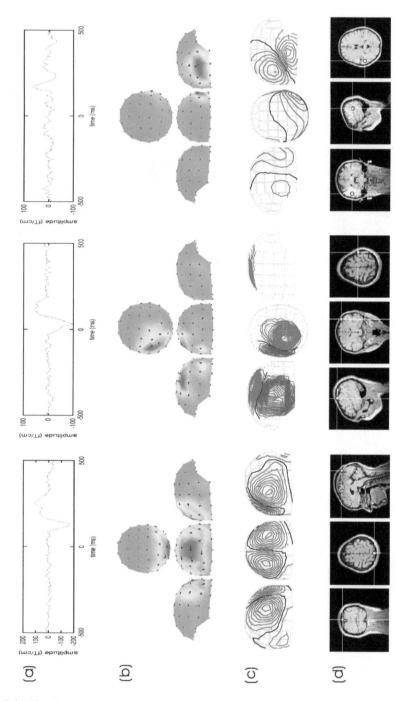

Color Plate B

even without channel selection/reduction.[5] Using the Neuromag software, one can simply load in the average sensor signals for a given component and use the "fit" button to get the dipole solution. The reduced subjectivity and time required to find dipole solutions can make data analysis and training of new researchers for MEG more cost effective.

## SOBI-Improved Detectability of Neuronal Sources

SOBI separation of the data resulted in a greater detectability of somatosensory sources but did not increase the detectability of visual sources. This modality specific improvement in source detectability depended on the $S/N$ ratio in the sensor data. Given this specific set of experiments, visual responses could be clearly identified from the raw sensor data even without the aid of SOBI; there was no room for further improvement in detectability by SOBI. In contrast, the relatively poor $S/N$ ratio in the raw sensor data for the somatosensory responses caused many failures in identifying a sensor at which a peak response could be found and in determining the peak response time. Under this poor signal-to-noise condition, in all but two cases SOBI resulted in components with the characteristic field map, characteristic temporal response profile, and the correct dipole location for a somatosensory source. These findings suggest another advantage that ICA algorithms can offer: improving the ability to detect and localize neuronal sources that are otherwise difficult to detect or are undetectable under relatively poor signal-to-noise conditions.

This improvement has significant practical implications. First, brain regions involved in higher level cognitive processing tend to show greater trial-to-trial variability in their activation and therefore have a lower signal-to-noise ratio in the average response. Second, behavioral tasks that bear greater resemblance to real-world situations tend to involve greater variability in both stimulus presentation and subsequent processing. Finally, studies of clinical patients and children are often limited by the length of the experiment and therefore often provide data from a limited number of trials. Our results suggest that ICA may offer an improved capability to detect and localize neuronal source activations in these difficult situations.

We should mention that fICA-separated components have been shown to yield localization results qualitatively similar to those arrived at without ICA preprocessing (Vigário et al., 1999). It may appear from this study that no substantial benefits of ICA could be found for neuro-

---

[5]SOBI also separated out many complex components that have multiple patches or very broad field activation. These components reflect synchronized activation in multiple brains. Functional connectivity among these brain regions may be inferred.

magnetic source localization. In comparison to our findings, Vigário et al.'s study was optimally designed to produce strong and focal activation of a small number of neuromagnetic sources, and the $S/N$ was high. Under such an optimal condition, the advantages of ICA algorithms are likely to be masked by a ceiling effect.

### Summary

We identified and localized visual and somatosensory sources activated in 4 subjects during four cognitive tasks. Because of the relatively large variability involved in highly cognitive tasks and the small number of trials collected, these tasks were characterized by relatively poor signal-to-noise ratios in the sensor data and therefore were ideal for evaluating differential localization performance. Our results showed that despite the large variability associated with the visual and somatosensory activations during these particular tasks, SOBI was able to separate and identify visual and somatosensory components that were localized to expected cortical regions. Most important is that, for the most variable somatosensory activation evoked by incidental stimulation during button presses, SOBI preprocessing resulted in a greater rate of detection and localization for the expected somatosensory sources than that obtained from localization using the raw sensor data. Furthermore, the process of generating dipole solutions for SOBI components was simpler, more efficient, and less subjective.

## SINGLE-TRIAL RESPONSE ONSET TIME DETECTION[6]

Single-trial response onset time detection is performed only when there is an evoked response that clearly deviates from the baseline in the averaged component data. For all identified neuronal sources, we estimated response-onset times by the leading edge of the response rather than the time of the peak response. This measure is more robust against noise and also better captures the intuitive goal of detecting the time of the earliest detectable response rather than of the maximal response.

The process of single-trial response onset detection is iterative: Both the threshold and detection windows are adjusted until no further reduction in false detection can be achieved. An initial threshold was set between the peak amplitude and one half of the peak amplitude in the event-triggered average plot (not shown). The beginning of the detection window initially was set at the time the event-triggered averages first ex-

---

[6]For more recent results, see Tang et al., 2002b.

ceeded the range of baseline fluctuation. Typically, the baseline window is approximately 100 msec to 200 msec prior to stimulus onset. The detection window ended when the event-triggered averages first returned to the same level as when the detection window began because the detection windows should be sufficiently large to capture the entire distribution of response-onset times. (These initial values are not critical because they will be adjusted in both directions as we described later).

Because single-trial responses can be very different from the event-triggered averages, the threshold and detection windows were adjusted through an iterative process to ensure that no responses were excluded. Using the initial threshold and detection window, response- onset times were determined and graphically superimposed on the MEG image (detected response time [DRT] curve) to allow visual verification of the detected onset times. The DRT curve should be smooth, indicating a unimodal distribution. When multiple events were detected exactly at the beginning of the detection window, it is most likely that the signal amplitude of the component has crossed the threshold *before* the beginning of the detection window. Therefore, these events were considered false detections and were not marked by and removed from the DRT curve. For components showing biphasic responses, most of the single-trial response time analysis presented here was performed on the initial phase of the response, when the amplitude of the initial response was sufficiently large. Some results pertaining to the later phases are shown when the early phase response had such low amplitude as to make them difficult to detect using the method presented here. For a more updated procedural description, see Tang et al., 2002b.

**Threshold**

If the threshold is set too high, not only can many trials remain undetected, but also one will overestimate the onset times by missing the initial onset. Such an overestimation of onset times is easily seen as a right shift in the DRT curve from the leading edge of color change associated with the responses (Fig. 6.9a). Because the threshold is set too high, many single-trial responses were missed (detection rate: 177/350). Because all trials with responses detected are displayed on top of the MEG image and sorted by detected response latency, and trials with no responses detected are displayed at the bottom, missing responses are apparent under visual inspection, as shown at the bottom of Fig. 6.9a. If the threshold is set too low, false detection can occur when the amplitude of baseline fluctuation is relatively large. In this case, many false detections would be made at the beginning of the detection window (253/350), resulting in a low detection rate (97/350 after automatic removal of such false detention), as shown in Fig. 6.9b. In both cases, the threshold could be either lowered or raised accordingly in the next iteration until the DRT curve captures the edge of the color change associated with all apparent response-onset times.

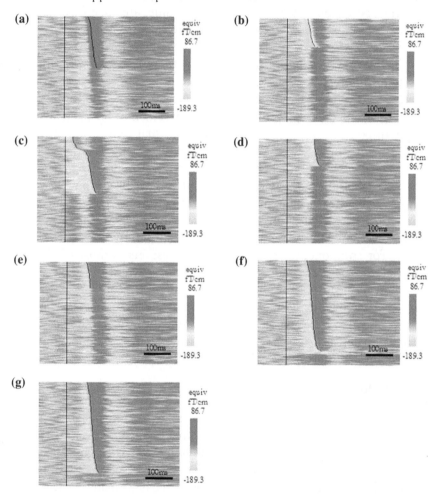

FIG. 6.9. Examples, all from the same component, of suboptimal detection due to (Panel a) too high a threshold (Panel b) too low a threshold, (Panel c) too early a beginning window (wb), (Panel d) too late a beginning window (wb), (Panel e) too early an end window (we), (Panel f) too late an end window (we), (Panel g) an optimal detection is shown. See Table 6.1 for associated detection parameters and results. equiv = equivalent. Ventrical lines: stimulus onset. Rows = trials. N = 350 trials. Sorted by increasing onset times. From "Independent components of magnetoencephalography: Single-trial onset times," by A. C. Tang et al., 2002b, *NeuroImage, 17*(4). Copyright © 2002 by Elsevier. Reprinted with permission.

**Detection Window**

Once the detection threshold is determined, one further examines the MEG image for false detections associated with incorrect settings of the beginning and ending of the detection window $wb$, and $we$. If $wb$ is too early, then the response window will include a part of the baseline. As a result, the DRT curve shows a discontinuity, with the point of discontinuity separating trials of false detection (left portion) from trials of correct detection (right portion), as in Fig. 6.9c. If $wb$ is too late, then many single-trial responses are excluded from detection (Fig. 6.9d).

If $we$ is too early, later response onsets may be missing (see bottom portion of Fig. 6.9e). This case is apparent on visual inspection. If $we$ is too late, then the later portion of a biphasic response will be falsely detected as the initial response. This form of false detection is easily seen near the tail end of the DRT curve (Fig. 6.9f). In any of the preceding cases, one can adjust the detection window parameters for the next iteration.

For each neuronal component, this iterative process continues until no further reduction in the frequency of false detections or missing responses can be achieved. The final result is shown in Fig. 6.9g. See Table 6.1 for a summary of parameters and results of the sample detection (Fig. 6.9). Statistics on the detected onset times (mean ± se) are then computed and reported along with the resulting MEG image (Fig. 6.9g). The same procedure can be performed on a control window of equal size either prior to or following the actual detection window. The resulting number of detected onsets within the control windows can be compared statically with that obtained for the detection window.

**Effect of Filter Length on Detected Onset Times**

Because filtering can affect response onset times, we first investigated the effect of a low-pass filter, as such a filter is often used to remove noise unrelated to the evoked responses. Figures 6.10 and 6.11 display the result of response-onset time detection using different low-pass filter parameters for a SOBI component with auditory evoked responses. Filtering visibly reduced the amount of background noise, thus highlighting the evoked responses (Fig. 6.10). There was no apparent change in the detected onset times or in the number of detections as the low-pass filter

**TABLE 6.1**

**Detection Parameters and Results**

| | Detection Parameters | | | Detection Results | |
|---|---|---|---|---|---|
| Cases | Threshold | wb | we | Rate | Quality |
| high threshold | 150 | 70 | 120 | 177 / 350 | missing onsets |
| low threshold | −100 | 70 | 120 | 97 / 350 | missing onsets |
| early wb | 10 | 25 | 120 | 189 / 350 | missing & false onsets |
| late wb | 10 | 95 | 120 | 91 / 350 | missing onsets |
| early we | 10 | 70 | 85 | 90 / 350 | missing onsets |
| late we | 10 | 70 | 320 | 313 / 350 | false onsets |
| optimal | 10 | 70 | 120 | 305 / 350 | |

*Note:* Detection parameters (threshold and detection window) and detection results for the examples given in Fig 6.9. Thresholds are relative to a per-trial 100 msec prestimulus baseline.

was changed from no filter, to 40 Hz, 20 Hz and 10 Hz (Fig. 6.10) and as the roll off parameter was changed from 0.5 Hz to 5 Hz (Fig. 6.11). A quantitative comparison between the detected onset times using different low-pass filter parameters revealed very small changes in the number of onsets detected. When a more aggressive low-pass filter was used, the number of events detected was reduced from to 145 to 141 (4 from a total of 150 trials).

If an onset time is detectable only when no filter is used, it is possible that such a detected response is a result of false detection due to noisy on-going background activity. Therefore, by using a more aggressive low-pass filter one can reduce the chance of false detection. On the other hand, a more aggressive filter can change the detected onset times. Thus, a change in the number of onsets detected that are caused by different low-pass filters could be a result of better onset-time estimation associated with a reduction in false detection or worse estimation due to temporal smearing after filtering. To ensure that temporal smearing was not the cause of the change in the detected onset times, we always performed the detection procedure both with and without filtering and examined graphically whether the filtering altered the temporal profile of the evoked response. As shown in Fig. 6.10, filtering with a 10-Hz low-pass

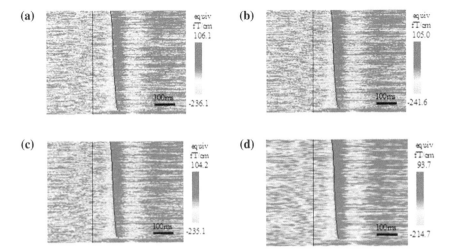

FIG. 6.10.    Effect of a low-pass filter on response-onset time detection (onset times, percentage response detected). Panel a: no filter: 90 ± 1 msec; 96.7%; Panel b: low-pass at 40 Hz: 91 ± 1 msec; 96%; Panel c: low-pass at 20 Hz: 92 ± 1 msec; 95.3%; Panel d: low-pass at 10 Hz: 92 ± 1 msec; 94%. For all panels, a rolloff of 5 Hz was used. $N$ = 150 trials. From "Independent components of magnetoencephalography: Single-trial onset times," by A. C. Tang et al., 2002b, *NeuroImage, 17*(4). Copyright © 2002 by Elsevier. Reprinted with permission.

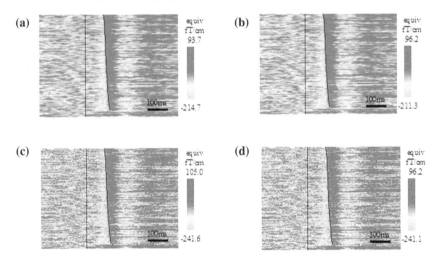

FIG. 6.11.    Effect of filter rolloff on response-onset time detection (onset times, percentage response detected). Panel a: 10-Hz low pass and 5-Hz rolloff: 92 ± 1 msec, 94%. Panel b: 10-Hz low pass and 0.5-Hz rolloff: 92 ± 1msec, 94%. Panel c: 40-Hz low pass and 5-Hz rolloff: 91 ± 1 msec, 96%. Panel d: 40-Hz low pass and 0.5-Hz rolloff: 91 ± 1 msec, 96%. $N$ = 150 trials. equiv = equivalent. From "Independent components of magnetoencephalography: Single-trial onset times," by A. C. Tang et al., 2002b, *NeuroImage, 17*(4). Copyright © 2002 by Elsevier. Reprinted with permission.

filter changed the estimated onset times by less than 2 msec, and did not distort the profile of the evoked responses.

A more aggressive low-pass filter can reduce the influence of ongoing background activity, and thereby minimize false detection, without significantly altering the temporal profile of the evoked responses. Therefore, in the following analysis, a low-pass filter of 10 Hz with a rolloff of 5 Hz was used unless otherwise specified. It is important to note that, for different neuronal sources, the effect of a given filter on response-onset times will be different. When a filter significantly changes the temporal profile of the evoked responses, a less aggressive filter should be used for an accurate estimation of response onsets.

## Response-Onset Time Detection Across Sensory Modalities

In this section we demonstrate that single-trial response-onset time detection can be achieved in three major sensory modalities and under experimental conditions of both large and small trial-to-trial variability. Single-trial onset time detection with *large* trial-to-trial variability was performed for the visual and somatosensory evoked responses recorded during the four cognitive tasks. Single-trial onset time detection with *small* trial-to-trial variability was performed for the auditory evoked responses recorded during the simple binaural pure tone presentation.

The detected response-onset times are shown in MEG image (Fig. 6.12b), with the evoked responses aligned to the stimulus onset (time 0, marked by the vertical line on the left side of the MEG image) and the DRT marked as a curve to the right of the stimulus-onset line (DRT curve). The detection results are shown sorted by latency from stimulus to detected response onset. The corresponding stimulus triggered average (Fig. 6.12a), sensor projections or field maps (Fig. 6.12c), and dipole location superimposed on the subject's structural MRI images (e.g., Fig. 6.12d) are also provided, for comparison with results from standard analysis. For the visual source shown in Fig. 6.12a–d, the single-trial response onsets were detected in 64 of 90 trials (71.1%). The estimated onset times were 111 ± 1 msec. Its temporal profile in the average response, the field map, the contour plot, and the dipole location were characteristic of typical visual sources from the occipito–parietal lobes. For comparison with typical visually evoked responses, see Brenner, Williamson, & Kaufman (1975); Hari (1994); and Supek et al. (1999).

For the somatosensory source shown in Fig. 6.13a–f, the single-trial response onsets were detected in 129 of 150 trials (86%) when the contra-

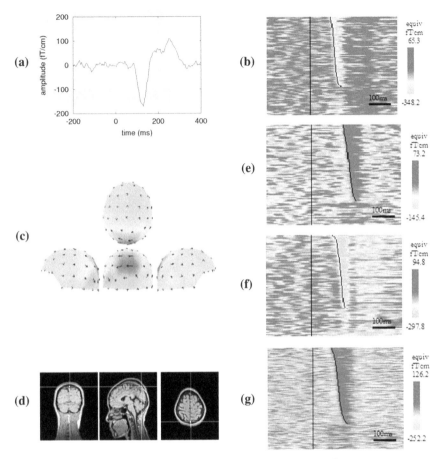

FIG. 6.12. Panels a–d: Detection of single-trial response-onset times from a occipito–parietal source that responded to a visual stimulus. Panel a: Visual-stimulus-locked average response (unfiltered), Panel b: detected single-trial response times marked on a magnetoencephalography (MEG) image, Panel c: field map of the parietal source activation, Panel d: fitted equivalent current dipole (ECD) superimposed on the subject's structural magnetic resonance (MRI). Panels e–g: single-trial visual response-onset detection in visual sources across 3 additional subjects, sorted by onset latency. Panels b and e–g: subjects 1–4. $N = 90$ trials, except for (d). $N = 270$ trials. equiv = equivalent. From "Independent components of magnetoencephalography: Single-trial onset times," by A. C. Tang et al., 2002b, *NeuroImage, 17*(4). Copyright © 2002 by Elsevier. Reprinted with permission.

lateral thumb pressed the mouse button and in 105 of 120 trials (87.5%) when the ipsilateral thumb pressed the mouse button. The response-onset times from the time when the button press was detected on the trigger line were –1 ± 2 msec and 15 ± 1 msec for the contra- and ipsilateral activation, respectively. These numbers indicate that the somatosensory responses

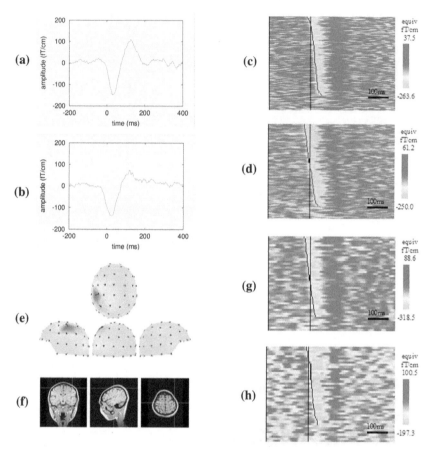

FIG. 6.13.   Detection of single-trial response-onset times from a somatosensory source that responded to left (Panel a) and right (Panel b) button presses. Panels a and b: Left and right button-press-triggered average responses (unfiltered). Panels c and d: Detected single-trial response-onset times triggered by left and right button presses respectively, marked on magnetoencephalography (MEG) images. Panel e: field map of the somatosensory source. Panel f: fitted equivalent current diploe (ECD) superimposed on the subject's structural magnetic resonance (MRI). Panels g and h: single-trial somatosensory response-onset detection across 2 additional subjects, sorted by onset latency. Panels c, g, and h: subjects 1–3. Data are shown for contralateral activation only. The number of trials varied from subject to subject. equiv = equivalent. From "Independent components of magnetoencephalography: Single-trial onset times," by A. C. Tang et al., 2002b, *NeuroImage, 17*(4). Copyright © 2002 by Elsevier. Reprinted with permission.

could start as soon as the thumb movement was initiated—as soon as, or even before, the mouse button was completely depressed. The temporal profile in the average responses was slower to rise and broader in width than the typical responses evoked by electrical stimulation (Brenner,

Lipton, Kaufman, & Williamson, 1978; Hari & Forss, 1999; Karhu & Tesche, 1999). This was expected, because somatosensory stimulation due to button press movement and feedback is much more prolonged and variable than stimulation by the brief and well-controlled median nerve shock. The field map, contour plot, and dipole location are consistent with activation of the hand region of the somatosensory cortex.

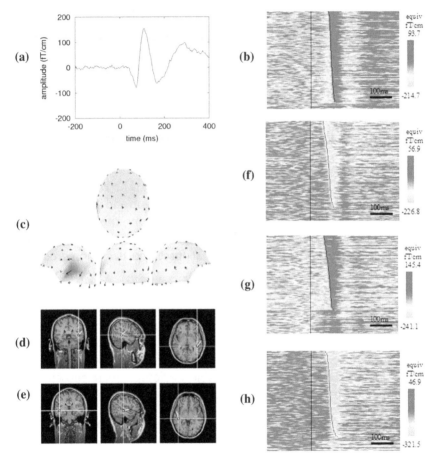

FIG. 6.14.    Detection of single-trial response-onset times from an auditory source. Panel a: auditory stimulus triggered average response (unfiltered). Panel b: detected single-trial response times marked on a magnetoencephalography (MEG) image. Panel c: field map of the temporal source. Panels d and e: fitted equivalent current dipoles (ECD) superimposed on the subject's structural magnetic resonance (MRI) images. Panles f–h: single-trial auditory response-onset detection across 3 additional subjects, sorted by onset latency. Panels b, f–h: Subjects 1–4. $N = 150$ trials. equiv = equivalent. From "Independent components of magnetoencephalography: Single-trial onset times," by A. C. Tang et al., 2002b, *NeuroImage, 17*(4). Copyright © 2002 by Elsevier. Reprinted with permission.

For the auditory source shown in Fig. 6.14a–e, the single-trial response onsets were detected in 141 of 150 trials (94%). The estimated response onset times were $92 \pm 1$ msec. The temporal profile in the average response, field map, contour plot, and dipole location were characteristic of typical auditory sources. This particular auditory SOBI component had a two-dipole solution, one in each of the two hemispheres, and (necessarily, because of the SOBI decomposition) both having the same time course of response. This is consistent with the binaural stimulation used in this experiment.[6] The temporal profile in the average response, the field map, the contour plot, and the dipole location were characteristic of typical auditory sources in the temporal lobes. For comparison with typical auditory evoked responses, see Hari, Aittoniemi, Jarvinen, and Varpula (1980); Roberts, Ferrari, Stufflebeam, and Poeppel (2000); Romani, Williamson, and Kaufman (1982).

### Cross-Subject Response Onset Detection: Visual

As previously discussed (Tang et al., 2000b), visual sources were identifiable along both the ventral and dorsal streams. The occipito–parietal sources along the dorsal stream varied less in location and in response profile. In contrast, the occipito-temporal sources along the ventral stream showed greater variability in response profile and precise location. To give readers a sense of how well the single-trial onset time detection procedure can perform across a variety of visual sources, we show detection for the visual responses from a variety of visual areas from multiple subjects. In 13 of 16 (81%) expected visual sources along the ventral processing stream,[7] single-trial onset time detection could be performed. The detection rate was $69 \pm 2\%$, and the estimated response-onset times were $139 \pm 9$ msec ($N = 13$). Figure 6.12E, F, and G show results of onset time detection for the visual sources from three additional subjects. Sources were chosen to reflect variability in the responses and in the detection.

### Cross-Subject Response Onset Detection: Somatosensory

Somatosensory sources were identified in all subjects who made button press responses during the four cognitive tasks. Single-trial response-on-

---

[6]It is possible to obtain two separate components from the left and right hemisphere if there is sufficient hemispherical asymmetry in the temporal details of neuronal responses from the left and right auditory cortices.

[7]Given the tasks involved memory of visual forms, we expected at least one visual source to be activated along the ventral processing pathway. A total of 16 such sources were expected for 4 experiments in 4 subjects.

set time detection was attempted on one of the SOBI somatosensory components for each subject in at least one of the four tasks. Because the activation of these somatosensory sources was highly variable, in only 7 of 24 (29%) of the somatosensory sources could single-trial onset time detection be performed. Among these sources, for the contralateral button presses, single-trial onset times were estimated to be 0 ± 3 msec with a detection rate of 81 ± 2% ($N = 7$). For the ipsilateral button presses, single-trial onset times were estimated to be 5 ± 3 ms with a detection rate of 76 ± 5% ($N = 3$). Figure 6.13g and h show results of onset time detection for the latter source in 2 additional subjects.

## Cross-Subject Response Onset Detection: Auditory

Auditory evoked responses from the presentation of a pure tone were the least variable compared with the visual and somatosensory responses from the cognitive tasks just discussed. In all 6 subjects, auditory sources can be identified and localized from the SOBI-separated components. Single-trial response-onset time detection could be performed in 6 of 6 expected auditory sources[8] with a detection rate of 80 ± 5% and estimated response-onset times of 85 ± 1 msec ($N = 6$).

Figure 6.14f, g and H show results of onset detection for the auditory source from 3 additional subjects. Because the trial-to-trial variability in auditory stimulation was very low compared with the variability in the visual and somatosensory stimulation during the cognitive tasks, the average detection rate was higher for these auditory sources. Furthermore, single-trial response-onset time detection could be performed among a higher percentage of expected sources (100%) for the auditory responses than for the visual (81%) and somatosensory (29%) responses.

## Statistical Analysis

To determine quantitatively whether the detected responses are due to baseline ongoing activity, we performed the detection procedure on a baseline or control window of equal length immediately before or sometime after the response window (defined by *wb* and *we)* using otherwise-identical parameters. When a post response control window was selected, we made sure that the background fluctuation was comparable to or greater than that of the prestimulus baseline. To determine whether

---

[8]Given that the tasks involved auditory stimulation, we expected at least one auditory source to be activated in each subject. A total of six auditory sources were therefore expected for the 6 subjects.

the detected response onsets were more numerous than those detected in the control windows, we performed a *t* test on the difference between the number of detections during the response window and the number of detections during the control windows. This test result, from all components studied, indicates that our method is capable of detecting evoked responses from single-trial MEG data that are above background ongoing activity (t(16) = 16.145, $p < .0005$). Figure 6.15 shows examples of response-onset time detection for the response window, a preresponse control window, and a postresponse control window. The trials are sorted according to the detected onset times in Fig. 6.15a, b, and e and the same detection results are also shown in chronological.

For sources with good apparent signal-to-noise ratios across multiple subjects, we applied the detection procedure to both a detection window

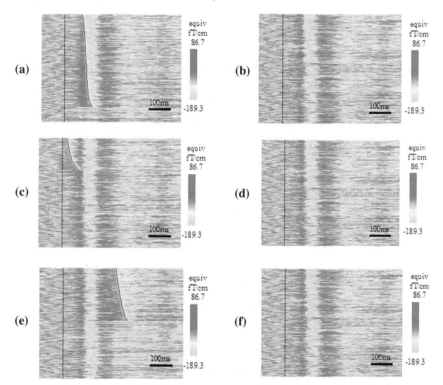

FIG. 6.15.   Detected response onsets for the response and pre- and postresponse control windows, in (Panel a) response window, sorted; (Panel b) response window, unsorted; (Panel c) precontrol window, sorted; (Panel d) precontrol window, unsorted; (Panel e) postcontrol window, sorted; (Panel f) postcontrol window, unsorted.

(*wb* and *we*) and a control window. The detection rates for the response windows were $78 \pm 2\%$ ($N = 8$) for the somatosensory components $69 \pm 2\%$ ($N = 13$) for the visual components, and $80 \pm 5\%$ ($N = 6$) for the auditory components. When all sources were pooled, the detection rate within the detection window across all modalities was $74 \pm 2\%$. The detection rates obtained for the control windows using otherwise-identical parameters were much lower $27 \pm 4$ for the somatosensory components, $27 \pm 3\%$ for the visual components, and $23 \pm 3\%$ for the auditory components. When all sources were pooled, the detection rate across all modalities within the control window was $26 \pm 2\%$. The numbers of detections that were above the background activity were $52 \pm 6\%$ for somatosensory components, $42 \pm 4\%$ for the visual components, and $57 \pm 6\%$ for the auditory components. When all sources were pooled across modalities, the rate of detection that was above the false detection rate was $48 \pm 3\%$. These results indicate that our method is capable of detecting evoked responses from single-trial MEG data that are above background ongoing activity.

Because these components were obtained during different experiments, a number of factors could contribute to the large variation, including differences in stimulus presentation, task complexity, different stages of processing (early vs. later), pathways (e.g., ventral vs. dorsal), modalities of sensory processing (visual, auditory, and somatosensory), different states of alertness (amount of alpha oscillation), and different levels of power in the background brain activity. The detection for the visual components seemed to be particularly poor in comparison to those for the somatosensory and auditory components. It is important to point out that the visual components included here have a greater intrinsic variability due to the number of brain regions from which visual components can be localized. In addition, the visual cortex tends to have more alpha band background activity than any of the other sensory cortices (Williamson et al., 1996). Greater alpha band background activity can contribute to the higher detection rate during the control window.

## DISCUSSION

We conclude this chapter with a brief discussion of the independence assumption made by all ICA methods, a summary of state-of-art ICA capabilities, and an outline of future directions.

## Assumptions

SOBI shares a number of weaknesses with all ICA methods: They all assume that there are as many sensors as sources, they all make some kind of independence assumption, they all assume that the mixing process is linear, and they all assume that the mixing process is stable. In this section, we discuss assumptions of particular relevance to SOBI and MEG rather than general issues in ICA. Like all ICA algorithms, SOBI assumes that the mixing process is stable. In the context of MEG, a stable mixing process corresponds to assuming that the head is motionless relative to the sensors. For this reason head stabilization can be particularly important in MEG when ICA is used. SOBI also assumes that there are at least as many sensors as sources. For us, this is not a serious problem, as our MEG device has 122 sensors, yet we recover only a few dozen sources that show task-related evoked responses. The observation that only a small number of sources are active during typical cognitive and sensory activation tasks is consistent with the results of studies using both EEG (Makeig et al., 1999) and MEG (Vigário et al., 2000). The crucial assumption in ICA is that of independence. For a thorough discussion of the independence assumption as it pertains to MEG, see Vigário et al. (2000). Here we discuss independence only in the context of the particular measure of independence used by SOBI.

## The SOBI Independence Assumption

The major concern that EEG and MEG researchers have regarding the independence assumption arises from the fact that if one computes correlations between EEG or MEG sensor readings over multiple brain regions during behavioral tasks, one would find that some brain regions have non-zero correlations. A good example of correlated brain activity is the apparently correlated evoked responses, due to common input, from neuronal populations in multiple visual areas along the processing pathway during a visual stimulus presentation. On the basis of such an observation, one could conclude that because the statistical independence assumed by ICA is clearly violated, the results of ICA must not be trusted. Yet we have shown that SOBI was able to separate visual components that clearly correspond to neuronal responses from early and later visual processing stages that are correlated because of common input (Tang et al., 2000a, 2000b). Others (Makeig et al., 1999; Vigário et al., 2000) have produced behaviorally and neurophysiologically meaningful components under a variety of task conditions.

Because different ICA algorithms use the independence assumption differently, we offer the following explanation that applies specifically to SOBI. One needs to recognize that correlation is not a binary quantity. As a consequence, neither is violation of the independence assumption. The important question is not whether the assumption is violated but whether the assumption is *sufficiently* violated such that the estimated neuronal sources by SOBI are no longer meaningful. The way SOBI uses the independence assumption is to minimize the total correlations computed with a set of time delays. As such, each delay-correlation matrix $\mathbf{R}_t$ generally makes only a small contribution to the objective function. For example, the correlation one would observe between V1 and V2 responses could be high only at or around one particular time delay, say in **R20ms**. In optimizing its objective function, SOBI can leave a particularly large non-zero off-diagonal element, say the one corresponding to the 20 msec delayed correlation between V1 and V2, in order to minimize the sum squared off-diagonal elements across all the components and time delays. Therefore, this particular method of maximizing independence is not necessarily incompatible with a large correlation at a particular time delay between two sources sharing common inputs.

Most ICA algorithms, including SOBI, minimize some objective function. It is possible for the optimization process to find a poor local minimum. In general, poor results can result from many underlying causes: poor experimental design, poorly conducted experiments, poor head stabilization, poor optimization within the ICA algorithm, violation of assumptions, and so on. No amount of attention to any one possible problem can validate ICA-based methods for processing functional brain imaging data. As with any statistical procedure, the real issue here should not be whether assumptions are violated at all but whether the algorithms can robustly produce components that are behaviorally, neuroanatomically, and physiologically interpretable, despite some violation of the assumptions under which the algorithms were derived. For example, $t$ tests are very robust against the violation of normality assumption and are therefore regularly performed on data that are not guaranteed to be Gaussian. Only empirical results can give confidence that a method is correctly separating the MEG data.

### ICA Advantages

Applying SOBI, one particular ICA algorithm to data from a total of 10 subjects (4 tested on four cognitive tasks and 6 from one auditory sensory activation task), we provided a step-by-step demonstration of how to apply ICA to MEG data, how to identify neuromagnetic sources of interest, how to localize the identified sources, and how to measure single-trial response onset times from the identified neuronal sources. Through this process, we have demonstrated that ICA offers the following:

- automatic separation of neuronal sources from noise sources (ocular artifacts, 60 Hz, and sensor noise); automatic separation of neuronal sources from different modalities (visual, somatosensory, and auditory),
- automatic separation of neuronal sources within the same sensory modality (left and right somatosensory sources),
- reduction in subjectivity and simplification of the source modeling process (no need to set the dipole fitting time and or to select channels),
- increased probability of neuronal source detection and localization under poor $S/N$ conditions with over 90% detection rate in single-trial response-onset time measurement.

## Future Directions

A number of important methodological issues remain. The first concerns with the effect of varying the delays used in the calculation of the correlation matrix and the interaction between the selection of delays and the temporal property of the neuronal source activation. The second concerns with the amount of the data needed for good separation results. The third has to do with how SOBI may interface with other source modeling methods to generate the best localization results. The last but perhaps the most urgent one is to develop software systems that integrate the preceding outlined analysis steps in a seamless fashion to support users with a wide range of computer experience.

## ACKNOWLEDGMENTS

This work was supported by a DARPA Augmented Cognition grant given to ACT and grants from the NFFBI and MIND institute given to ACT and BAP. A special thanks to Natalie A. Malaszenko and Bethany C. Reeb for their help with the production of this manuscript.

## REFERENCES

Aine, C., Huang, M., Stephen, J., & Christner, R. (2000). Multistart algorithms for MEG empirical data analysis reliably characterize locations and time courses of multiple sources. *NeuroImage, 12*(2), 159–172.

Amari, S.-I., & Cichocki, A. (1998). Adaptive blind signal processing-neural network approaches. *Proceedings of the Institute of Electrical and Electronics Engineers, 9*, 2026–2048.

Bell, A. J., & Sejnowski, T. J. (1995). An information-maximization approach to blind separation and blind deconvolution. *Neural Computation, 7*(6), 1129–1159.

Belouchrani, A., Meraim, K. A., Cardoso, J. F., & Moulines, E. (1993). Second-order blind separation of correlated sources. In *Proceedings of the International Conference on Digital Signaling* (pp. 346–351), Cyprus.

Brenner, D., Lipton, J., Kaufman, L., & Williamson, S. J. (1978). Somatically evoked magnetic fields of the human brain. *Science, 199*(4324), 81–83.

Brenner, D., Williamson, S. J., & Kaufman, L. (1975). Visually evoked magnetic fields of the human brain. *Science, 190*(4213), 480–482.

Cao, J. T., Murata, N., Amari, S., Cichocki, A., Takeda, T., Endo, H., & Harada, N. (2000). Single-trial magnetoencephalographic data decomposition and localization based on independent component analysis approach. *Institute of Electronics, Information and Communication Engineers Transactions on Fundamentals of Electronics, Communications and Computer Sciences, E83A*(9), 1757–1766.

Cardoso, J. F. (1994). On the performance of orthogonal source separation algorithms. In *European Signal Processing Conference* (pp. 776–779), Edinburgh, Scotland.

Cardoso, J. F. (1998). Blind signal separation: Statistical principles. *Proceedings of the Institute of Electrical and Electronics Engineers, 9*(10), 2009–2025.

Comon, P. (1994). Independent component analysis: A new concept. *Signal Processing, 36*, 287–314.

Ermer, J. J., Mosher, J. C., Huang, M. X., & Leahy, R. M. (2000). Paired MEG data set source localization using recursively applied and projected (RAP) MUSIC. *Institute of Electrical and Electronics Engineers Transactions on Biomedical Engineering, 47*(9), 1248–1260.

Gavit, L., Baillet, S., Mangin, J., Pescatore, J., & Garnero, L. (2001). A multiresolution framework to MEG/EEG source imaging. *Institute of Electrical and Electronics Engineers: Transactions on Biomedical Engineering, 48*(10) 1080–1087.

Hari, R. (1994). Human cortical functions revealed by magnetoencephalography. *Progress in Brain Research, 100*, 163–168.

Hari, R., Aittoniemi, K., Jarvinen, M.-L., & Varpula, T. (1980). Auditory evoked transient and sustained magnetic fields of the human brain. *Experimental Brain Research, 40*, 237–240.

Hari, R., & Forss, N. (1999). Magnetoencephalography in the study of human somatosensory cortical processing. *Philosophical Transactions of the Royal Society London Series B, 354*, 1145–1154.

Hotelling, H. (1933). Analysis of a complex of statistical variables into principal components. *Journal of Educational Psychology, 24*, 417–441, 498–520.

Huang, M. X., Aine, C., Davis, L., Butman, J., Christner, R., Weisend, M., Stephen, J., et al. (2000). Sources on the anterior and posterior banks of the central sulcus identified from magnetic somatosensory evoked responses using multi-start spatio-temporal localization. *Human Brain Mapping, 11*(2), 59–76.

Hyvärinen, A. (1999). Survey on independent component analysis. *Neural Computing Surveys, 2*, 94–128.

Hyvärinen, A., & Oja, E. (1997). A fast fixed-point algorithm for independent component analysis. *Neural Computation, 9*(7), 1483–1492.

Ioannides, A. A., Liu, M. J., Liu, L. C., Bamidis, P. D., Hellstrand, E., & Stephan, K. M. (1995). Magnetic-field tomography of cortical and deep processes: Examples of real-time mapping of averaged and single trial MEG signals. *International Journal of Psychophysiology, 20*(3), 161–175.

Jung, T. P., Humphries, C., Lee, T. W., Makeig, S., McKeown, M. J., Iragui, V., & Sejnowski, T. J. (1999). Removing electroencephalographic artifacts: comparison between ICA and PCA. In *Neural networks for signal processing VIII* (pp. 63–72). Institute of Electrical and Electronics Engineers Press.

Jung, T. P., Humphries, C., Lee, T. W., McKeown, M. J., Iragui, V., Makeig, S., & Sejnowski, T. J. (2000). Removing electroencephalographic artifacts by blind source separation. *Psychophysiology, 37*, 163–178.

Jung, T. P., Makeig, S., Westerfield, M., Townsend, J., Courchesne, E., & Sejnowski, T. J. (2000). Removal of eye activity artifacts from visual event-related potentials in normal and clinical subjects. *Clinical Neurophysiology, 111*(10), 1745–1758.

Karhu, J., & Tesche, C. D. (1999). Simultaneous early processing of sensory input in human primary (SI) and secondary (SII) somatosensory cortices. *Journal of Neurophysiology, 81*, 2017–2025.

Kinouchi, Y., Ohara, G., Nagashino, H., Soga, T., Shichijo, F., & Matsumoto, K. (1996). Dipole source localization of MEG by BP neural networks. *Brain Topography, 8*(3), 317–321.

Lewine, J. D., & Orrison, W. W. (1995). Magnetoencephalography and magnetic source imaging. In W. W. Orrison, J. D. Lewine, J. A. Sanders, & M. F. Hartshorne (Eds.), *Functional Brain Imaging* (pp. 369–417). St. Louis, MO: Mosby.

Makeig, S., Bell, A. J., Jung, T. P., & Sejnowski, T. J. (1996). Independent component analysis of electroencephalographic data. In *Advances in Neural Information Processing Systems, 8* (pp. 145–151). Cambridge, MA: MIT Press.

Makeig, S., Jung, T. P., Bell, A. J., Ghahremani, D., & Sejnowski, T. J. (1997). Blind separation of auditory event-related brain responses into independent components. *Proceedings of the National Academy of Science USA, 94*(20), 10979–10984.

Makeig, S., Westerfield, M., Jung, T. P., Covington, J., Townsend, J., Sejnwoski, T. J., & Courchesne, E. (1999). Functionally independent components of the late positive event-related potential during visual spatial attention. *Journal of Neuroscience, 19*(7), 2665–2680.

Mosher, J. C., & Leahy, R. M. (1998). Recursive music: A frame-work for EEG and MEG source localization. *Institute of Electrical and Electronics Engineers Transactions on Biomedical Engineering, 45*(11), 1342–1354.

Mosher, J. C., & Leahy, R. M. (1999). Source localization using recursively applied projected (RAP) MUSIC. *Institute of Electrical and Electronics Engineers Transactions on Signal Processing, 47*(2), 332–340.

Mosher, J. C., Lewis, P. S., & Leahy, R. M. (1992). Multiple dipole modeling and localization from spatiotemporal MEG data. *Institute of Electrical and Electronics Engineers Transactions on Biomedical Engineering, 39*(6), 541–557.

Nagano, T., Ohno, Y., Uesugi, N., Ikeda, H., Ishiyama, A., & Kasai, N. (1998). Multi-source localization by genetic algorithm using MEG. *Institute of Electrical and Electronics Engineers Transactions on Magnetics, 34*(5/pt.1), 2976–2979.

Roberts, T., Ferrari, P., Stufflebeam, S., & Poeppel, D. (2000). Latency of the auditory evoked neuromagnetic field components: Stimulus dependence and insights toward perception. *Journal of Clinical Neurophysiology, 17*(2), 114–129.

Romani, G., Williamson, S., & Kaufman, L. (1982, June). Tonotopic organization of the human auditory cortex. *Science, 216*(4552), 1339–1340.

Schmidt, D. M., George, J. S., & Wood, C. C. (1999). Bayesian inference applied to the electromagnetic inverse problem. *Human Brain Mapping, 7*(3), 195–212.

Schwartz, D. P., Badier, J. M., Bihoue, P., & Bouliou, A. (1999). Evaluation of a new MEG-EEG spatio-temporal localization approach using a realistic source model. *Brain Topography, 11*(4), 279–289.

Sekihara, K., Nagarajan, S. S., Poeppel, D., Miyauchi, S., Fujimaki, N., Koizumi, H., & Miyashita, Y. (2000). Estimating neural sources from each time-frequency component of magnetoencephalographic data. *Institute of Electrical and Electronics Engineers Transactions on Biomedical Engineering, 47*(5), 642–653.

Sekihara, K., Poeppel, D., Marantz, A., Koizumi, H., & Miyashita, Y. (1997). Noise covariance incorporated MEG-MUSIC algorithm: A method for multiple-dipole estimation tolerant of the influence of background brain activity. *Institute of Electrical and Electronics Engineers Transactions on Biomedical Engineering, 44*(9), 839–847.

Supek, S., Aine, C. J., Ranken, D., Best, E., Flynn, E. R., & Wood, C. C. (1999). Single vs. paired visual stimulation: superposition of early neuromagnetic responses and retinotopy in extrastriate cortex in humans. *Brain Research, 830*(1), 43–55.

Tang, A. C., Pearlmutter, B. A., Malaszenko, N. A., Phung, D. B., & Reeb, B. C. (2002a). Localization of independent components of magnetoencephalography in cognitive tasks. *Neural Computation, 14*(8), 1827–1858.

Tang, A. C., Pearlmutter, B. A., Malaszenko, N. A., & Phung, D. B. (2002b). Independent components of magnetoencephalography: Single-trial response onset times. *NeuroImage, 17*(4), 233–240.

Tang, A. C., Pearlmutter, B. A., & Zibulevsky, M. (2000a). Blind separation of multichannel neuromagnetic responses. *Neural Computing, 32–33*, 1115–1120.

Tang, A. C., Pearlmutter, B. A., Zibulevsky, M., Hely, T. A., & Weisend, M. P. (2000b). An MEG study of response latency and variability in the human visual system during a visual-motor integration task. In *Advances in Neural Information Processing Systems, 12*, (pp.185–191). Cambridge, MA: MIT Press.

Tang, A. C., Phung, D., Pearlmutter, B. A., & Christner, R. (2000c). Localization of independent components from magnetoencephalography. In P. Pajunen & J. Karhunen (Eds.), *International Workshop on Independent Component Analysis and Blind Signal Separation* (pp. 387–392), Helsinki, Finland.

Uutela, K., Hämäläinen, M., & Salmelin, R. (1998). Global optimization in the localization of neuromagnetic sources. *Institute of Electrical and Electronics Engineers Transactions on Biomedical Engineering, 45*(6), 716–723.

Vigário, R., Jousmäki, V., Hämäläinen, M., Hari, R., & Oja, E. (1998). Independent component analysis for identification of artifacts in magnetoencephalographic recordings. In *Advances in Neural Information Processing Systems, 10* (pp. 229–235). Cambridge, MA: MIT Press.

Vigário, R., Särelä, J., Jousmäki, V., Hämäläinen, M., & Oja, E. (2000). Independent component approach to the analysis of EEG and MEG recordings. *Institute of Electrical and Electronics Engineers Transactions on Biomedical Engineering, 47*(5), 589–593.

Vigário, R., Sarela, J., Jousmaki, V., & Oja, E. (1999). Independent component analysis in decomposition of auditory and somatosensory evoked fields. In *Proceedings of the First International Conference on Independent Component Analysis and Blind Signal Separation ICA '99* (pp. 167–172), Aussois, France.

Williamson, S., Kaufman, L., Curtis, S., Lu, Z., Michel, C., & Wang, J. (1996). Neural substrates of working memories are revealed magnetically by the local suppression of alpha rhythm. *Electroencephalography and Clinical Neurophysiology Supplement, 47*, 163–180.

Wübbeler, G., Ziehe, A., Mackert, B. M., Müller, K. R., Trahms, L., & Curio, G. (2000). Independent component analysis of non-invasively recorded cortical magnetic DC-fields in humans. *Institute of Electrical and Electronics Engineers Transactions on Biomedical Engineering, 47*(5), 594–599.

Ziehe, A., Müller, K. R., Nolte, G., Mackert, B. M., & Curio, G. (2000). Artifact reduction in magnetoneurography based on time-delayed second order correlations. *Institute of Electrical and Electronics Engineers Transactions on Biomedical Engineering, 47*(1), 75–87.

# 7

# Toward Noise-Immune Magnetoencephalography Instrumentation

J. Vrba
S. E. Robinson
A. A. Fife
*CTF Systems, Inc.*

Whole-cortex magnetoencephalography (MEG) and fetal MEG (fMEG) systems produced by CTF Systems Inc. are described. These systems are operated with digitally based superconducting quantum interference device electronics with a 32-bit dynamic range and excellent linearity. The primary sensors are radial gradiometers with baselines selected for optimum signal-to-noise ratio. These systems are equipped with a powerful synthetic noise cancellation, which in combination with conventional biomagnetic shielded rooms provides noise cancellation in excess of 7 orders of magnitude and superior vibrational immunity.

CTF Systems Inc. has developed and produced superconducting quantum interference device (SQUID) sensors and instrumentation since 1970, and its experience encompasses both low- and high critical temperature (high-Tc) superconductors. Instruments developed during the early years include vector and tensor gradiometers for mobile applications, rock magnetometers, geomagnetometers, single-channel biomagnetometers, and hardware third-order gradiometers. In 1992 (Vrba et al., 1993), CTF was one of the first companies to introduce a whole-cortex magnetoencephalo-graphy (MEG) system, and in 1999 CTF developed a MEG system for measuring the extremely weak signals from the fetal cortex (Robinson et al., 2000). CTF's MEG systems incorporate a highly effective noise cancellation method that is based on higher order gradiometers. These instruments exhibit the best low-frequency noise characteristics available at present. CTF manufactures whole-cortex MEG systems with a wide range of MEG sensor channels, for example, 64, 143, 151, 275, where the system architecture is compatible with more than 740 channels. The system also allows inclusion of up to 128 electroencephalography (EEG) channels. CTF's digital SQUID electronics provides a 32-bit dynamic range, and its resident Digital Signal Processors (DSPs) and Programmable Gate Arrays (PGAs) can perform computationally expensive tasks in real time.

In this chapter we focus on CTF's MEG systems and describe the hardware, the noise cancellation methods, the software capabilities, and examples of measurements.

## HARDWARE

A schematic diagram of CTF's MEG system is shown in Fig. 7.1, and a photograph of the system with a supine patient is shown in Fig. 7.2a. The MEG system is usually sited within a magnetically shielded room (or it may be operated unshielded if the environmental noise is not too harsh). The MEG liquid helium dewar and the patient support operate with the patient in any position between seated and supine. The MEG and EEG

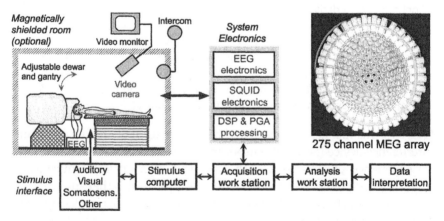

FIG. 7.1. A schematic diagram of CTF's magnetoencephalography (MEG; or fetal MEG) systems. A MEG sensor array with 275 channels is shown in the inset (for more information, see www.vsmmedtech.com).

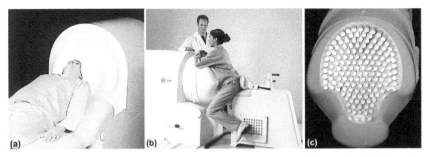

FIG. 7.2. Photographs of the CTF whole-cortex magnetoencephalography (MEG) and fetal MEG (fMEG) systems. Panel a: whole-cortex MEG system in position for supine measurement, Panel b: fMEG system in which mothers straddle and lean against the fMEG sensor array, Panel c: cutaway view of the 151-channel fMEG sensor array.

signals are connected to electronics outside the shielded room and are preprocessed before collection by a computer workstation.

The whole-cortex primary sensors are radial gradiometers with 5-cm baselines and 2-cm diameter coils, coupled to integrated, all-Nb DC SQUIDs based on $Nb-Al_2O_3-Nb$ trilayer junctions. These DC SQUIDs typically exhibit white energy sensitivities in the range of 1 to $4 \times 10^{-31}$ J/Hz. The system is also equipped with 29 reference SQUID sensors, located far from the subject head. The system white noise sensitivity is in the range of 3 to 7 fT rms/√Hz and, depending on the site, the onset of the observed low-frequency noise is in the range of 0.5 to 2 Hz.

CTF recently introduced a fetal MEG (fMEG) system. In this system, the dewar is horizontal, and the mother straddles the sensing region and leans her abdomen against the curved sensing surface (covering an area of about 1300 $cm^2$ extending from the perineal area to approximately the lower ribs). The fMEG primary sensors are radial gradiometers with 8-cm baselines and 2-cm diameters, and the system is also provided with 29 references for higher order gradiometer synthesis. A photograph of the mother seated on the system is shown in Fig. 7.2b, and a cutaway view of the sensors is shown in Fig. 7.2c.

The SQUID electronics (Fig. 7.3) operate each SQUID sensor in an analogue mode. After amplification, the SQUID outputs are digitized, and the feedback loop is closed digitally. The feedback loop is locked at an extremum of the SQUID transfer function and remains locked while the SQUID input is in the $\pm 1 \Phi_o$ range (Vrba, 2000). When this range is exceeded, the locking point is shifted along the transfer function, and the flux transitions along the transfer function are counted and used to extend the dynamic range to 32 bits. The measured nonlinearity is less than $10^{-6}$ at

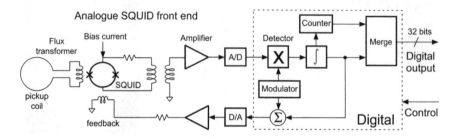

FIG. 7.3. A schematic diagram of CTF's digital superconducting interference device (SQUID) electronics for magnetoencephalography (MEG) and fetal MEG applications. The SQUID sensors are operated in analogue mode. The amplified SQUID signals are digitized, and the feedback loop is closed digitally.

1,000 $\Phi_o$ peak-to-peak input signal, and it is not known whether this is due to the measuring system or due to the SQUID and its electronics.

The electronics are stable and are based on "set and forget" tuning. The system architecture allows sample rates of up to 4 kHz for up to 384 channels. The electronics also provide for signal preprocessing (e.g., filtering, gradiometer synthesis, etc.), before data collection by computer, and the DSP and PGA computational power can be used for real time (or off-line) execution of computationally expensive tasks (e.g., covariance and crosspower updates, coherence calculations, spatial filtering, etc.). The system also allows for a maximum of 128 simultaneous EEG channels with $\leq 2$ $\mu$V rms noise in a 1-kHz bandwidth (dc or ac coupled).

The MEG system incorporates provisions to determine head position. For this, small coils are affixed to the nasion and preauricular points. These coils are energized at predetermined frequencies, and their magnetic signals are detected by the SQUID sensors. The positions of the coils can be determined with accuracy better than a fraction of a millimeter; determination of head position is limited only by the accuracy of coil placement. The system is also coupled to a stimulus delivery computer, which can control auditory, visual, somatosensory, and other stimuli.

## NOISE CANCELLATION

The noise in CTF's MEG systems is eliminated by the joint action of various additive methods: magnetic shielding, primary sensors with optimized signal-to-noise ratio (SNR), synthetic higher order gradiometers, frequency-independent and -dependent adaptation, and signal space methods. The shielding is accomplished by conventional magnetically shielded rooms for biomagnetism (Vacuumschmelze GmbH, Hanau, Germany, AK3b). Additional noise cancellation methods are used because even within shielded rooms, the residual environmental noise is large.

In this section we first discuss the synthetic higher order gradiometers and then describe the primary sensor design for optimum noise cancellation. We conclude the section with a discussion of methods for adaptive and signal space noise cancellation. Synthetic higher order gradiometers rely on low-order sensors (magnetometers or first-order gradiometers) and references sufficient for synthesis of the required gradiometer order (Vrba, 1996). An example of first-order gradiometer synthesis, using a magnetometer sensor and a reference vector magnetometer, is illustrated in Fig. 7.4a (Becker et al., 1993). If the vector of the applied magnetic field is denoted by **B,** and if the primary sensor magnetometer orientation is **p**, then the primary sensor output is $s = \alpha_s \mathbf{p} \cdot \mathbf{B}$, where $\alpha_s$ is the sensor gain. Assume that the reference vector magnetometer gains are the same and equal to $\alpha_r$. Then the reference outputs are $r_i = \alpha_r B_i$, $i = 1, 2, 3$. The first-order gradiometer can then be synthesized by subtracting from the sensor signal the properly scaled reference output projected to the vector **p**:

$$g^{(1)} = s - \frac{\alpha_s}{\alpha_r}(\mathbf{p} \cdot \mathbf{r}) = \alpha_s \mathit{p} G b_1 \quad , \tag{7.1}$$

where **G** is the first gradient tensor and $\mathbf{b}_1$ is the synthetic gradiometer baseline. The righthand side of Equation 7.1 indicates that the synthetic gradiometer is a projection of the first gradient tensor onto the magnetometer orientation vector **p** and the baseline $\mathbf{b}_1$.

The second-order gradiometers can be synthesized in an analogous manner. Assume that the primary sensor is a first-order hardware gradiometer with baseline $\mathbf{b}_1$ and coil orientation **p**. The reference is a first gradiometer tensor detector positioned at a distance $\mathbf{b}_2$ from the primary sensor, as in Fig. 7.4b. The second-order gradiometer can again be synthesized by subtracting from the primary sensor, a properly scaled reference projection. The result can be expressed as

$$g^{(2)} = \alpha_{G1} \mathit{p} G^{(2)} b_1 b_2 \quad , \tag{7.2}$$

where $\alpha_{G1}$ is the primary gradiometer gain and $G^{(2)}$ is the second gradient tensor. The synthetic second-order gradiometer output is a projection of the second gradient tensor onto the vectors **p**, $\mathbf{b}_1$, and $\mathbf{b}_2$.

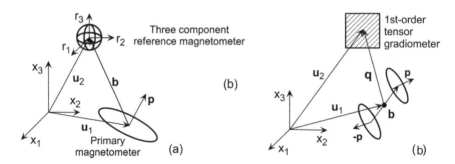

FIG. 7.4.    Illustration of gradiometer synthesis. Panel a: synthesis of a first-order gradiometer from a primary magnetometer sensor and a vector magnetometer reference. From "Signal Processing in Magnetoencephalography" by J. Vrba and S. E. Robinson, 2001, *Methods, 25,* p. 262. Copyright 2001 by Academic Press. Adapted by permission. Panel b: synthesis of a second-order gradiometer from a hardware first-order gradiometer and a first-order gradiometer tensor reference.

The procedure just described is readily generalized to synthetic gradiometers of any order and may be based on primary sensors of any order. In a general case, the references contain a mixture of magnetometers and gradiometers and, in addition to gradiometer synthesis, they are also used to cancel the common mode errors of the primary sensors.

Unlike adaptive noise cancellation methods, the synthetic gradiometer subtraction coefficients, between the references and the primary sensors, are fixed and predetermined at the time of manufacture; that is, they are independent of time, the noise character, and the dewar orientation. When the reference sensors are properly designed, the synthetic gradiometers do not significantly reduce signal; in fact, they can slightly increase or reduce it (see Fig. 7.5a; (Vrba, Cheung, Taylor, & Robinson, 1999). Synthetic gradiometers provide significant noise cancellation; however, they do not introduce white noise. This property is illustrated in Fig. 7.5b, where above about 5 Hz, the hardware (first-) and synthetic third-order gradiometer white noise levels are the same. The third-order gradiometers eliminate frequency lines above about 10 Hz. At low frequencies, third-order gradiometers detect about four orders of magnitude lower noise than magnetometers, and the combination of the AK3b shielded room and synthetic third-order gradiometers provides overall noise attenuation of nearly six orders of magnitude.

In addition to the noise attenuation by synthetic gradiometers, environmental noise can be canceled adaptively. If the noise is stationary, and the dewar is not moved, adaptive noise cancellation performs slightly

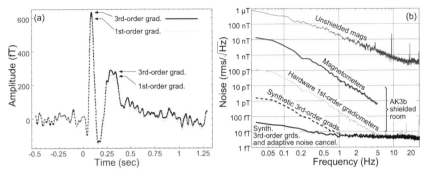

FIG. 7.5.    Illustration of synthetic higher order gradiometer performance. Panel a: synthetic gradiometers do not reduce the detected signal. For the auditory evoked fields, the signal of the synthetic third-order gradiometer is *larger* than the signal of its hardware first-order gradiometer primary sensor. From "Signal Processing in Magnetoencephalography" by J. Vrba and S. E. Robinson, 2001, *Methods, 25,* p. 263. Copyright 2001 by Academic Press. Adapted by permission. Panel b: synthetic gradiometers do not increase white noise levels, although they provide dramatic reduction of the environmental noise. The lower four curves indicate environmental noise detected within an AK3b shielded room (Vacuumschmelze GmbH, Hanau, Germany) by magnetometers, hardware first-order gradiometers, and synthetic third-order gradiometers with and without adaptive noise cancellation. The upper curve indicates unshielded noise at the same site. From "Magnetoencephalography: The Art of Finding a Needle in a Haystack" by J. Vrba, 2002, *Physica C,* 368, p. 4. Copyright 2002 by Elsevier Science. Adapted by permission.

better than with gradiometers with respect to the environmental noise but not relative to the white noise (Vrba, 2000). However, as commonly observed at MEG laboratories, the time intervals during which the noise remains stationary are short, often only a few seconds or minutes. Only if the noise is due to a well-defined process (e.g. a train moving along a fixed track), and the periods of stationarity are long, can the same adaptive coefficients be used as long as the dewar orientation is unchanged. However, if the character of the environmental noise changes, then the adaptive coefficients must be re-evaluated. Figure 7.5b illustrates that, within the shielded room, the noise of third-order gradiometers with additional adaptive noise cancellation is about 5.5 orders of magnitude lower than that of the magnetometers, and the combined noise attenuation by the synthetic gradiometers, adaptive noise cancellation, and the shielded room is about 7.5 orders of magnitude lower. This performance matches or exceeds the noise cancellation for magnetometers in the best shielded room available at present (Bork, Hahlbohm, Klein, & Schnabel, 2001). Adaptation can also be performed in a frequency-dependent fashion.

We have discussed the noise cancellation by synthetic gradiometers and by adaptation for arbitrarily defined primary sensors. However, the primary sensors themselves can also be optimized to improve the overall SNR.

First, consider radial gradiometer or magnetometer primary sensors. *Radial gradiometers* in this context refers to differential magnetometers with finite baselines. The analysis also includes magnetometers that are equivalent to gradiometers with infinite baselines. The SNR of these devices can be optimized by the proper choice of the baseline length. The magnetic signal detected from a near-field source increases with increasing baseline, while the environmental noise due to distant sources also increases with baseline (Figs. 7.6a and b, respectively). Because the near-field source and interference are at different distances from the sensor, it follows that there is an optimum baseline for which SNR is maximized (Fig. 7.6c). Based on the noise measured within shielded rooms at various MEG sites (Fig. 7.5b), we show that the optimum baselines are short, usually in the range of 3 cm to 8 cm (Vrba, 1997) and, as a result, short-baseline radial gradiometers yield better results than magnetometers or long-baseline gradiometers.

The choice between radial and planar primary gradiometers was made by comparing their respective dipole reconstruction accuracy. The re-

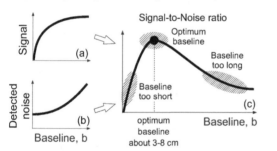
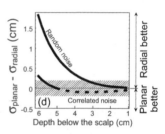

FIG. 7.6.  Optimization of the primary flux transformers. Panels a–c: optimization of the radial gradiometer baseline. Panel a: detected brain signal increases with increasing baseline, Panel b: detected environmental noise also increases with increasing baseline, Panel c: the SNR exhibits a maximum at some optimum baseline, Panel d: the difference of the standard deviations σ of the dipole localization error for planar and radial gradiometers in the presence of random or correlated noise as a function of the depth below the scalp. Solid lines represent radial gradiometers, which yield smaller localization errors; dashed lines represent planar gradiometers, which yield smaller localization errors; the shaded band represents mechanical uncertainty of the head localization. Random noise calculations: bandwidth = 100 Hz, white noise of planar and radial gradiometers, $n_w$ = 5 fT rms/√Hz. Correlated noise calculation: bandwidth = 100 Hz, number of averages = 100, brain noise density detected by radial gradiometers $n_{br}$ = 30 fT rms/√Hz and by planar gradiometers $n_{bp}$ = 15 fT rms/√Hz. From "Signal Processing in Magnetoencephalography" by J. Vrba and S. E. Robinson, 2001, *Methods, 25,* p. 256. Copyright 2001 by Academic Press. Adapted by permission.

sults are shown in Fig. 7.6d. When random noise is the dominant noise source, radial gradiometers clearly yield better results, because the planar gradiometer depth resolution is worse than that for radial gradiometers. Also, the information content of the planar gradiometer array is smaller (per channel) than that of the radial gradiometer array (Knuutila et al., 1993). For uncorrelated and environmental noise, radial gradiometers with synthetic third-order gradiometer noise cancellation produce significantly better results than planar gradiometers (Vrba & Robinson, 1999). For correlated noise (e.g., brain noise from the regions that are of no interest), the planar gradiometers produce slightly better results for more superficial sources (Knuutila et al., 1993). However, this advantage is smaller than the usual inaccuracy of head localization or registration with magnetic resonance imaging (MRI). Overall, radial gradiometers represent a better design choice in more measurement situations and for these reasons were chosen for the CTF MEG systems.

In addition to synthetic gradiometers, adaptive techniques, and primary sensor optimization, the CTF instrumentation also includes an option to eliminate the noise by signal space methods. Once the signal space noise vectors have been determined (e.g., Parkkonen, Simola, Tuoriniemi, & Ahonen, 1999), they can be used to form the noise vector matrix $\mathbf{V}$, and projected out from the signal using the projection operator $\mathbf{I} - \mathbf{V}(\mathbf{V}^T\mathbf{V})^{-1}\mathbf{V}^T$. Alternatively, the environmental noise can be eliminated by beamforming methods, for example, synthetic aperture magnetometry (SAM) (Robinson & Vrba, 1999).

The ability of synthetic gradiometers to provide a vibrationally stable system is illustrated in Figs. 7.7a and b, where synthetic gradiometers eliminate vibrational noise due to head motion. The noise cancellation by synthetic gradiometers is further illustrated in Fig. 7.7c, where interictal epilepsy spikes were measured in an unshielded environment (Fife et al., 1999; Vrba, Cheung, et al., 1999).

## SOFTWARE AND EXAMPLES OF RESULTS

A flow diagram of CTF's MEG software in Fig. 7.8 shows two principal modes of operation: (a) the SQUID electronics setup mode and (b) data acquisition and processing. The noise cancellation, as outlined in the preceding section, is embedded in this CTF software and is an important prerequisite for signal processing. In addition, the CTF software provides a range of display and interpretational techniques, including maps, traces, integration with MRI, dipole analysis, beamformers (SAM or conventional linearly con-

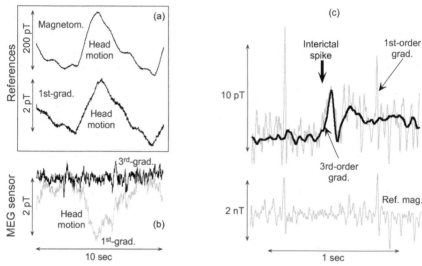

FIG. 7.7. Vibrational stability of and noise cancellation by synthetic third-order gradiometers. Panels a and b: demonstration of vibrational stability during the measurement of an epileptic patient with head motion (Vrba, McCubbin, & Robinson, 1999), shielded environment, bandwidth DC to 70 Hz, head motion approximately 10 sec before the onset of the seizure. Panel a: a reference magnetometer and a gradiometer; Panel b: sensor SR26 in hardware first-order gradiometer and synthetic third-order gradiometer modes. From "Signal Processing in Magnetoencephalography" by J. Vrba and S. E. Robinson, 2001, *Methods, 25,* p. 263. Copyright 2001 by Academic Press. Adapted by permission. Panel c: interictal epilepsy spike measured in an unshielded environment (Fife et al., 1999; Vrba, Cheung, et al., 1999). The patient was an 8-year-old boy with a small head, resulting in 3- to 4-cm gaps between the scalp and the helmet surfaces. Bandwidth DC to 40 Hz, channel MRO22. Gray lines represent the hardware first-order gradiometer primary sensor and the reference magnetometer; the black line represents synthetic third-order gradiometer.

strained minimum variance beamformers), multiple signal classification (MUSIC), minimum norm, and so on. The software also allows for batch processing and scripting of both the collection and processing procedures.

Examples of MEG results and processing methods are shown in Figs. 7.9a–e. The somatosensory evoked field (SEF) due to the mechanical stimulation of the right index finger collected in an unshielded environment is shown in Fig. 7.9a and b. Figure 7.9a shows that large environmental noise exists even after the data averaging (the data were low-pass filtered to eliminate the power lines and their harmonics). The environmental noise is eliminated by the synthesis of third-order gradiometers (Fig. 7.9b).

The software allows for standard single- and multiple-dipole analyses as indicated in Fig. 7.9c and for more sophisticated array processing methods such as MUSIC, linear beamformers, and SAM. An example of

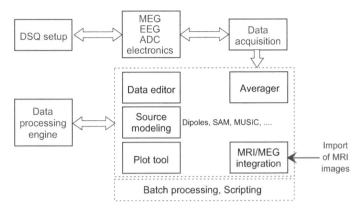

FIG. 7.8. Schematic diagram of CTF System's Inc.'s magnetoencephalography software.

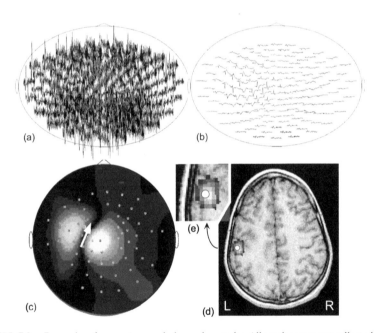

FIG. 7.9. Examples of magnetoencephalography results. All results were not collected at the same location. Panel a: SEF data measured in an unshielded environment with first-order gradiometers. Mechanical stimulation of the right index finger tip, randomized interstimulus interval = 0.6–0.9 sec, 300 averages, trial duration = 0.41 sec, bandwidth dc to 50 Hz. Panel b: the same SEF data after noise cancellation by synthetic third-order gradiometer; Panel c: dipole analysis of SEF data; Panel d: synthetic aperture magnetometry (SAM) and dipole analyses of SEF data evoked by electrical stimulation of the right median nerve, bandwidth 30–100 Hz. The dipole is represented by a black-rimmed white dot overlaid on the SAM result. Panel e: enlarged region around the source in Panel d. For more information, visit www.vsmmedtech.com

the electrically stimulated median nerve analysis is shown in Fig. 7.9d. The unaveraged signals were analyzed by SAM and are superposed on an MRI axial slice. The active region outlined by SAM corresponds well with the P50 dipole analysis of the averaged signals (3.4% fit error), which is shown by a black-rimmed white dot.

## CONCLUSIONS

During the last 10 years, CTF Systems Inc. has developed a range of whole-cortex and MEG instrumentation with robust performance and with little need for maintenance or periodic retuning. These systems exhibit high sensitivity, and their unique noise cancellation, based on synthetic higher order gradiometers, provide excellent noise immunity and stability against vibrations. The primary sensors are radial gradiometers with baselines selected for optimum SNR. The system electronics operate on digital principles and provide wide dynamic range and the capability of real-time processing of computationally expensive tasks.

## ACKNOWLEDGMENT

We thank D. Cheyne for providing the data for Figs. 7.9a and 7.9b, G. Haid for providing the photographs in Fig. 7.2, and S. Lee and K. Betts for clarifying software and electronics issues.

## REFERENCES

Becker, W., Diekmann, V., Jurgens, R., & Kornhuber, C. (1993). First experiences with a multi-channel software gradiometer recording normal and tangential components of MEG. *Physiological Measurement 14,* A45–A50.

Bork, J., Hahlbohm, H.-D., Klein, R., & Schnabel, A. (2001). The 8-layered magnetically shielded room of the PTB: Design and construction In J. Nenonen, R. Ilmoniemi, & T. Katila (Eds.), *Preeedings of the 12th International Conference on Biomagnetism* (pp. 970–973). Finland: Helsinki University of Technology.

Fife, A. A., Vrba, J., Robinson, S. E., Anderson, G., Betts, K., Burbank, M. B., Cheyne, D., Cheung, T., Govorkow, S., Haid, G., Haid, V., Hunter, C., Kubik, P. R., Lee, S., McKay, J., Reichl, E., Schroyen, C., Sekachev, I., Spear, P., Taylor, B., Tillotson, M., & Sutherling, W. (1999). Synthetic gradiometer systems for MEG. *IEEE Transactions on Applied Superconductivity, 9,* 4063–4068.

Knuutila, K. E. T., Ahonen, A. I., Hamalainen, M. S., Kajola, M. J., Laine, P. P., Lounasmaa, O. V., et al. (1993). A 122-channel whole-cortex SQUID system for measuring the brain's magnetic fields. *IEEE Transactions on Magnetics, 29,* 3315–3320.

Parkkonen, L. T., Simola, J. T., Tuoriniemi, J. T., & Ahonen, A. I. (1999). An interference suppression system for multichannel magnetic field detector arrays. In T. Yoshimoto, M. Kotani, S. Kuriki, H. Karibe, & N. Nakasato (Eds.), *Recent advances in biomagnetism* (pp. 13–16). Tohoku, Japan: Tohoku University Press.

Robinson, S. E., Burbank, M. B., Fife, A. A., Haid, G., Kubik, P. R., Sekachev, I., Taylor, B., Tillotson, M., Vrba, J., Wong, G., Lowery, C., Eswaran, H., Wilson, D., Murphy, P., & Preissl, H. (2000). A biomagnetic system for human reproductive assessment. In J. Nenonen, R.

Ilmoniemi, & T. Katila (Eds.), *Biomag2000, Proc. 12th Int. Conf. on Biomagnetism* (pp. 919–922). Espoo, Finland: Helsinki University of Technology.

Robinson, S. E., & Vrba, J. (1999). Functional neuroimaging by synthetic aperture magnetometry (SAM). In T. Yoshimoto, M. Kotani, S. Kuriki, H. Karibe, & N. Nakasato (Eds.), *Recent advances in biomagnetism* (pp. 302–305). Tohoku, Japan: Tohoku University Press.

Vrba, J. (1996). SQUID gradiometers in real environments. In H. Weinstock (Ed.), *SQUID sensors: Fundamentals, fabrication and applications* (pp. 117–178). Dordrecht, the Netherlands: Kluwer Academic.

Vrba, J. (1997). Baseline optimization for noise cancellation systems. In *Proceedings of the 19th International Conference of IEEE-EMBS*, B. Feinberg (Ed.), CD-ROM (pp.1240–1243).

Vrba, J. (2000). Multichannel SQUID biomagnetic systems. In H. Weinstock (Ed.), *Applications of superconductivity* (pp. 61–138). Dordrecht, the Netherlands: Kluwer Academic.

Vrba, J. (2002). Magnetoencephalography: The art of finding a needle in a haystack. *Physica C, 368,* 1–9.

Vrba, J., Betts, K., Burbank, M. B., Cheung, T., Fife, A. A., Haid, G., Kubik, P. R., Lee, S., McCubbin, J., McKay, J., McKenzie, D., Spear, P., Taylor, B., Tillotson, M., Cheyne, D., & Weinberg, H. (1993). Whole cortex 64 channel SQUID biomagnetometer system. *IEEE Transactions on Applied Superconductivity, 3,* 1878–1882.

Vrba, J., Cheung, T., Taylor, B., & Robinson, S. E. (1999). Synthetic higher-order gradiometers reduce environmental noise, not the measured brain signals. In T. Yoshimoto, M. Kotami, S. Kuriki, H. Karibe, & N. Nakasato (Eds.), *Recent advances in biomagnetism* (pp. 105–108). Tohoku, Japan: Tohoku University Press.

Vrba, J., McCubbin, J., & Robinson, S. E. (1999). Vibration analysis of MEG systems. In T. Yoshimoto, M. Kotami, S. Kuriki, H. Karibe, & N. Nakasato (Eds.), *Recent advances in biomagnetism* (pp. 109–112). Tohoku, Japan: Tohoku University Press.

Vrba, J., & Robinson, S. E. (1999). Detection probability curves for evaluating localization algorithms and comparing sensor array types. In T. Yoshimoto, M. Kotami, S. Kuriki, H. Karibe, & N. Nakasato (Eds.), *Recent advances in biomagnetism* (pp. 97–100). Tohoku, Japan: Tohoku University Press.

Vrba, J., & Robinson, S. E. (2001). Signal processing in magnetoencephalography. *Methods 25,* 249–271.

# 8

---

# Full-Sensitivity Biomagnetometers: Sam Williamson's Vision Brought to Life

R. T. Johnson
E. C. Hirschkoff
D. S. Buchanan
*4-D Neuroimaging*

The advent of superconducting magnetometers in the 1960s enabled for the first time the practical detection of the minute magnetic fields produced by the natural functioning of the human brain and neurologic system. In this chapter we review the evolution of the first primitive magnetometers into the practical whole-head recording systems available today. Sam Williamson, a pioneer in this science, urged commercial developers of these systems to strive for the maximum sensitivity that the superconducting quantum interference device would allow and to never "hardwire" in sensitivity reductions. This impetus led 4-D Neuroimaging to focus its development on the use of magnetometer-style signal coils that met Williamson's standard. Starting with basic physics arguments, continuing with implementation techniques, and concluding with samples of actual data, we present the case for the use of these signal coils (as opposed to gradiometers).

## THE HISTORY

Sam Williamson has influenced 4-D Neuroimaging from the very early days of the company; one could reasonably say that Sam helped to create 4-D. The company started in 1970 as S.H.E. (Superconductivity, Helium, Electronics) Corporation, manufacturing instruments and systems based on important advances in low-temperature physics. SHE manufactured the first commercial superconducting quantum interference device (SQUID) sensors and built them into a variety of standard and special scientific systems—for example, dilution refrigerators, variable-temperature susceptometers, geomagnetic sensors, biomagnetic sensors. In the mid 1970s, Sam and his close colleague Lloyd Kaufman asked SHE to build for them a single-channel magnetometer that could be used to detect the magnetic fields produced by the natural functioning of the human body. After agreeing on a system that could realistically be designed and built, they placed an order for that first system. In 1976, SHE delivered a single-channel second-order axial gradiometer sensor. Shortly thereafter, Sam and Lloyd used this magnetometer for measurements of brain activity associated with the stimulation of the fingers of the hand, demonstrating the localizing capability of magnetic measurements (see Brenner, Lipton, Kaufman, & Williamson, 1978).

In the early 1980s, Sam and Lloyd again came to SHE—this time to ask the company to design and build a multichannel biomagnetometer system. It had become very apparent that measuring the magnetic field over the head at one location at a time placed very stringent limits on what practical localization recordings were possible. Their experience to that point convinced company officials not only to share the costs of designing and building a five-channel system for them but also that measuring biomagnetic signals had a potentially large commercial future. On the basis of this assessment, SHE's officials switched the company's focus to biomagnetism—changing its name to Biomagnetic Technologies, Inc. (BTi)—and started the development of multichannel biomagnetometer systems. BTi provided the five-channel system to Sam and Lloyd at Washington Square, New York University, in 1985. Shortly thereafter, BTi supplied two 7-channel systems to Bellevue Hospital of the New York University Medical Center. Even as BTi pursued the commercial development of biomagnetism, Sam continued to prod and poke the company in new technical directions. In the late 1980s, Sam and BTi worked together to develop the first commercial mechanically cooled biomagnetometer: CryoSQUID™.

A dual CryoSQUID™ system was installed in Sam's laboratory and used in conjunction with the existing five-channel system.

From that time on, BTi has developed systems with much greater numbers of channels and much greater data-processing capabilities. The company has continually worked to provide top-quality, user-friendly systems for clinical users while still maintaining the flexibility and system control demanded by researchers. In the late 1980s, a system with 37 signal channels in a circular pattern on a concave surface was introduced for the BTi line of biomagnetometers; the name Magnes® was introduced for this sensor. By its shape, this 37-channel sensor was useful for the measurement of brain, cardiac, gastrointestinal, fetal cardiac, and spinal cord signals. The company collaborated with researchers to understand and facilitate their work in each of these areas; it also worked with medical sites at hospitals to assist in the development of clinical applications. The next step in Magnes sensor technology was the development of a second 37-signal channel sensor wherein the signal channels were oriented vertically upward; thus, the two 37-channel sensors could be used in a single system (called Magnes–II), allowing simultaneous measurement of signals from

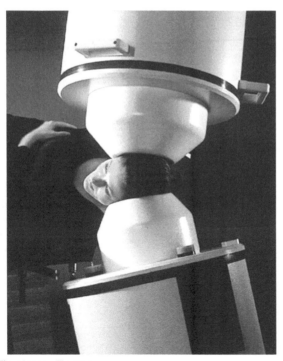

FIG. 8.1.   The Magnes–II system.

both sides of the brain (see Fig. 8.1). This pair of sensors provided measurement capability for most of the biomagnetic signals of interest, although positioning the patient between the sensors took time. The Magnes–II system provided the primary instrument for the initial development of the clinical use of magnetoencephalography for epilepsy.

As the field of magnetoencephalography advanced, the development of a whole-head sensor specifically designed to measure the biomagnetic activity in the human brain received greater focus. In 1996, BTi came out with its first whole-head system, the Magnes 2500 WH, with 148 magnetometer signal channels and 8 reference coils for noise reduction (see Fig. 8.2). This was followed in 1999 by the Magnes 3600 WH, a 248-signal channel system with 14 reference coils. Concurrently with these system developments, the company has worked with regulatory agencies to ensure that it meets the requirements for a clinical medical device manufacturer, and it has championed the technology with clinicians and insurance companies to establish reimbursement for various clinical measurement protocols. (In the spring of 2001, the American Medical Association approved reimbursement codes [Current Procedural Terminology codes] for two neuromagnetic procedures: (a) presurgical evaluation of patients with epilepsy and (b) functional mapping for surgical planning. These codes

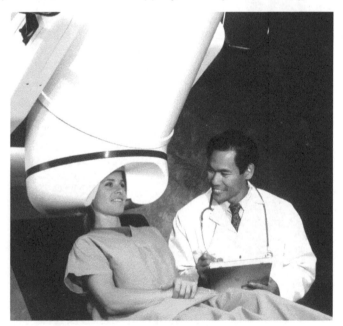

FIG. 8.2.   The Magnes 2500 WH in seated position.

were published in November 2001.) In December 1999, BTi merged with one of its chief competitors, Neuromag Oy, based in Finland (see chap. 9). This merger created 4-D Neuroimaging. The biomagnetometers developed by both BTi and Neuromag Oy continue to be manufactured, improved, and serviced by 4-D Neuroimaging.

## THE LEGACY

One lesson that Sam always stressed to BTi was that the maximum detector sensitivity should always be sought to enable ultimate recording of deep brain activity. Although there are often compromises in system design that trade off basic detector sensitivity against the practicalities of operating in a hospital environment, if at all possible do not hard wire into the system limits on using the full sensitivity of a SQUID; instead, apply desensitizing measures required for reliable operation in a way that can be "turned off" as other software methods or external measures for noise reduction become available, thus preserving the basic capability for full SQUID sensitivity.

To date, manufacturers have provided three types of sensing coils for sensor signal channels: (a) magnetometers, (b) axial first-order gradiometers, and (c) planar first-order gradiometers (see chap. 1). The signal-to-noise of the data from these signal channels have been enhanced with various environmental noise reduction techniques. There has been much discussion about which of these types of signal coils provides the optimum system. 4-D has chosen to offer systems with any of the three types of signal coils. Users can choose the type that best meets their needs. As specific clinical applications develop, an optimum system may be revealed. Perhaps, depending on the application, the optimum system will use a combination of signal coil types—as offered in the 4-D Vectorview system, which uses both magnetometer and planar gradiometer signal coils, or the 4-D Magnes systems, which offer combinations of magnetometer and axial gradiometer coils.

However, based on first principles, on basic physics, magnetometer signal coils provide the full SQUID sensitivity that Sam urged the company to preserve. First-order gradiometer signal coils by their very design, either axial or planar, measure only the difference between the magnetic fields at two nearby locations, not the values of those fields themselves. Because the magnetic field produced by an environmental noise source located far away is very nearly the same at these two locations, the difference between them is very nearly zero; thus, the effect of the noise source is eliminated from the output. For the sources of interest in the brain, however, these gradiometer coils also measure the difference in the magnetic field at the two locations, and that difference is both small and decreases very rapidly with distance from the source, so such sensor coils are much less sensitive to deeper sources in the brain.

By contrast, a magnetometer signal coil detects the value of the field itself at the location of the coil. The output of such a signal coil obviously contains signals from both the source of interest in the brain and from all the environmental noise sources as well, all mixed together. However, by using a separate set of detecting coils (called *reference coils*) located far from the magnetometer signal coils themselves to measure the environmental noise alone, and then subtracting the contribution of the noise source from the signal coil output, 4-D has been able to retain the maximum possible sensitivity for measuring sources throughout the brain. We describe in detail this noise elimination process (commercially called *noise reduction*) later.

A useful measure of system performance is a well-defined quantity called *detectability*. Detectability is basically the magnitude of a current dipole source at a specified location within a volume conductor that will have a signal-to-noise ratio of 1 when measured with a given sensor comprising an array of $N$ detection coils. The details of detectability were given by Johnson, Black, and Buchanan (2000). Figure 8.3 is a reproduction from their article. In this figure, M is a 160-channel system with magnetometer signal coils, AG is a 160-channel axial gradiometer system (5-cm baseline), and PG is a 136-channel planar gradiometer system (1.65-cm baseline) with 2 orthogonal planar gradiometers located at each of 68 sites. All three systems have comparable areas of coverage. The minimum detectable dipole is determined from this plot by multiplying the plotted values by the SQUID noise for the signal channels. At present, all commercial systems have comparable system white noise levels, approximately 5 fT/√Hz in magnetic field units. This noise level is after application of the noise reduction techniques referred to earlier which, in a magnetically shielded room (MSR), removed essentially all of the environmental noise above the SQUID noise in the typical installation. It is clear from Fig. 8.3 that the optimum system, particularly when dealing with deep signal sources and sophisticated noise reduction technology, is one with magnetometer signal coils.

Deep, or distant, signal sources often occur in practice. For example, epileptic signal sources often occur in the mesial temporal region of the brain. Distant sources are even more relevant with the current fixed-shell whole-head systems, which must be sized to accept the

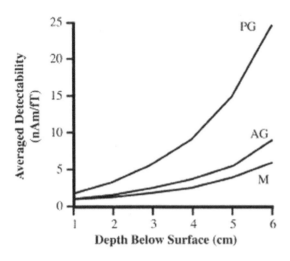

FIG. 8.3. Detectability for three arrays averaged over polar angles between 0 and 60° in the mid-coronal (Y–Z) plane as a function of depth below the surface of the head sphere. The source current is oriented along the $X$ axis (anterior direction). The three sensor arrays are described in the text: PG, planar gradiometer; AG, axial gradiometer; m, magnetometer. From Source Detectability for Multichannel Biomagnetic Sensors, by R. T. Johnson, W. C. Black, & D. S. Buchanan, 2000, in *Biomag 96, Proceedings of the Tenth International Conference on Biomagnetism, Volume 1* (pp. 59–62), edited by C. J. Aine, Y. Okada, G. Stroink, S. J. Swithenby, & C. C. Wood. New York: Springer-Verlag. Copyright © 2000. Reprinted with permission.

largest head of interest. In such an instance, the head of a young child would be much smaller than the whole-head sensor shell, and regions in the child's brain, even when near the brain surface, might be rather far from the signal coils; this is particularly true if the region of interest is not known or if simultaneous brain activity on both sides of the head is of interest.

## CONTROLLING THE ENVIRONMENT

It is desirable to remove as much of the noise of the environment as possible from the measured signals, to maximize the available sensitivity. Environmental noise is a major limitation in all real environments, especially hospitals. This noise includes signals from a variety of sources, prominent among which are magnetic signals from nearby motor and hospital conveyance vehicle traffic (e.g., automobiles, elevators); pumps and other electric motors; power line frequency signals; and high-frequency noise from communication, radio, and TV transmitters. High frequency noise is handled well by MSRs that are manufactured using high-permeability and high electrical conductivity materials; because of the inclusion of high-permeability materials, MSRs also reduce environmental noise down to low frequencies, including DC. However, the reduction of magnetic noise at frequencies below ~200 Hz (which includes the third harmonic of line-frequency signals) requires additional efforts. For this reason, a novel magnetic noise reduction approach was developed for the 4-D Magnes systems with magnetometer signal coils.

Magnes systems have eight or more reference coils that are used to measure the environmental magnetic noise. For the purposes of this discussion, consider the minimum configuration of eight coils: three orthogonal magnetometer coils and five first-order gradiometer coils. These coils are located in a space above the signal coil array, approximately 20–40 cm from the signal coils. The location of the reference coils is chosen as an optimum compromise between two competing factors: (a) being far enough away so that the signals of interest detected by the signal coils are minimally detected by the reference coils and (b) being close enough that the environmental magnetic noise seen by the reference coils is very similar to that seen by the signal coils. The five gradiometer reference coils are sufficient to determine all nine first derivatives of the magnetic field at the location of these coils; this follows from two of Maxwell's equations: $\nabla \times \mathbf{B} = \mathbf{0}$ in free space, and $\nabla \cdot \mathbf{B} = 0$. Thus, using the signals measured in the reference coils we can estimate the magnetic field at any signal coil. This estimation is then subtracted from the signal-channel signals to remove the environmental noise it represents. The reference coils measure the magnetic field and its first-order spatial derivatives, providing accurate estimations of environmental noise to first order. The use of an MSR tends to make the internal magnetic fields more uniform so that the assumption of linearly varying environmental noise signals is quite accurate. In practice, a very significant reduction in environmental noise signals is obtained. In typical environments, the SQUID noise is the limiting factor of the measurements.

## THE DETAILS

In all currently implemented noise reduction schemes that use reference channels, a weighted sum of the reference channel signals is created specific to each signal channel to estimate the size of the interfering environmental noise. This can be expressed as:

$$S_j'(t) = S_j(t) - \sum_i a_{ji} R_i(t) \qquad\qquad 8.1$$

where $S_j'(t)$ is the noise reduced signal for the $j$th channel, $S_j(t)$ is the signal before noise reduction, $R_i(t)$ is the measurement of the environmental noise by the $i^{th}$ reference channel, and the $a_{ji}$ are the weights coupling the $j^{th}$ signal channel with the $i^{th}$ reference channel—as indicated, the $a_{ji}$ are independent of time. Because this reduction term can be interpreted as a geometrical expression for the field at the location of signal coil $j$ based on the value of the field and field gradients at another point (the location of the reference array), the weights $a_{ji}$ could in principle be calculated from the relative locations and orientations of the reference coils and the signal coils. However, the locations, orientations, and sensitivities of the signal and reference coils are not generally known to sufficient precision to allow a sufficiently precise calculation of the optimum values of the weights.

To determine the weights, an *expectation approach* is used, based on the observation that the optimum set of weights—that is, those weights that minimize the noise in the signal channels—will minimize the total power present in the signal channels in the absence of signals from the brain or body. Using a broad spectrum of noise measurements made with no patient in the MSR, an algorithm is used to determine the set of weights that minimizes the power in the signal-channel signals. Within the limits of the known geometry, the weight values determined in this way qualitatively agree with their expected values. Given the stability of the system, both structurally and electronically, one would not expect the weights to vary from week to week or with the position of the sensor inside the MSR. Both of these properties are qualitatively observed in practice. Because of specific noise sources at sites, one often determines slight variations in weights for the different sensor positions that provide improved performance. To account for variations in the environment over time, these optimized weights can be rapidly and easily recalculated as needed.

If doing so would be beneficial for specific experimental conditions, the same software just described can be used to further reduce the noise in the data collected during a subject measurement. Weights optimized to unusual noise sources that are active during an acquisition can be determined, and then these weights may be applied to the acquired data in a postprocessing step. This is a completely safe noise reduction step as long as the signals of interest are below the noise, as is the case when using the system to measure very small brain signals. The weights determined will then be chosen to minimize the remnant noise and will have minimal effect on the signals of interest. After the application of these postprocessing weights, signals would be further processed using filtering, averaging, and so on.

This noise reduction technique has, at times, been considered equivalent to a long-baseline gradiometer. Although this analogy has some in-structural value, it can be highly misleading if extended too far. In fact, significantly higher levels of noise reduction are produced by this scheme compared with a simple long-baseline gradiometer because of its adaptive and multidimensional nature.

An axial gradiometer can be viewed as a signal coil and a reference coil with a fixed weight. Each coil measures a signal, and the signal in the reference coil is subtracted from the signal in the signal coil. In the Magnes approach, however, the weight can be adjusted, and very slight variations in weight can significantly improve the noise reduction. Obviously, there is also increased flexibility in the Magnes approach, because the "equivalent" long baseline "bucking coil" is actually eight coils, each with a separately determined weight. As a simplified example of the difference between a long-baseline axial gradiometer and the magnetometer-plus-reference-array approach, consider Fig. 8.4, in which an axial gradiometer has two coils separated by a 20-cm baseline distance and a noise source represented as a coil in the plane of the signal coil at a distance $d$ from the signal coil. The graph in Fig. 8.4 shows the weight factor that would perfectly cancel a noise signal produced by the coil a distance $d$ away. A hard-wired axial gradiometer uses a fixed-weight factor of –1.0. The 4-D method can select a weight factor to minimize noise. The figure shows that for a signal source

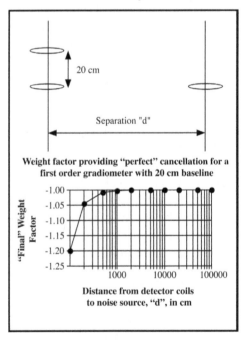

FIG. 8.4.

5 m from the signal coil, altering the bucking coil weight from –1.0 to –1.007 produces perfect (complete) cancellation of the noise signal with clearly minimal effects on any signal of interest. For larger distances, the bucking coil weight is even closer to –1.0. In this way, weights determined using the acquired data, as mentioned earlier, can greatly improve the noise reduction for specific distant noise sources active during the acquisition. Also, because, as indicated in this example, these weights represent very small variations from the weights representing a perfect gradiometer, their effect on any signals of interest will be minimal.

One cannot develop noise reduction techniques that will reduce noise below the white noise level of the SQUID and electronics themselves. This is the limit that ultimately determines system performance. Once this limit has been reached, all further enhancements to the technique basically only add extra complexity to the system. To illustrate this point, auditory evoked response data from a Magnes 2500 magnetometer based system are presented in Figs. 8.5 through 8.8; these are from an auditory experiment in which pure tones were presented to a human subject.

Figures 8.5 and 8.6 show the raw epoch data both as collected (Panel a) and noise reduced (Panel b); each figure shows two epochs from two different data acquisitions. In these acquisitions, only real-time reference

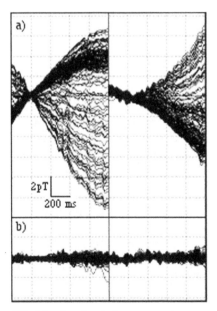

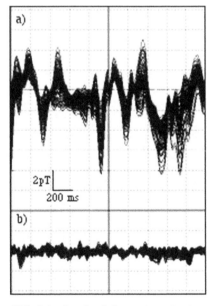

FIG. 8.5.    Panel a: before noise reduction; Panel b: after noise reduction.

FIG. 8.6.    Panel a: before noise reduction; Panel b: after noise reduction.

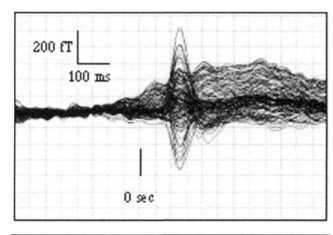

FIG. 8.7.   Average of data in Fig. 8.5 before noise reduction.

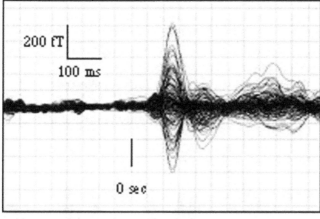

FIG. 8.8.   Average of data in Fig. 8.5 after noise reduction.

magnetometer weights were used during the collection of the data. This accounts for the large amount of noise present in the as-collected data. After postprocessing noise reduction was applied this noise is greatly reduced, as shown in the bottom half of the figures. Figure 8.7 shows the average of 155 epochs of auditory evoked response before noise reduction, and Figure 8.8 shows the very clean evoked response with an excellent signal-to-noise ratio down to low frequencies, which results after noise reduction is applied to the same data.

These data show that a very good signal-to-noise ratio is obtained with this system. Using noise measurements taken with the system when no patient is present, calculated power spectra show that the system reaches the SQUID white noise level. Thus, Magnes systems with magnetometer signal coils handle environmental noise very well; because magnetometer signal coils are optimum when environmental noise is excluded, they are also optimum when including environmental noise using the methods developed for the Magnes systems.

For an axial gradiometer, the signal coil and bucking coil are wound in series, both part of the same single coil. Thus, any signal that is removed by the bucking coil is lost forever; it cannot be recovered. For the Magnes magnetometer coil system, some signal may be removed in the noise reduction calculation (although much less, because of the greater separation between the reference and signal coils); however, this signal is still present in the separate reference coil recordings and is potentially recoverable if needed. The raw output from the magnetometer coils and from the reference coils are all collected, saved, and available for later processing. This lost signal may not be negligible. The magnetic field from a current dipole, which is the frequently used model for signals of interest in neuromagnetic measurements, falls off as $1/r^2$. Thus, for a signal source 5 cm from the signal coil on a 5-cm axial gradiometer, 25% of the signal detected by the signal coil is removed by the bucking coil. This decreases to 15% for an 8-cm axial gradiometer and to 0.4% for a 20-cm axial gradiometer.

Magnetometer signal coils in systems installed inside MSRs provide the largest signals possible from the object of interest: the brain. With today's noise reduction techniques, these systems can be made to operate at the SQUID noise level with the result that the best possible signal-to-noise performance is achieved. 4-D Magnetometer based systems are in daily use around the world today in both the most demanding research environments and clinical environments. Looking back at the history of the field, and the company, we at 4-D are thankful to Sam Williamson, his vision, and his helpful prods and pokes.

## REFERENCES

Brenner, D., Lipton, J., Kaufman, L., & Williamson, S. J. (1978, January). Somatically evoked magnetic fields of the human brain. *Science, 199*, 81–83.

Johnson, R. T., Black, W. C., & Buchanan, D. S. (2000). Source detectability for multichannel biomagnetic sensors. In C. J. Aine, Y. Okada, G. Stroink, S. J. Swithenby, & C. C. Wood (Eds.), *Biomag 96, Proceedings of the Tenth International Conference on Biomagnetism Vol. I* (pp. 59–62). New York: Springer.

# 9

## From 1- to 306-Channel Magnetoencephalography in 15 Years: Highlights of Neuromagnetic Brain Research in Finland

Olli V. Lounasmaa*
Riitta Hari
*Helsinki University of Technology*

We first present a brief summary of the development of magneto-encephalography (MEG) hard- and software in the Low Temperature Laboratory since the 1980s. In spite of important technical advances in instrumentation during that period, the early MEG data, recorded with single-channel devices by Samuel Williamson and others, are still relevant, as evidenced by later research. However, the whole-head covering MEG instruments with up to 306 superconducting quantum interference device sensors have opened totally new possibilities for studies of temporal aspects of signal processing simultaneously in both hemispheres of the human brain. We

*Editors' Note*: We were informed that Academician Olli Lounasmaa died suddenly on December 27, 2002. By then he had already finished work on this chapter, which may have been his final contribution to the scientific literature.

Dr. Lounasmaa is a major historical figure in the field of low temperature physics. His pioneering work on superfluid helium-3 won international acclaim. In the early 1980s he became interested in neuromagnetism. He established a major neuromagnetism unit in his low-temperature physics laboratory in Helsinki. The field benefited greatly from the fact that so imaginative and creative an experimenter turned his attention to studying the human brain. He played a major role in developing systems for measuring the brain's magnetic field at hundreds of places about the scalp at the same time. His many talented students were drawn to MSI because of Dr. Lounasmaa's involvement. We are extremely grateful for this chapter. It is not a sufficient memorial to so great a scientist, but it may well awaken in non-physicists a desire to study his work and emulate his energy and creativity.

briefly review work carried out by our research team on action viewing, cortex–muscle coherence, language functions, activation of subcortical structures, and clinical applications of MEG.

We are honored to contribute to this book, compiled to celebrate the 60th birthday of Professor Samuel J. Williamson who has been our friend and colleague for almost 20 years. When we started our neuromagnetic brain research in Finland, Sam and his colleagues had already pioneered the field by publishing papers on both visually and somatically evoked brain activations (Brenner, Lipton, Kaufman, & Williamson, 1978; Brenner, Williamson, & Kaufman, 1975). The insightful review on biomagnetism, very clearly and didactically written by Sam with Lloyd Kaufman (Williamson & Kaufman, 1981) served for us as the "bible" of neuromagnetism for the first decade of our research in this field. We also carefully studied in our lab meetings the textbook on Biomagnetism by Williamson, Romani, Kaufman, and Modena (1983).

In our Brain Research Unit (BRU), we are studying human brain functions, with a special emphasis on temporal aspects of cortical information processing. Over the years, our interdisciplinary team has developed the MEG method on a wide scale; the group consists at present of over 30 neuroscientists, including physicians, physicists, engineers, psychologists, and linguists. The work has comprised developments of instrumentation, mathematical signal analysis, and applications of MEG to studies of human brain functions in health and disease (Hämäläinen, Hari, Ilmoniemi, Knuutila, & Lounasmaa, 1993; Hari, 1998; Hari, Levänen, & Raij, 2000; Lounasmaa, Hämäläinen, Hari, & Salmelin, 1996). Neuromag Ltd., the spin-off company of our research, now manufactures whole-head neuromagnetometers on commercial basis.

Supported by systematic methodological development, our MEG studies have covered all major senses—audition, somatosensation, vision, olfaction, and pain—as well as voluntary movements and the neural basis of cognitive functions. The present subprojects focus on auditory, tactile, and visual processing in the human cerebral cortex, multimodal integrative functions, language perception and production, functional significance of spontaneous brain rhythms, and activation of subcortical brain structures. Much progress has been made in developing clinical applications of MEG. Some of these projects will be briefly described in this review.

## DEVELOPMENT OF HARDWARE

The first magnetoencephalography (MEG) measurements were made with one-superconducting quantum interference device (SQUID) systems, and the number of sensors increased only slowly. In the LTL, the sequence of progress was $1 \rightarrow 4 \rightarrow 7 \rightarrow 24 \rightarrow 122 \rightarrow 306$ channels. The first multichannel device, with four SQUIDs, was built in 1983 (Ilmoniemi, Hari, & Reinikainen, 1984), and the prototype of the first whole-head-covering device with 122 channels, manufactured by Neuromag Ltd. in our laboratory, became operational in September 1992 (Ahonen et al., 1993).

Figure 9.1 illustrates the 122-channel device. The concave bottom of the helium dewar houses the 122 flux transformers, wired in the form of planar first-order gradiometers. The two figure-of-eight coils at 61 locations around the subject's scalp record the orthogonal tangential derivatives $\partial B_r / \partial x$ and $\partial B_r / \partial y$ of the magnetic field component $B_r$ normal to the dewar bottom. The two independent gradient components give together both the magnitude and direction of the local current in the brain.

The prototype of the latest model of whole-scalp covering instruments, the Vectorview with 306 SQUID sensors, was installed in our laboratory in the summer of 1998. The 102 measuring sites of the device are each equipped with two gradient coils, again recording the derivatives $\partial B_r / \partial x$ and $\partial B_r / \partial y$, and a magnetometer coil, measuring the $z$-component of $B_r$ and sensitive even to deep sources.

Figure 9.2 shows the subject sitting under the instrument. The dewar can be tilted around its horizontal axis if a prone or supine position of the subject is preferred. Figure 9.3 illustrates auditory evoked responses obtained with this 306-channel device.

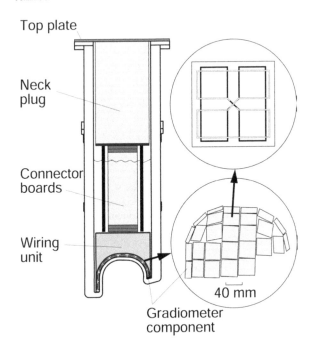

Top plate

Neck plug

Connector boards

Wiring unit

40 mm

Gradiometer component

FIG. 9.1. Schematic drawing of the Neuromag 122-channel instrument. Left: The neuromagnetometer probe comprising the dewar and the modular insert structure with the SQUID sensors. Right: Dual gradiometer unit (above) and the 61-chip array (below). From "122-channel SQUID instrument for investigating the magnetic signals from the human brain," by A. I. Ahonen et al., 1993, *Physica Scripta, T49*, p. 198–205. Copyright © 1993 by Physica Scripta. Adapted with permission.

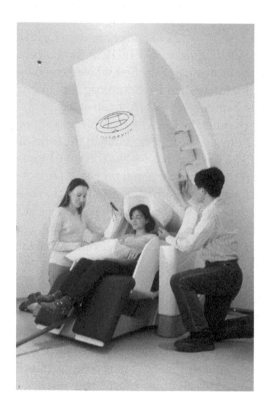

FIG. 9.2. Photograph of the 306-channel neuromagnetometer manufactured by Neuromag Ltd. and installed in the LTL. Copyright © by Low Temperature Laboratory. Reprinted with permission.

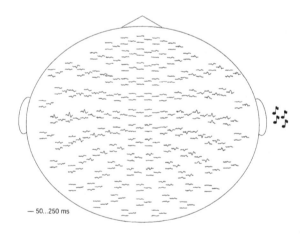

— 50...250 ms

FIG. 9.3. Auditory responses recorded with the 306-channel neuromagnetometer. In each triplet of curves, the two gradiometer signals are shown on the left and the magnetometer signal on the right. Figure provided by R. Salmelin. Reprinted with permission.

## DEVELOPMENT OF SOFTWARE

The increase of measurement channels in MEG devices has required new and more efficient methods for data handling. Our present analysis software includes both the standard time-varying multidipole models and distributed-source models developed in the LTL. The *minimum-norm estimate*, first used in 1984 (Hämäläinen & Ilmoniemi, 1994), has motivated the development of many similar distributed source models in other laboratories.

More recently, we have introduced the *minimum current estimate* (MCE; Uutela, Hämäläinen, & Somersalo, 1999). This method can be used to recover several local or extended sources, even if their activities overlap in time. In many MEG measurements, such as studies of sensory evoked responses, the extent of the activated brain region is relatively small. Whereas the traditional minimum-norm estimate works best with smooth, extended sources, the assumptions underlying the MCE are in accordance with focal sources. The traditional dipole model may be able to locate some source configurations more accurately than the MCE.

However, even then the MCE visualization can help the experimenter to find the proper multidipole model. The advantages of the MCE are (a) a minimal need for user intervention and (b) fast calculation.

## ACTION VIEWING

The monkey frontal cortex contains "mirror" neurons that discharge during the execution of actions and during observation of movements made by others (Rizzolatti, Fadiga, Gallese, & Fogassi, 1996). These neurons may form a system that allows an individual to understand the actions and intentions of another person. We have studied the human action observation/action execution matching system by recording neuromagnetic oscillatory and evoked signals when humans either themselves performed movements or were observing similar actions made by another individual.

Figure 9.4 shows the experimental conditions used in one study. The human primary motor cortex was activated not only during execution of finger manipulations but also during observation of similar movements made by another subject (Hari et al., 1998).

In a more recent study, Broca's region became activated both during execution and viewing of pinching movements (Nishitani & Hari 2000). Activation started earlier in Broca's region than in the motor cortex, and

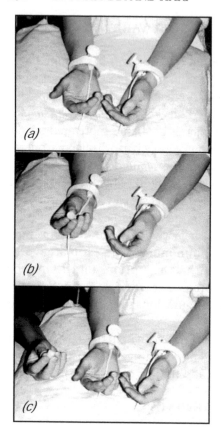

FIG. 9.4.   Experimental setup used in the action viewing experiment of Hari et al. (1998). The subject was studied when she kept her hands at rest (a), manipulated a small object with her right-hand fingers (b), or when she just viewed another person who was performing similar finger movements (c). From "Activation of human primary motor cortex during action observation: A neuromagnetic study," by R. Hari et al., 1998, *Proceedings of the National Academy of Science, USA, 95.* Copyright © 1998 by PNAS. Reprinted with permission.

both these areas were responding significantly stronger during imitation of action than during execution or observation. These findings confirm the existence of an action observation–execution matching network in humans and suggest that Broca's region plays a central role in this system. Recently we have observed the human mirror–neuron system to activate in a nice sequence during observation and imitation of lip forms: The activation progressed from visual cortex to superior temporal sulcus, then via inferior parietal cortex to Broca's area, and finally to the primary motor cortex; the whole activation sequence occurred in about 250 msec (Nishitani & Hari, 2002).

## CORTEX–MUSCLE COHERENCE

All cortical sensory projection areas seem to have their own rhythms, which can be modified independently of the other areas (for a review, see Hari & Salmelin, 1997). During recent years, we have become interested in *motor cortex–muscle* coherence (Hari & Salenius 1999; Salenius, Portin, Kajola, Salmelin, & Hari, 1997). The studies comprise simultaneous measurements of MEG signals and of a surface electromyogram from a muscle, which is kept isometrically contracted. Calculations of the coherence spectra between the two signals give information about the cortex–muscle communication.

Figure 9.5 shows a surface electromyogram from the contracting foot muscle and the simultaneously recorded MEG over the motor cortex. Both signals are rhythmic but display different waveforms. The coherence spectra between the cortical and muscular signals peak around 20 Hz, as is shown separately for isometric contractions of left and right upper and lower limb muscles. The coherence has a clear somatotopic organization so that the site of maximum signal differs for upper and lower limb contractions and for left and right limbs. It is interesting that cortical signals always preceded the motor unit firing and, in line with the different conduction distances, the delay was 15 to 20 msec longer for lower than for upper limb muscles. It is thus likely that the coherent cortical signals reflect direct corticospinal drive to the motor units of the contracting muscle. The rhythmic modulation apparently facilitates efficient interplay of the motor units.

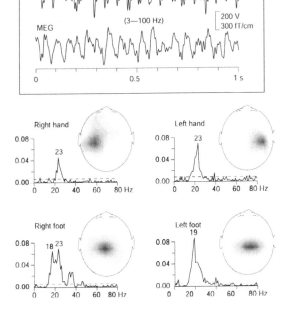

FIG. 9.5. Top: Simultaneous recordings of the surface electromyogram (EMG) from a contracting muscle and the MEG signal from the corresponding part of the motor cortex. Bottom: Coherence spectra between MEG and EMG and the sites of maximum coherence illustrated on schematic heads. From "Cortical control of human motorneuron firing during isometric contraction," by S. Salenius et al., 1997, *Journal of Neurophysiology,* 77(6). Copyright © 1997 by American Physiological Society. Reprinted with permission.

Cortex–muscle coherence is a good example of the power of MEG, that is, of excellent temporal resolution combined with reasonable spatial accuracy. The phenomenon is of interest for understanding cortical control of voluntary movements and the pathophysiology of various motor disorders as well as for unraveling the significance of cortical rhythms.

## LANGUAGE FUNCTIONS

One aim in our Brain Research Unit is to unravel brain mechanisms underlying the perception and production of language in healthy subjects and to find out how these processes may go wrong, for example, in dyslexia, stuttering, and aphasia. In our recent MEG experiments we have used written and spoken single words and complete sentences to characterize time windows and brain areas that are critical for fluent reading and speech.

Our original characterization of cortical dynamics during picture naming showed that it was possible to track the processing stages from perception to speech production in individual subjects (Salmelin, Hari, Lounasmaa, & Sams, 1994).

Figure 9.6 depicts results from recent MEG studies of the reading process in normal and dyslexic readers (Helenius, Salmelin, Service, & Connolly, 1998; Helenius, Tarkiainen, Cornelissen, Hansen, & Salmelin, 1999; Salmelin, Service, Kiesilä, Uutela, & Salonen, 1996; Tarkiainen, Helenius, Hansen, Cornelissen, & Salmelin, 1999). The sequence of cortical activation proceeds via visual feature analysis to letter-string specific processing and further to comprehension of word and sentence meaning.

The visual feature analysis occurs rather similarly in both groups, but in dyslexic subjects the process is disrupted at the level of the letter-string specific analysis, about 150 msec after seeing a word, and thereafter the activation is weak and delayed. The adequate description of language function obviously requires accurate monitoring of both sites and time sequences of brain activations; such information can be obtained by means of whole-scalp MEG recordings.

## ACTIVATION OF SUBCORTICAL BRAIN STRUCTURES

Although most MEG studies have focused on cortical functions, there has been continuous interest in picking up signals also from deep brain structures, such as the thalamus, hippocampus, and cerebellum. All these regions are essential for normal brain function. The thalamus is an im-

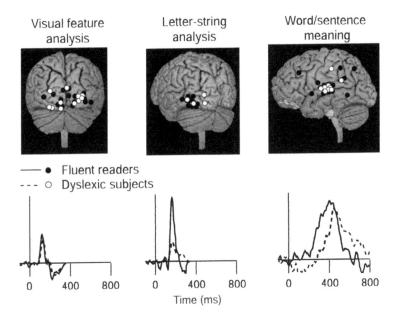

Visual feature analysis    Letter-string analysis    Word/sentence meaning

———— ● Fluent readers
- - - ○ Dyslexic subjects

Time (ms)

FIG. 9.6.    Comparison of brain activations in fluent and dyslexic readers. See text for details. Figure compiled by R. Salmelin.

portant relay station for sensory input from the periphery to the cerebral cortex; the hippocampus is essential for normal memory function; and the cerebellum, classically considered as a motor timing machine, is involved in several cognitive functions.

Because MEG's spatial accuracy is relatively poor for deep brain regions, direct localization of signal sources in subcortical structures has been rare. However, one can put source currents to brain areas of interest—for example, in the hippocampus—and then calculate how the signal pattern could be accounted for by these sources. The result of the calculation is a set of waveforms that represent the time-varying strengths of the assumed source regions. This type of forward approach (see Fig. 9.7) has been used in our group to interpret both evoked and spontaneous MEG signals by activations in the human thalamus and hippocampus (Tesche, 1996, 1997; Tesche & Karhu, 1999).

## CLINICAL APPLICATIONS OF MEG

The CliniMEG group of our Brain Research Unit has been developing MEG routines for diagnosis of neurological patients in hospital environ-

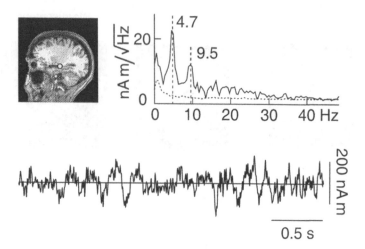

FIG. 9.7.    Slow theta waves (bottom panel) and their frequency spectrum (top panel) recorded from the human hippocampus by the forward approach. The 4.7-Hz peak was observed when the subject was doing mental calculations but not when he was watching a picture. From "Non-invasive detection of ongoing neuronal population activity in normal human hippocampus" by C. D. Tesche, 1997, *Brain Research, 749.* Copyright © 1997. Adapted by permission of the author.

ment; the work is based on our previous extensive studies of the functional brain organization in healthy subjects and of the pathophysiology of different neurological diseases.

Figure 9.8 shows preoperative MEG localization of functionally important cortical areas in a patient with a brain tumor. This noninvasive procedure helps the neurosurgeon navigate during the operation, and the display of cortical vessels on the magnetic resonance imaging reconstructions is also extremely helpful. The combined use of anatomical and functional information in preoperative evaluation has now been tested by our CliniMEG group with very encouraging results on more than 30 operated patients, with preoperative confirmation of the localization results.

## CONCLUSION

MEG, with its superb temporal and reasonable spatial resolution, has evolved during the last 20 years to an important noninvasive tool to explore the dynamics of human brain activation during various tasks and stimuli. With improved instrumentation and analysis methods, MEG has also found its way to hospitals. In the near future, the combination of MEG and functional magnetic resonance imaging fMRI will become com-

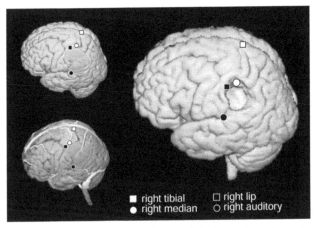

FIG. 9.8. Magnetic resonance surface renderings of the brain of a patient with a tumor close to the central sulcus, before (left) and after (right) surgery. Pre- and postoperatively identified functional landmarks to somatosensory and auditory stimulation are illustrated by symbols. The lower left figure also shows the blood vessels on the brain surface. From "Three-dimensional integration of brain anatomy and function to facilitate intraoperative navigation around the sensorymotor strip," by J. Mäkelä et al., 2001, *Human Brain Mapping*, 12, pp. 180-192. Copyright © 2001 by Wiley. Adapted with permission.

mon in identifying brain activations with high accuracy both in space and in time. The MEG method, pioneered by Samuel Williamson, is slowly bearing fruit.

## ACKNOWLEDGMENTS

We thank Nina Forss, Matti Hämäläinen, Riitta Salmelin, and Claudia Tesche for contributions to this chapter.

## REFERENCES

Ahonen, A. I., Hämäläinen, M. S., Kajola, M. J., Knuutila, J. E. T., Laine, P. P., Lounasmaa, O. V., Parkkonen, L. T., Simola, J. T., & Tesche, C. D. (1993). 122-channel SQUID instrument for investigating the magnetic signals from the human brain. *Physica Scripta, T49*, 198–205.
Brenner, D., Lipton, J., Kaufman, L., & Williamson, S. (1978). Somatically evoked magnetic fields of the human brain. *Science, 199*, 81–83.
Brenner, D., Williamson, S. J., & Kaufman, L. (1975). Visually evoked magnetic fields of the human brain. *Science, 190*, 480–481.
Hämäläinen, M., Hari, R., Ilmoniemi, R., Knuutila, J., & Lounasmaa, O. V. (1993). Magnetoencephalography—theory, instrumentation, and applications to noninvasive studies of the working human brain. *Reviews of Modern Physics, 65*, 413–497.
Hämäläinen, M. S., & Ilmoniemi, R. J. (1994). Interpreting magnetic fields of the brain: Minimum-norm estimates. *IEEE Transactions in Biomedical Engineering, 32*, 35–42.
Hari, R. (1998). Magnetoencephalography as a tool of clinical neurophysiology. In E. Niedermeyer & F. Lopes da Silva (Eds.), *Electroencephalography: Basic principles, clinical applications and related fields* (4th ed., pp. 1107–1134). Baltimore: Williams & Wilkins.

Hari, R., Levänen, S., & Raij, T. (2000). Timing of human cortical functions during cognition: Role of MEG. *Trends in Cognitive Science, 12,* 455–462.

Hari, R., & Salenius, S. (1999). Rhythmical corticomotoneuronal communication. *NeuroReport, 10,* R1–R10.

Hari, R., & Salmelin, R. (1997). Human cortical rhythms: A neuromagnetic view through the skull. *Trends in Neuroscience, 20,* 44–49.

Hari, R., Forss, N., Avikainen, S., Kirveskari, E., Salenius, S., & Rizzolatti, G. (1998). Activation of human primary motor cortex during action observation: A neuromagnetic study. *Proceedings of the National Academy of Science, 95,* 15061–15065.

Helenius, P., Salmelin, R., Service, E., & Connolly, J. F. (1998). Distinct time courses of word and context comprehension in the left temporal cortex. *Brain, 121,* 1133–1142.

Helenius, P., Tarkiainen, A., Cornelissen, P., Hansen, P. C., & Salmelin, R. (1999). Dissociation of normal feature analysis and deficient processing of letter-strings in dyslexic adults. *Cerebral Cortex, 9,* 476–483.

Ilmoniemi, R., Hari, R., & Reinikainen, K. (1984). A four-channel SQUID magnetometer for brain research. *Electroencephalography and Clinical Neurophysiology, 58,* 467–473.

Lounasmaa, O. V., Hämäläinen, M., Hari, R., & Salmelin, R. (1996). Information processing in the human brain—magnetoencephalographic approach. *Proceedings of the National Academy of Science, 93,* 8809–8815.

Mäkelä, J., Kirveskari, E., Seppä, M., Hämäläinen, M., Forss, N., Avikainen, S., Salonen, O., Salenius, S., Kovala, T., Randell, T., Jääskeläinen, J., & Hari, R. (2001). Three-dimensional integration of brain anatomy and function to facilitate intraoperative navigation around the sensorymotor strip. *Human Brain Mapping, 12,* 180–192.

Nishitani, N., & Hari, R. (2000). Temporal dynamics of cortical representation for action. *PNAS, 97,* 913–918.

Nishitani, N., & Hari, R. (2002). Viewing lip forms: Cortical activation. *Neuron, 19,* 1211–1220.

Rizzolatti, G., Fadiga, L., Gallese, V., & Fogassi, L. (1996). Premotor cortex and recognition of motor actions. *Cognitive Brain Research, 3,* 131–141.

Salenius, S., Portin, K., Kajola, M., Salmelin, R., & Hari, R. (1997). Cortical control of human motorneuron firing during isometric contraction. *Journal of Neurophysiology, 77,* 3401–3405.

Salmelin, R., Hari, R., Lounasmaa, O. V., & Sams, M. (1994). Dynamics of brain activation during picture naming. *Nature, 368,* 463–465.

Salmelin, R., Service, E., Kiesilä, P., Uutela, K., & Salonen, O. (1996). Impaired visual word processing in dyslexia revealed with magnetoencephalography. *Annals of Neurology, 40,* 157–162.

Tarkiainen, A., Helenius, P., Hansen, P., Cornelissen, P., & Salmelin, R. (1999). Dynamics of letter string perception in the human occipitotemporal cortex. *Brain, 122,* 2119–2132.

Tesche, C. D. (1996). MEG imaging of neuronal population dynamics in the human thalamus. *Electroencephalography and Clinical Neurophysiology, S47,* 81–90.

Tesche, C. D. (1997). Non-invasive detection of ongoing neuronal population activity in normal human hippocampus. *Brain Research, 749,* 53–60.

Tesche, C. D., & Karhu, J. (1999). Interactive processing of sensory input and motor output in the human hippocampus. *Journal of Cognitive Neuroscience, 11,* 424–436.

Uutela, K., Hämäläinen, M., & Somersalo, E. (1999). Visualization of magnetoencephalographic data using minimum current estimates. *Neuroimage, 10,* 173–180.

Williamson, S., Romani, G.-L., Kaufman, L., & Modena, I. (Eds.). (1983). *Biomagnetism—An Interdisciplinary Approach.* New York: Plenum.

Williamson, S. J., & Kaufman, L. (1981). Biomagnetism. *Journal of Magnetism and Magnetic Materials, 22,* 129–202.

# 10

## Magnetoencephalography: From Pioneering Studies to Functional Brain Imaging

Cosimo Del Gratta
Gian Luca Romani
*Università G. D'Annunzio*
*Istituto Nazionale di Fisica della Materia*

In the first part of this chapter we want to stress that the most important features of present-day neuromagnetic technique directly stem from the seminal work of the pioneering days of biomagnetism in the late 1970s and early 1980s. We describe as an example the pioneering studies undertaken at that time at New York University, because they constitute the personal exciting and rewarding experience of Gian Luca Romani. Several other groups around the world were working in biomagnetism at that time and made important contributions to the field; they are mentioned elsewhere in this volume. In the second part of this chapter we report for comparison some recent studies in biomagnetism that show how this technique has undergone impressive progress and has gained an important place among present-day neuroimaging techniques.

The aim of this chapter is to outline the link between the early days of neuromagnetism and current experimental and clinical work. This link is the ability of magnetoencephalography (MEG) to perform functional imaging. This was first recognized in the early 1980s and is now evident in the work of many laboratories all over the world. We believe that the success of MEG as a functional imaging tool for the brain is largely due to the advances achieved in those pioneering studies, which laid the foundations for future work.

The electrical activity of cells has been known since the work of Galvani in 1791 and the first electroencephalogram (EEG) recording, made by Berger in 1929. On the other hand, the magnetic effect of electrical currents was discovered by Oersted in 1820, while the brain magnetic field was first revealed by Cohen in 1968, and in fact the first direct recording of brain alpha waves without signal averaging was performed in 1972 using a superconducting quantum interference device (SQUID) in a magnetically shielded room (Cohen, 1972). In both cases, approximately 150 years elapsed between the time of the fundamental discovery and the possibility of its application to brain studies. This was largely due to the weakness of brain signals. In particular, the magnetic field of the brain is about 10 orders of magnitude weaker than the Earth's static field. Indeed, it was only with the advent of SQUID-based magnetometers that MEG could be performed. Another well-known difficulty in MEG, in addition to the weakness of the signals, is that measurements are disturbed by many sources of ambient magnetic fields that are much stronger than the field of the brain. These ambient fields are rejected either by performing the measurement inside a shielded room or using a gradiometric pickup coil, or by using a combination of both techniques.

After having demonstrated that it was indeed possible to record magnetic fields from the brain, researchers quickly recognized that the magnetic field is only weakly affected by the tissues—brain, skull, and scalp—intervening between the neuronal currents and the field sensors. If neural activity is localized in a small region of the brain, then mapping the magnetic field over the scalp leads to sharp field patterns. This is in contrast to EEG, in which volume conduction distorts the scalp potentials, resulting in much more blurred patterns. This superiority over EEG provided the impetus for the development of a theoretical background for the modeling of the neural sources of the field, and of the head as a volume conductor, while an intense experimental activity was pursued. The ability of MEG to localize in three-dimensional space a small active region of the cortex was soon demonstrated, and the localization of evoked fields, elicited by a variety of peripheral stimulation—sensory, visual, and auditory—was performed. Localization of an active brain tissue requires the mapping, with appropriate density, of a scalp area with a size proportional to the depth of the active tissue below the scalp. Because the first neuromagnetometers were equipped with just one SQUID sensor, a complete map could be obtained only by repositioning the sensor several times and by synchronizing the detected magnetic signal to the same cerebral event, in the optimistic hypothesis that the brain response could be regarded as stationary. With this method, instantaneous maps of brain activity could not be recorded. The need for multichannel instruments was therefore quickly recognized. This posed several problems, such as the fabrication of an appropriate nonmagnetic cryostat, the availability of a large number of reliable and easy-to-handle SQUIDs, and the acquisition of a large number of signals with a high sampling rate. Nevertheless, the number of channels in MEG systems slowly increased, progressively reducing the time needed to collect a complete magnetic field map. In the second half of the 1990s, whole-head coverage systems were developed that allowed the recording of instantaneous maps and, as a consequence, the dynamic study of brain activity. Parallel to this evolution of the instrumentation, experimental work was conducted and the theoretical background was improved, for example, by extending the modeling to realistic volume conductors and distributed sources, or by using magnetic resonance imaging (MRI) for model construction and data rendering.

To date, MEG is a well-established technology for brain investigation. Whole-head neuromagnetometers are operating in several laboratories in the United States, Japan, and Europe, and more and more often they are used for fundamental as well as clinical studies and, in some cases, even as a diagnostic tool. For a review on MEG see, for example, Del Gratta, Pizzella, Tecchio, and Romani (2001) and Hämäläinen, Hari, Ilmoniemi, Knuutila, and Lounasmaa (1993). For a review on the instrumentation for biomagnetism, see, for example, Pizzella, Della Penna, Del Gratta, and Romani (2001). Several achievements in the field of neurophysiology have marked the evolution of MEG, from the early studies of the primary areas of the brain to the more recent cognitive studies and studies on brain plasticity. Future perspectives see MEG as one of the main characters in the field of brain imaging, acting together with other imaging techniques, such as functional MRI and positron emission tomography.

## PIONEERING WORK IN THE LATE 1970S AND EARLY 1980S

We believe that the most important contribution of MEG to quantitative brain investigation is neither the fabrication of powerful brain imaging instruments nor its relative merits compared to EEG; rather, it is the fact that its foundations were established in a rigorous scientific way, both experimentally and theoretically. This fact allowed the subsequent successful evolution of MEG and greatly influenced the progress in EEG. We would like to recall here that these foundations were laid mainly by Sam Williamson.

The early days of neuromagnetism, 1975–1983, were characterized by an impressive evolution, from basic measurements of the neuromagnetic field—aimed only at demonstrating their feasibility—to complete experimental brain studies performed outside the cryogenics laboratory with only limited technical support.

Looking back at the works published in these days, we note three main themes that characterize the research that was carried out:

1. *Clarify the electromagnetism of neuromagnetic field generation and detection.* This required, on the one hand, finding the link between neural activity and the measured field. Which electrical events are responsible for the neuromagnetic fields? How large should an active neural population be so that its magnetic field can be detected? On the other hand, this required finding a model for neuromagnetic field generation that is able to calculate the field of a specific source in the brain, and, conversely, given a measured field, to estimate the characteristics of the electric source underlying it. From the point of view of field detection, the issue of flux transformer geometry is a central one. What are the optimal sizes for a pickup coil radius, or gradiometer baseline in various given situations, high or low ambient noise, shallow or deep sources, and so on? In other words, what is the relation between the geometrical parameters of the flux transformer and its sensitivity profile?

2. *Bring the neuromagnetometers out of the shielded room, because the first shielded rooms were uncomfortable and expensive—and out of the cryogenics laboratory.* This is so the neuromagnetometers could be used for experiments in a larger number of, and a variety of neurological, psychological laboratories. This involved in particular the design and the fabrication of appropriate flux transformers to be coupled to the SQUIDs' second-order gradiometers to allow them to operate in an unshielded environment.

3. *Test the neuromagnetic techniques in experimental brain studies, to evaluate its capabilities.* This means finding the areas of neurophysiology, neurology, neuropsychology, and so on, where the neuromagnetic technique may contribute new results or improve the level of knowledge.

Sam Williamson gave answers to the preceding questions and solved many of the problems, but we should stress that in doing so he was always oriented toward practical and effective methods, such as the handy formulas for dipole localization in the homogeneous half-space and in the homogeneous sphere, where the depth of the dipole was worked out as a function of distance or angular distance, respectively, between the two extremes of the magnetic field map, including the corrections for the finite pickup coil size and gradiometer baseline (Romani et al., 1982a; Williamson & Kaufman, 1981, 1981b). Although mathematically accessible, and of practical use, these formulas were extremely useful in the interpretation of neuromagnetic data in important studies of primary areas, as we discuss later. Last, but not least, applying a method formerly suggested by Tripp (1981), Williamson introduced a simple model to estimate the intensity of the current dipole moment of a neuron (Williamson & Kaufman, 1990) that gives an idea of how neuromagnetic signals are generated, and what kind of neural activity we are able to observe. Indeed, the figure that he evaluated, namely $Q \approx 3 \times 10^{-14}$Am, demonstrated that an ordinary neuromagnetic signal, such as an evoked auditory field, is likely to be due to the simultaneous firing of about 50,000 neurons: Thus, MEG is a means of investigating macroscopic brain activity.

Among the experimental brain studies achieved in that time was the first demonstration of the tonotopic organization of the human auditory cortex. This finding had a profound impact on the progress of biomagnetism, in that it opened the way to source localization and, in perspective, to functional imaging. Furthermore, it proved that it was possible to perform functional imaging with the theoretical modeling introduced by Williamson.

The investigation of the human auditory cortex by neuromagnetic measurements gave the first noninvasive confirmation that human neurons, similar to animal neurons, are tuned to different tonal frequencies and serially located along the floor and roof of the Sylvian fissure (Romani, Williamson, & Kaufman, 1982b, 1982c). Romani et al. (1982b, 1982c) used a single-channel neuromagnetometer equipped with a second-order gradiometer coupled to a SQUID and suited for operation in a magnetically unshielded environment. They mapped the temporo–parietal area of the hemisphere of 2 subjects by positioning the probe orthogonally at about 40 locations on the scalp. For each probe location the subjects were binaurally presented pure tones with different frequencies, sinusoidally modulated at low frequency (32 Hz), and the amplitude and phase of the response at the modulation frequency were recorded. Maps of magnetic field distribution over the scalp, corresponding to the above-mentioned steady-state stimulation modality, were analyzed by modeling the source as an equivalent current dipole (ECD) and the head as a homogeneously conducting sphere. Locations of the ECDs were estimated for each stimulation frequency from the angle subtended at the center of the sphere by the two extrema of the maps, taking into account the correction for finite gradiometer baseline and pickup coil area. ECDs showed progressively deeper localization with respect to the delivery of acoustic stimuli containing more acute frequencies. The variation of depth for both subjects was adequately represented by a logarithmic function of frequency. Such a logarithmic progression—namely, a tonotopic organization—strictly reproduces that of the acoustic epithelium within the cochlea.

Romani et al.'s (1982b, 1982c) study is interesting not only in its own right but also from the point of view of this chapter, which aims to link "new" and "old" neuromagnetism. Indeed, all current topics of the theory and practice of neuromagnetism are present in Romani et al's (1982b, 1982c) study, for example, the inverse-problem solution and the problem of positioning the probe with respect to subject anatomy. It is striking not only how simply these problems are dealt with but also how effectively. As mentioned earlier, this problem solving technique was created from the point of view of Sam Williamson.

In conclusion, we stress that this result has been replicated in several studies performed successively during the late 1980s and 1990s but with a different stimulation modality, that is, transient rather than steady state. A recent study performed using one of the most advanced source modeling and multimodal integration procedures BESA (Megis Software, Munich, Germany) and Brain Voyager (Brain Innovation, Maastricht, The Netherlands), demonstrated that a pure tonotopic progression characterizes more prominently the short latency (40 msec) component rather than the 100-msec one (M. Scherg, personal communication, August 15, 2000), thus confirming the result achieved 20 years earlier and closing a loop between new and old neuromagnetism.

Recent advances in brain imaging were experienced in Rome and Chieti, Italy. The work we describe in the following sections was performed at the Neurology Center of Fatebenefratelli Hospital, Isola Tiberina, Rome, and the Institute of Advanced Biomedical Technologies, at Chieti University, Chieti. The former is equipped with a 28-channel system with vertical first-order gradiometers and magnetometers with software noise rejection, operating in a shielded room. This instrument was formerly developed at the Institute of Solid State Electronics National Research Council (CNR), in Rome (Foglietti et al., 1991), and was later transferred into a clinical environment at the Neurology Center of Fatebenefratelli Hospital. In the second center, a whole-head 165-channel helmet system (AtB, Pescara, Italy) was recently acquired (Della Penna et al., 2000). This system is operating in a highly shielded room, with four layers of mu-metal. Each sensor is a SQUID-integrated magnetometer; in addition to 153 sensors distributed over the scalp, four triplets of mutually orthogonal sensors are located in the upper part of the Dewar and used for software noise rejection. This system is located in the university campus, near the hospital. The Institute for Advanced Biomedical Technologies also has acquired a Siemens Vision MRI scanner with 1.5 T-static field, to be used for structural and functional MRI as well as for data integration with MEG.

One of the most promising fields of research is the so-called *multimodal approach*, that is, the application of different imaging techniques to a specific problem to possibly get a synergic effect for the comprehension of the problem itself. Several studies of this kind have appeared recently in the literature (Babiloni et al., 1999; Grimm et al., 1998).

## FUNCTIONAL IMAGING
## OF THE SENSORY–MOTOR AREAS

In the last few years, we have paid much attention to the investigation of the sensory–motor areas, in particular, Kristeva-Feige and colleagues, who performed recordings of the motor evoked field due to finger movement as compared with stimulation of the same finger, with the aim at investigating whether it is possible to noninvasively discriminate in humans the different projections of proprioceptive and cutaneous fibers in the primary somatosensory area. The results showed that the equivalent dipolar source for the first component of the motor evoked field was significantly deeper (area 3a) than that associated with the first component of the somatosensory evoked field; the latter was consistent with a generator located in the posterior bank of the central sulcus (area 3b). This study well demonstrated MEG's capability of discriminating subareas inside the primary cortices in man.

As another example, we report on a neurophysiological study in which the somatotopy of the secondary somatosensory area was investigated with both MEG and fMRI during electrical stimulation of the median nerve at the wrist and the tibial nerve at the medial malleolous. Although Hari et al. (1993) had already observed the somatotopic organization of secondary somatosensory (SII) with MEG, it had not been studied with fMRI. Bilateral activations were observed in the perisylvian area with fMRI showing a clear somatotopic organization, where the median nerve representation was more lower–anterior, and the tibial nerve representation was more superior–posterior (Del Gratta et al., 2000). The same measurements were successively repeated in combination with MEG: ECDs were localized in the same area presenting mutual spatial relationships consistent with the fMRI findings, as shown in Fig. 10.1 (Del Gratta et al., 2002).

In more recent work, Torquati et al. (2002) investigated the differences in responses to somatosensory electrical stimuli in the primary and secondary sensory cortices using different levels of stimulus intensity. Ten different levels were used, starting from below the sensory threshold up to a weak painful level. Primary somatosensory area (SI) response linearly increased in amplitude as the stimulus intensity raised up to a strong motor level and then saturated at higher stimulation intensities. The contra-

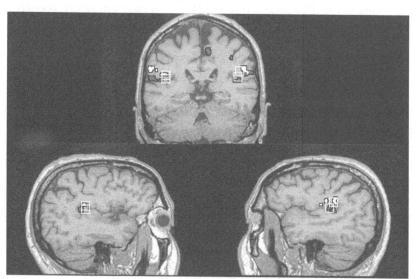

FIG. 10.1. A combined MEG–fMRI study of the somatotopic organization of the secondary somatosensory cortex. Co-registered to the anatomical MRI, are shown bilaterally in the SII areas, the fMRI activations, and the ECD locations and error boxes (white squares), during left median (dark grey) and left tibial (light grey) nerve electric stimulation. Both methods indicate approximately the same spatial relationship between median and tibial areas. Note, in the coronal view, the activation of the supplementary motor area for median nerve stimulation.

lateral and ipsilateral SII source strengths increased with stimulus intensity up to the motor threshold, then decreased at the strong motor level, and again increased at the weak painful threshold. These results suggest that different areas of the SII cortices are activated as the intensity of stimulation increases from not painful to painful.

## PRESURGICAL INVESTIGATION IN EPILEPSY

The neuromagnetic approach was applied to the study of focal epilepsy almost 20 years ago (Barth, Sutherling, Engel, & Beatty, 1982). After a first series of findings (Barth, Sutherling, Engel, & Beatty, 1984; Ricci et al., 1987) that focused on the possibility of identifying the location of foci of interictal activity, efforts were diminished because of the lack of an instrumentation adequate for a routine clinical trial. More recently, the development of large multichannel systems has given new impulse to the field, and the presurgical investigation of epileptic patients is being carried on in various laboratories in many countries. There has been an impressive development in this area, and the current trend relies strongly on the combination of MEG with other techniques, both invasive and noninvasive. We have recently started a multimodal approach to this topic in the frame of a national project, involving several groups and several imaging techniques applied in a blind test procedure.

As an example, we cite the case of a 35-year-old woman affected by temporal lobe epilepsy. The noninvasive source analysis obtained with MEG was compared with the presence of lesions suggested by MRI. A good agreement was found between the two. In Fig. 10.2 are shown, superimposed on MRI, the ECD localization from interictal spike activity (sagittal view, lower right), the ECD localization from activity elicited by median nerve stimulation (sagittal view, upper left, and other views).

We should stress, however, that the main contribution of the neuromagnetic approach is provided in cases where no lesion is revealed by computerized tomography and MRI, and therefore no suggestions for surgeons are available. These are the most crucial cases, in which only a combination of MEG with electrocorticography (EcoG) or stereo EEG, plus clinical evidence from video EEG, will decide whether to proceed to surgical excision.

## PRESURGICAL MAPPING

The possibility of accurately identifying the location of the equivalent generators elicited during sensory stimulation, simple motor tasks inside

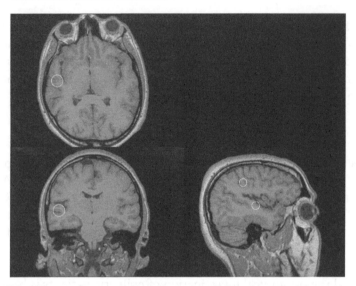

FIG. 10.2.   The case of a patient affected by temporal lobe epilepsy. Superimposed on the magnetic resonance image are the locations of the equivalent current dipoles corresponding to median nerve stimulation (indicated only in the sagittal view, the circle in the upper left of the figure) and to interictal spike activity (the other circle in the three views).

primary areas (somatomotor, visual, auditory), or both, is another interesting feature of the neuromagnetic method.

Whenever the standard anatomic topography is modified by an enlarging neoplastic mass or a trauma (Nakasato et al., 1996), the a priori knowledge of functional landmarks of eloquent areas to be preserved during surgical excision is of fundamental aid to the surgeon. With modern technology, such information can be directly integrated with the best neuronavigator apparatuses to obtain maximum benefit for the patient. Figure 10.3 shows an example of a 67-year-old patient affected by an astrocytoma that was studied with MEG and median nerve stimulation and with fMRI while he performed a complex motor task.

## CEREBRAL PLASTICITY

In 1994, Rossini et al. conducted a study in which they aimed to verify the existence of a short-term functional rearrangement of single-finger representation in the primary somato–sensory cortex of man during temporary sensory deprivation, similar to what had been previously observed in animals (Merzenich et al., 1983). By producing a relatively brief

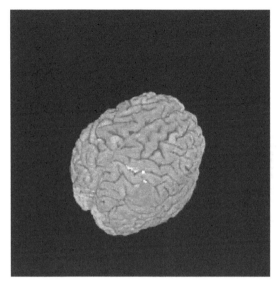

FIG. 10.3. An example of a combined presurgical study with functional magnetic resonance and magnetoencephalography. The case of a patient affected by astrocytoma. Superimposed on the rendered magnetic resonance image are the locations of functional magnetic resonance activation during the performance of a complex hand movement (leftmost activation-primary motor area; lowermost activation-primary somatosensory area), and the equivalent current dipole (location represented by a square) corresponding to the magnetic field elicited by median nerve electric stimulation. The lesion area appears as a uniform (no sulci visible) patch just inferior to the activation in the primary somatosensory area.

(20-min) anesthetic block of the sensory information from adjacent fingers, Rossini et al. (1994) demonstrated that the location and strength of the equivalent generators responsible for cortical responses N20m and P30m from the nonanesthetized finger were significantly modified. This is shown in Fig. 10.4 for the little finger, median, and thumb.

These first results induced the same group of researchers to begin a systematic investigation of hemispheric asymmetries in a population of patients with focal hemispheric vascular lesions (Rossini, Tecchio, et al., 1998). The aim of the study was to establish whether the neuromagnetic method was suitable for identifying parameters associated with cerebral plasticity during recovery of sensory–motor functions after a stroke. Rossini, Tecchio, et al. (1998) studied the location and strength of the equivalent sources activated in the primary somatosensory cortex after stimulation of the left and right median nerve and of the first and fifth digits of each hand. After identifying in a population of normal subjects as relevant parameters (a) the location asymmetry of the digits and of the median nerve with respect to their projection in the two hemispheres, and (b) the extension of the hand area in the right and left hemispheres, the authors demonstrated that either one or both parameters were altered in stroke patients whenever the lost somatic function was being recovered during rehabilitation. They also observed that cortical reorganization following a subcortical lesion was larger than that occur-

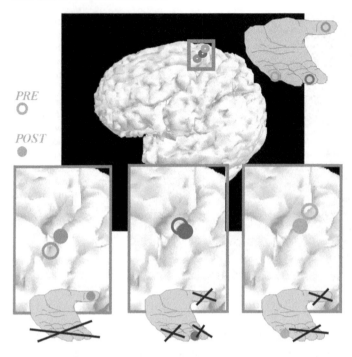

FIG. 10.4.   Short-term plasticity induced by transient ischemia. The location of the equivalent current dipoles elicited by stimulation of the median, thumb, and little finger are indicated before (pre) and after (post) ischemia of the other fingers (indicated by crosses).

ring after a cortical damage and that ECD strength from the damaged side was more intense than normal. Last, the selective reorganization of N20m and P30m observed in some patients suggested at least a partial independence of the sources active during these two components.

As an example of a clinical application, we mention a study recently conducted by Rossini, Caltagirone, et al., (1998) that used MEG, fMRI, and transcranial magnetic stimulation (TMS) to investigate a stroke patient with a malacic lesion in the left fronto–parieto–temporal cortex that had produced hemiplegia and motor aphasia. At the time of the study, 12 months after the event, the patient had satisfactorily recovered hand motor control, with only a minimal residual paresis in the right forearm, whereas no recovery from aphasia was observable. The investigation of the somatosensory functions was performed by means of MEG under single-digit and median-nerve stimulation; the efferent pathway was studied by means of TMS, and the extension and location of the hand motor area were studied by means of fMRI during execution of a simple motor task. All three techniques evidenced an asymmetrical enlargement and posterior shift of the sensorimotor areas localized in the affected hemisphere. This supports the idea that fMRI, TMS, and MEG rely on similar functional substrates and therefore may be safely combined in studying patients with the aim of testing the presence and amount of plasticity phenomena underlying partial or total clinical recovery of the lost function.

As a final example of plasticity, we mention a result recently obtained by Tecchio et al. (2000) who studied a population of 10 patients suffering from an otosclerosis process of the stapes, before and after stapes substitution. The authors observed that in all 10 patients the tonotopic organization of the auditory cortex was missing, in contrast with what was commonly seen in normal subjects. After surgery, and recovery of the auditory perception, in a subset of patients the tonotopic structure was recovered as well. It is interesting that the recovery of cortical organization was significantly better in younger patients, who suffered a shorter period of hearing impairment.

## CONCLUSION

The ability of MEG to perform functional localization was assessed in the early 1980s by a few pioneering groups working in biomagnetism. The role of their early studies was invaluable in providing the impetus for experimental and theoretical work in biomagnetism in that it showed, with simple but rigorous methods and practice, that functional localization was indeed possible. Today, with the outgrowth of experimental apparatuses, MEG has become one of the methods of choice for the investigation of neural function with very high time resolution. Furthermore, it is commonly accepted as a powerful tool complementary to positron emission tomography and to fMRI for the investigation of fundamental brain functioning and as an additional diagnostic procedure for the study of several diseases.

## ACKNOWLEDGMENTS

We acknowledge all the members of the groups in Chieti and Rome who contributed to the work presented in this chapter.

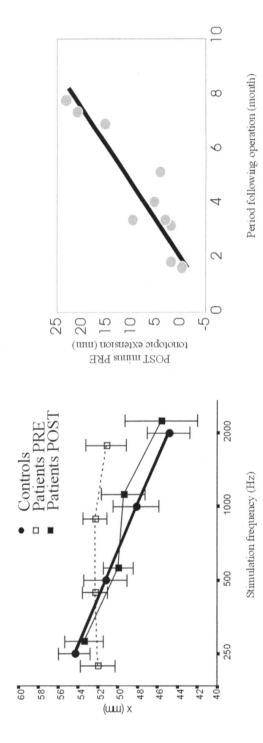

FIG. 10.5.   Tonotopic organization of the auditory cortex in patients with othosclerosis undergoing stapes substitution. Left panel: equivalent current dipole depth versus tone burst frequency (larger values indicate more superficial dipoles) in normal subjects (filled circles), patients before surgery (empty squares), and patients after surgery (filled squares). Right panel: difference in the tonotpic extension between pre- and postsurgery in relation with the time elapsed after surgery.

# REFERENCES

Babiloni, F., Carducci, F., Del Gratta, C., Babiloni, C., Roberti, G. M., Cincotti, F., Bagni, O., Romani, G. L., & Rossini, P. M. (1999). Multimodal integration of high resolution EEG, MEG and functional magnetic resonance data. *International Journal of Bioelectromagnetism, 1,* 1–19

Barth, D. S., Sutherling, W., Engel, J., Jr., & Beatty, J. (1982, November). Neuromagnetic localization of epileptiform spike activity in the human brain. *Science, 218,* 891–894.

Barth, D. S., Sutherling, W., Engel, J. Jr., & Beatty, J. (1984, January). Neuromagnetic evidence of spatially distributed sources underlying epileptiform spikes in the human brain. *Science, 223,* 293–296.

Cohen, D. (1972, February). Magnetoencephalography: Detection of the brain's electrical activity with a superconducting magnetometer. *Science, 175,* 664–666.

Del Gratta, C., Della Penna, S., Tartaro, A., Ferretti, A., Torquati, K., Bonomo, L., Romani, G. L., & Rossini, P. M. (2000). Topographic organization of the human primary and secondary somatosensory areas: An fMRI study. *NeuroReport, 11,* 2035–2043.

Del Gratta, C., Della Penna, S., Ferretti, A., Franciotti, R., Pizzella, V., Tartaro, A., Torquati, K., Bonomo, L., Romani, G. L., & Rossini, P. M. (2002). Topographic organization of the human primary and secondary somatosensory cortices: Comparisons of fMRI and MEG findings. *NeuroImage, 17,* 1373–1383.

Del Gratta, C., Pizzella, V., Tecchio, F., & Romani, G. L. (2001). Magnetoencephalography—A noninvasive brain imaging method with 1 ms time resolution. *Reports on Progress in Physics, 64,* 1759–1814.

Della Penna, S., Del Gratta, C., Granata, C., Pasquarelli, A., Rossi, R., Russo, M., Torquati, K., & Erné, S. N. (2000). Biomagnetic systems for clinical use. *Philosophical Magazine B., 80,* 937–948.

Foglietti, V., Del Gratta, C., Pasquarelli, A., Pizzella, V., Torrioli, G., Romani, G. L., Gallagher, W. J., Ketchen, M. B., Kleinsasser, A. W., & Sandstrom, R. L. (1991). 28-channel hybrid system for neuromagnetic measurements. *IEEE Transactions on Magnetics, 27,* 2959–2962.

Grimm, C., Schreiber, A., Kristeva-Feige, R., Mergner, T., Hennig, J., & Lucking, C. H. (1998). Comparison between electric source localization and fMRI during somatosensory stimulation. *Electroencephalography and Clinical Neurophysiology, 106,* 22–29.

Hämäläinen, M., Hari, R., Ilmoniemi, R., Knuutila, J., & Lounasmaa, O. (1993). Magneto-encephalography—Theory, instrumentation, and applications to noninvasive studies of the working human brain. *Reviews of Modern Physics, 65,* 413–497.

Hari, R., Karhu, J., Hämäläinen, M., Knuutila, J., Salonen, O., Sama, M., & Vilkman, V. (1993). Functional organization of the first and second somatosensory cortices: A neuromagnetic study. *European Journal of Neuroscience, 5,* 724–734.

Kristeva-Feige, R., Rossi, S., Pizzella, V., Tecchio, F., Romani, G. L., Erné, S., Edrich, J., Orlacchio, A., & Rossini, P. M. (1995). Neuromagnetic fields of the brain evoked by voluntary movement and electrical stimulation of the index finger. *Brain Research, 682,* 22–28.

Merzenich, M. M., Kaas, J. H., Wall, J., Nelson, R. J., Sur, M., & Felleman, D. (1983). Topographic reorganization of somatosensory cortical areas 3b and 1 in adult monkeys following restricted deafferentation. *Neuroscience, 8,* 33–55.

Nakasato, N., Karou, S., Tsuyoshi, K., Satoshi, F., Akitake, K., Satoru, F., & Takashi, Y. (1996). Functional brain mapping using an MRI-linked whole head magnetoencephalography (MEG) system. In C. Barber, G. Celesia, G. C. Comi, & F. Mauguiere (Eds.), *Functional neuroscience* (pp. 119–126). Amsterdam: Elsevier.

Pizzella, V., Della Penna, S., Del Gratta, C., & Romani, G. L. (2001). SQUID systems for biomagnetic imaging. *Superconductor Science and Technology, 14,* R79–R114.

Ricci, G. B., Romani, G. L., Salustri, C., Pizzella, V., Torrioli, G., Buonomo, S., Peresson, M., & Modena, I. (1987). Study of focal epilepsy by multichannel neuromagnetic measurements. *Electroencephalography and Clinical Neurophysiology, 66,* 358–368.

Romani, G. L., Williamson, S. J., & Kaufman, L. (1982a). Biomagnetic instrumentation. *Review of Scientific Instruments, 53,* 1815–1845.

Romani, G. L., Williamson, S. J., & Kaufman, L. (1982b). Characterization of the human auditory cortex by the neuromagnetic method. *Experimental Brain Research, 47,* 381–393.

Romani, G. L., Williamson, S. J., & Kaufman, L. (1982c, June). Tonotopic organization of the human auditory cortex. *Science, 216*, 1339–1340.

Rossini, P. M., Caltagirone, C., Castriota-Scanderbeg, A., Cicinelli, P., Del Gratta, C., Demartin, M., Pizzella, V., Traversa, R., & Romani, G. L. (1998). Hand motor cortical area reorganization in stroke: A study with fMRI, MEG and TCS maps. *NeuroReport, 9*, 2141–2146.

Rossini, P. M., Martino, G., Narici, L., Pasquarelli, A., Peresson, M., Pizzella, V., Tecchio, F., Torrioli, G., & Romani, G. L. (1994). Short-term brain "plasticity" in humans: Transient finger representation changes in sensory cortex somatotopy following ischemic anaesthesia. *Brain Research, 642*, 169–177.

Rossini, P. M., Tecchio, F., Pizzella, V., Lupoi, D., Cassetta, E., Pasqualetti, P., Romani, G., L, & Orlacchio, A. (1998). On the reorganization of sensory hand areas after mono-hemispheric lesion: A functional (MEG)/anatomical (MRI) integrative study. *Brain Research, 782*, 153–166.

Tecchio, F., Bicciolo, G., De Campora, E., Pasqualetti, P., Pizzella, V., Indovina, I., Cassetta, E., Romani, G. L., & Rossini, P. M. (2000). Tonotopic cortical changes following stapes substitution in otosclerotic patients: A magnetoencephalographic study. *Human Brain Mapping, 10*, 28–38.

Torquati, K., Pizzella, V., Della Penna, S., Franciotti, R., Babiloni, C., Rossini, P. M., & Romani, G. L. (2002). Comparison between SI and SII responses as a function of stimulus intensity. *Neuroreport, 13*, 813–819.

Tripp, J. H. (1981). Biomagnetic fields and cellular current flows. In: S. N. Erné, H. D. Halbohom, & H. Lübbig (Eds.), *Biomagnetism* (pp. 207–215). Berlin, Germany: Walter de Gruyter.

Williamson, S. J., & Kaufman, L. (1981a). Biomagnetism. *Journal of Magnetism and Magnetic Materials, 22*, 129–201.

Williamson, S. J., & Kaufman, L. (1981b). Evoked cortical magnetic fields. In S. N. Erné, H. D. Halbohm, & H. Lübbig (Eds.), *Biomagnetism* (pp. 353–402). Berlin, Germany: Walter de Gruyter.

Williamson, S. J., & Kaufman, L. (1990). Theory of neuroelectric and neuromagnetic fields. In F. Grandori, M. Hoke, & G. L. Romani (Eds.), *Auditory evoked magnetic fields and electric potentials* (pp. 1–39). *Advances in audiology*. Basel, Switzerland: Karger.

# 11

## Optical Imaging of Brain Function and the Relation Between Neuronal Activity and Hemodynamics in Health and Disease

Edward L. Maclin
*The Beckman Institute and*
*University of Illinois at Urbana–Champaign*

Functional neuroimaging techniques based on hemodynamics (positron emission tomography, functional magnetic resonance imaging) and those based on electrophysiology (electroencephalography, magnetoencephalography, and their stimulus-related counterparts) provide complementary information regarding both normal and pathological brain function. Many details of the relation between neuronal activation and consequent changes of blood flow, volume, and oxygenation remain unclear. Hemodynamic regulation is also known to vary between brain regions and to be different in the very young and the elderly. This is particularly problematic when brain imaging techniques are applied to patients with cerebral infarct or stroke. In the diseased brain, the relation between neuronal and hemodynamic measures is particularly complicated, because mechanisms regulating various aspects of hemodynamic function are likely to be differentially affected by disease processes. An ability to quantitatively assess the relation of hemodynamic and functional states of cerebral tissue would be useful to both basic cognitive neuroscience and in the management of cerebral disease (see M. D. Ginsberg & J. Bogousslavsky, 1998, for an overview of current practice and research in the diagnosis and management of stroke). Among the currently available functional imaging modalities only noninvasive optical imaging, a relative newcomer to the field, has the potential to simultaneously measure both hemodynamic and neuronal aspects of cerebral physiology. This dual capability makes noninvasive optical imaging an exciting tool for investigating the relation between hemodynamics and neuronal activity. In this chapter I provide a brief introduction to some of the issues underlying functional neuroimaging studies of stroke as well as to recent work demonstrating the ability of optical imaging to simultaneously measure hemodynamic and neuronal phenomena in well-defined cortical regions.

## FUNCTIONAL NEUROIMAGING METHODS

The last two decades of the 20th century witnessed the birth of numerous new technologies for imaging the functioning human brain (Raichle, 1998). These functional neuroimaging techniques in turn spawned a new branch of science: cognitive neuroscience, whose ultimate goal is to understand just how the brain embodies the mind (Posner & Raichle, 1998). Some of these technologies—in particular, functional magnetic resonance imaging (fMRI)—are widely available, have been used to study a broad range of issues in cognitive neuroscience, and are increasingly being used to study diseases of the brain as well. Others, such as magnetoencephalography (MEG) and near infrared spectroscopy (NIRS), are less widely available and have been slower to be developed and widely adopted. Cognitive neuroscience (the functional part of functional neuroimaging) has yet to be systematically applied to medical practice, although much has been learned about how the brain is organized from studies of injured brains. In the future we can expect to see cognitive neuroscience playing an increasing role in clinical practice, both in diagnosis and rehabilitation.

It is important to distinguish two facets of functional neuroimaging as they relate to the study of ischemia. On the one hand are measures of the basal or spontaneous activity of the tissue, and on the other hand are measures of the degree to which the tissues can be activated by appropriate stimuli, cognitive tasks, or motor activity. Each imaging modality can provide both types of information; often the distinction is simply a matter of what the patient is asked to do during the measurements and how the resulting data are analyzed (e.g., electroencephalography [EEG]–MEG/EP–EF, MRI/fMRI, NIRS/event-related optical signal [EROS]). Two important dimensions of functional neuroimaging are (a) spatial and (b) temporal resolution. Most functional imaging modalities excel in only one dimension; one possible exception is near-infrared optical imaging, which holds the promise of high spatial and temporal resolution of both neuronal and hemodynamic activity.

In the next few years, great progress can be expected not only in the further development of each of the extant brain imaging methods but particularly in the simultaneous application of multiple methods to systematically combine the very different sorts of information each method provides to more fully illuminate the workings of the brain in both health and disease. In this chapter I briefly review the established functional neuroimaging methods and compare their strengths and weaknesses, and I discuss how infrared optical imaging may help illuminate the relation between functional brain activity and the brain's blood supply in both healthy and injured brains.

## PET

The first truly effective functional brain imaging modality was positron emission tomography (PET). In addition to inspiring the birth of cognitive neuroscience (Posner & Raichle, 1994), PET has provided the gold standard for the quantitative study of regional cerebral blood flow and oxygen and glucose metabolism (Frackowiak, Lenzi, Jones, & Heather, 1980). Subsequent PET studies were the first to show that the regulation of cerebral blood flow and metabolism is considerably more complex than was originally assumed (Fox, Raichle, Mintun, & Dence, 1988). PET's quantitative precision, and the continuing development of highly specific radio-labeled tracers for a wide range of metabolic and signaling pathways, will make PET an indispensable technique in the study of stroke for the foreseeable future (Heiss, 1998).

### MRI Studies of Perfusion and Metabolism

Since Lauterbur (1973) first described the possibility of MRI, it has developed to the point where virtually every hospital in the industrialized world has a system capable of rendering high-resolution (~1 mm) images of soft tissue in any part of the human body. These detailed anatomical images are essential for the accurate spatial interpretation of all functional neuroimaging data. MRI is rapidly becoming the method of choice for the acute diagnosis of stroke. In spite of difficulties in absolute quantification of MRI images, the ability to image both perfusion (blood flow) and diffusion (molecular movement along osmotic gradients) means

MRI will continue to play a central role in stroke diagnosis and management (Warach & Schlaug, 1998). Magnetic resonance spectroscopy holds great promise for localization and quantification of specific molecules in living tissue. Although currently far from ready for routine clinical application, magnetic resonance spectroscopy will undoubtedly also play an increasing role in both research and clinical practice (Pritchard, 1998). The recently demonstrated ability to map fiber paths through their effects on the diffusion tensor (Conturo et al., 1999) will aid greatly in the interpretation of functional neuroimaging data.

## fMRI

In the early 1990s, several groups demonstrated the ability of MRI to detect changes in blood oxygenation, the blood oxygenation level dependent (BOLD) signal (Kwong et al., 1992; Ogawa, Lee, Kay, & Tank, 1990; Schwarzbauer & Heinke, 1999; Turner, LeBihan, Moonen, Despres, & Frank, 1991). The wide availability, relatively noninvasive nature, and high spatial resolution of MRI have made fMRI the most widely applied functional neuroimaging technique. The development of echo planar imaging has made it possible to acquire a single image (slice) in a few hundred milliseconds on a typical medical scanner and even faster on state-of-the-art high field systems (Howseman, Thomas, Pell, Williams, & Ordidge, 1999; Kwong, 1995; Richter, 1999). However, the speed and linearity of the hemodynamic response to neural activation ultimately limit the temporal resolution of fMRI. It has been shown that this response is sufficiently linear, at least in healthy young brains, that temporally overlapping BOLD responses can be deconvolved, permitting the rapid serial presentation of randomly chosen stimuli (Boynton, Engel, Glover, & Heeger, 1996; Buckner et al., 1996; D'Esposito, Zarahn, & Aguirre, 1999; Hoge et al., 1999; Miezin, Maccotta, Ollinger, Petersen, & Buckner, 2000). This greatly expands the range of cognitive tasks that can be investigated. In an elegant series of invasive studies in monkeys, Logothetis, Pauls, Augath, Trinath, and Oeltermann (2001) showed that the response of the neurovascular system is specific both to individual animals and brain regions and that local field potentials yield better estimates of BOLD responses than do multi-unit responses. They concluded that the BOLD contrast mechanism reflects the input and intracortical processing of a given area rather than its output. Numerous questions remain concerning the relation of the BOLD signal to neuronal activity (Villringer & Dirnagl, 1995), particularly in conditions of compromised hemodynamic regulation, such as stroke or the aging brain. These questions can be addressed only using multiple independent, and preferably simultaneous, measures of different aspects of the neuronal and hemodynamic responses (Toronov et al., 2001).

## EEG

Cerebral ischemia, along with a wide range of other cerebral pathologies, has long been recognized to produce abnormalities in the EEG (Aminoff, 1986; Kitamura, Iwai, Tsumura, Ono, & Terashi, 1998; Murri et al., 1998). These abnormalities include diminished overall signal, decreases in alpha amplitude, decreases in alpha frequency, increases in low frequency (delta and theta) power, and periodic lateralizing epileptiform discharges. It is often stated that in clinical practice these phenomena, as currently interpreted, are of limited clinical utility (e.g., Aminoff, 1986, p. 56). A considerable body of evidence is accumulating that strongly suggests that improved methods of analysis can dramatically improve the usefulness of EEG for diagnosis and management of stroke patients.

Macdonell, Donnan, Bladin, Berkovic, and Wriedt (1988) were able to use visual interpretation of EEG to discriminate lacunar and cortical strokes, indicating the sensitivity of brain electrical activity to the physiological mechanisms of stroke. They studied 100 patients, clinically diagnosed with stroke, with computer tomography (CT) and EEG, and found that lateralized theta or delta activity (or both) predicted ipsilateral cortical infarction with a sensitivity of 76% and a specificity of 82%. Lacunar infarcts produced similar abnormalities in only 9% of cases. They also observed that EEG was particularly useful if the initial CT excludes hemorrhage but does not exclude infarction.

More recently, Kappelle, van Huffelen, and van Gijn (1990) were able to demonstrate, using both visual and computer (spectral) analysis of EEG, that lacunar infarcts exhibit a fairly specific pattern of EEG abnormalities. Asymmetries in alpha and mu rhythms were found to be especially important in diagnosing lacunar infarcts rather than abnormal slow-wave activity. They pointed out that these EEG signs were present in the earliest (poststroke) cases they were able to measure, whereas the CT scans were often still unremarkable.

Labar, Fisch, Pedley, Fink, and Solomon (1991) correlated trend analysis of total power, frequency centroid, alpha ratio, and percentage delta power with clinical and CT findings in 11 patients with subarachnoid hemorrhage. Overall, one or another index showed significant change in every patient. They found total power to be the most sensitive index

(91%), followed by alpha ratio (64%) and frequency centroid (55%). They concluded that trend analysis of EEG parameters is superior to CT and clinical assessment in predicting the course of illness in patients with cerebral ischemia, particularly in those with aneurysmal subarachnoid hemorrhage. Improved methods of spatial and temporal analysis EEG data clearly will continue to strengthen the role of EEG as a research and clinical tool.

## MEG

Juergen Vieth and colleagues at the University of Erlangen have been using MEG to study abnormal low-frequency magnetic activity for several years. In their initial work they studied 10 patients with either transient or permanent ischemic lesions (Vieth, Sack, Schueler, Grummich, & Schneider, 1989). Some patients were studied with a single-channel MEG system and simultaneous EEG. These data were analyzed by the *relative covariance* method of Chapman et al. (1983). Other patients were studied with a Siemans 37-channel Krenikon system, and conventional dipole-fitting methods were used. Vieth et al. (1989) found clearly dipolar field patterns in 4 patients, and moderately distorted patterns, suggestive of multiple sources, in 4 patients. In 2 cases the field maps were sufficiently distorted as to be unanalyzable. In all but 1 of the cases where equivalent source dipoles could be localized, the dipole appeared near the lesion. In 1 case the dipole fell within the lesion. They concluded that MEG would be valuable in the detection of clinically silent ischemic lesions, providing an indication for preventive treatments such as endarterectomy, platelet aggregation inhibitors, or anticoagulant drugs.

In subsequent studies, Vieth (1990) used a modeling procedure he called the *dipole pathway* (DPP) technique, which tracks the movement of an estimated dipole over time. This technique estimated a concentration of dipoles near the lesions but also found a significant number spreading away from the lesions.

More recently, Vieth et al. (1991) compared the dipole pathway technique with another approach he termed the *dipole-density-plot* (DDP). DDP accepts only dipoles with a signal-to-noise (S/N) ratio above a specified value, within a specified volume unit, and with a spatial density of estimated fits above a specified limit. They applied the DDP to data from 9 patients with abnormal low-frequency magnetic activity due to a variety of pathologies, including infarctions, hemorrhages, and tumors. They varied the three model parameters systematically and found that a higher signal-to-noise ratio, smaller volume unit, and higher density limit act together to concentrate dipole locations. In applying their dipole pathway model to the same data sets, they found that the pathways were located mainly within the dipole "clouds" estimated by the DDP. They concluded that the DDP is able to extract automatically a higher spatial density of estimated dipoles compared with the dipole pathway technique.

Another group, lead by Chris Gallen at the Scripps Clinic, has investigated both alteration of alpha activity (Gallen, Hampson, & Bloom, 1990) and slow waves (Gallen, Schwartz, Pantev, Hampson, Sobel, Hirschkoff, Rieke, Otis, & Bloom, 1992) in stroke patients. They have used a technique similar to the dipole pathway method of Vieth and his colleagues and have found slow-wave sources in 2 patients to "wander" through the penumbra. In 4 patients with occipital strokes, they have found substantial variations from the normal pattern of alpha reactivity to visual stimuli. They concluded that functional recovery from stroke might involve the redistribution of cortical activity into adjacent processing regions.

Taken together, these studies indicate the feasibility of using MEG to localize generators of individual slow waves and demonstrate the close association of slow wave generators with ischemic lesions and to provide quantitative, spatially resolved data on neuronal function and injury in individual patients.

### Evoked Potentials and Fields

Although there are notable exceptions (Kaufman, Curtis, Wang, & Williamson, 1991), the majority of "functional" electrophysiological studies use some form of (typically averaged) evoked response. There is a long history of research and application of evoked potentials, primarily somatosensory, in the diagnosis of stroke (e.g., Fierro, La Bua, Oliveri, Daniele, & Brighina, 1999; Pereon, Aubertin, & Guiheneuc, 1995; Stejskal & Sobota, 1985), although these spatially unresolved simple sensory responses are generally thought to be of limited clinical usefulness. A few studies have begun to investigate the effects of strokes on more cognitively related evoked potentials; these include studies of novelty (Knight & Nakada, 1998), anticipation (Oishi & Mochizuki, 1998), and memory (Rugg, 1998).

The relatively high spatial resolution of MEG has been used to map visual responses in the vicinity of occipital strokes (Maclin, Rose, & Paulson, 1991) as well as to demonstrate the apparent sparing of extrastriate responses in some patients (Maclin, Robinson, Knight, & Paulson, 1992). In another MEG study, Maclin, Rose, Knight, Orrison, and Davis (1994) demonstrated a linear relation between somatosensory evoked dipole strength (estimated from MEG) and degree of sensory impairment (graphesthesia). Toyoda, Ibayashi, Yamamoto, Kuwabara, & Fujishima (1998) recorded auditory evoked magnetic fields and cerebral blood flow (CBF, via PET) in 24 patients with temporal infarcts. They found that patients with abnormal P50 or N100 responses had decreased supratemporal and hemispheric blood flow when compared to patients with normal P50m responses.

## Optical Methods

Changes in the optical properties of the brain associated with mental activity can be observed with the naked eye, and advances in instrumentation have led to the development of a wide range of optical techniques for studying the brain (Bonhoeffer & Grinvald, 1996; Villringer & Chance, 1997). These techniques can be broadly divided along three dimensions: (a) wavelength (generally corresponding to invasive vs. noninvasive measures); (b) intrinsic versus extrinsic signals (i.e., "natural signals" vs. those relying on contrast agents); and (c) mechanism—absorption, scattering, or fluorescence. Although each of these techniques has much to offer in understanding brain function and physiology, noninvasive studies are possible only using near-infrared light to study intrinsic signals. Within these restrictions, two types of optical signals can be discerned in intact subjects: (a) a slow signal that corresponds quantitatively to hemodynamic parameters (NIRS; Frostig, Lieke, Ts'o, & Grinvald, 1990) and a fast signal whose origin is less clear but that correlates strongly with electrophysiological signals (EROS; Gratton, Corballis, Cho, Fabiani, & Hood, 1995).

### NIRS

Biological tissue absorbs most wavelengths of light quite efficiently but is remarkably transparent, although strongly scattering, in the near infrared (NIR). The NIR absorbance spectra of two of the most important molecules in the oxygen metabolism chain are strongly dependent on their oxidation state. These two facts form the basis for *in vivo* oximetry using NIRS (see Dujovny, Misra, & Widman, 1998; Madsen & Secher, 1999).

The first practical demonstration of NIRS was Millikan's (1942) earlobe oximeter, whereas the first cerebral measurements, in cats, were reported by Jobsis (1977). Although several tissue chromophores exhibit oxygenation-dependent absorbance (Giltvedt, Sira, & Helme, 1984), the observed signal is dominated by hemoglobin (Wray, Cope, Delpy, Wyatt, & Reynolds, 1988), with cytochrome oxidase providing a weak but detectable signal (Cooper & Springett, 1997).

The Beer–Lambert law (Beer, 1851) describes the absorption of light by a chromophore in a homogenous diffusing medium. Absorption is determined by the chromophore extinction coefficient; its concentration; and the "path length," or integrated distance the photons travel through the chromophore-containing region. Quantitative measurement of chromophore concentration therefore depends directly on accurate estimation of the path length (Cope & Delpy, 1988; Delpy & Cope, 1997; Delpy et al., 1988), which is known to vary with age (Duncan et al., 1996) and may vary as a function of pathology as well.

The fact that propagation of NIR photons in tissue is dominated by scattering rather than absorption means that measurement of photons entering an object at one point on its surface diffuse randomly throughout the object and are eventually either absorbed or emitted from a random point on the surface. The fact that photons diffuse deeply into tissue and then return to the surface is the basis of NIR imaging of the brain. The probability that photons emitted at any particular point on the surface have passed through any particular region in the interior of the object can be calculated given the diffusion and absorption coefficients at each point in the volume (Durduran et al., 1999). On the assumption of a homogeneous medium, photons traveling between two points on the surface are most likely to have traversed an arc-shaped region through the medium. The fact that the majority of photons have not simply traversed the region directly between the source and detector, as one might first assume, is due to the high probability that photons that wander near the surface will diffuse to the surface and be "lost," whereas photons that end up too deep are likely to be lost to absorption. The depth of this arc has been shown to be proportional to the distance between the source and measurement points (Cui, Kumar, & Chance, 1991; Gratton, Maier, Fabiani, Mantulin, & Gratton, 1994; Harris, Cowans, Wertheim, & Hamid, 1994; van der Zee, Arridge, Cope, & Delpy, 1990).

Just as in the interpretation of electrical and magnetic fields, the presence of anatomical inhomogeneities greatly complicates the tomographic interpretation of diffused photons. Considerable theoretical and experimental effort has been, and continues to be, devoted to determining the practical limits on spatial resolution in typically inhomogeneous living tissue. Substantial progress has been made in applications in relatively homogeneous tissues, particularly the breast, but the cranium presents a significantly more complex challenge (Firbank, Okada, & Delpy, 1998; Germon, Young, Manara, & Nelson, 1995).

Okada et al. (1997) reported an elaborate series of phantom studies in which they attempted to address some of the issues of cranial topography. They constructed a series of phantoms of increasing complexity, with up to four layers (scalp/skull, cerebrospinal fluid [CSF], gray matter, and white matter) whose absorbance, diffusion, and geometry they attempted to match to measured tissue values (Firbank, Hiraoka, Essenpries, & Delpy, 1993; van der Zee, Essenpries, & Delpy, 1993). Unfortunately, they used a clear (nonscattering) CSF layer with a uniform thickness of 1 mm, which almost certainly does not accurately reflect anatomical reality and which consequently overemphasizes the role of "ballistic" or radiatively transported photons. As a consequence of this almost certainly exaggerated clarity, thickness, and geometric uniformity of the CSF layer, both their measured and computed photon diffusion paths are very superficial, barely penetrating into the cortex at all.

In a series of studies with plastic phantoms, Kurth and Thayer (1999) found that infant- and childlike shells overlying the brain model did not adversely affect NIRS oximetry, whereas the adultlike shell yielded an error as high as 32%. They concluded that NIRS accurately measures $SO_2$ in their *in vitro* brain model, although low hemoglobin concentration and extracranial tissue of adult thickness may influence accuracy.

Totaro, Barattelli, Quaresima, Carolei, and Ferrari (1998) evaluated the effects of several factors (venous return, age, and sex) that might be expected to affect the reliability of NIRS to test $CO_2$ cerebrovascular reactivity. They found NIRS to be a reliable and reproducible method for the evaluation of cerebrovascular reactivity that should be validated for the assessment of patients with cerebrovascular disease.

The substantial body of literature on both clinical and cognitive NIRS studies of cerebral function clearly belies Okada et al.'s (1997) conclusions. Just as in the case of EEG and MEG, more work is needed to clarify the real role of tissue geometry in the interpretation of data collected at the surface of the head (Firbank, Elwell, Cooper, & Delpy, 1998; Firbank et al., 1998; Germon et al., 1998). One goal of this effort, particularly in clinical cases with abnormal tissue properties (e.g., tumors, abscesses, and hemangiomas), is to be able to derive these structural properties from MRI images.

***Time Resolved NIRS.***    Photons diffusing in a scattering medium may take quite different paths and different amounts of time to travel between two points. By restricting the accepted range of times of flight, the paths the photons are likely to have taken can be confined to a smaller volume, improving spatial resolution. Time-of-flight can be selected directly, by injecting a very brief pulse of light and gating the detector or indirectly by continuously modulating (at > 100 MHz) the input source and recording the phase of the detected modulation. This second approach allows integration over many modulation cycles, which substantially increases the signal-to-noise ratio. The use of heterodyning (cross-correlation) detectors permits use of relatively inexpensive low-frequency measurement circuits. The optimization and interpretation of these various approaches comprise an active area of research (Fishkin & Gratton, 1993; Fishkin, Fantini, van de Ven, & Gratton, 1996).

***Cognitive NIRS.***    Many groups have reported a variety of NIRS studies of cognitive brain activation (Danen, Wang, Li, Thayer, & Yodh, 1998; Hoshi & Tamura, 1993; Lichty et al., 1999). These include visual activation (Heekeren et al., 1999), somatosensory activation (Obrig et al., 1996), motor activation (Hirth, Obrig, Valdueza, Dirnagl, & Villringer, 1997), language studies (Fallgatter, Muller, & Strik, 1998; Hock et al., 1997; Sakatani, Lichty, Xie, Li, & Zuo, 1999; Watanabe et al., 1998), and executive functions (Fallgatter & Strik, 1998). Several recent articles have described real-time optical imaging of cerebral hemodynamics with temporal resolution of 160 msec (Franceschini, Toronov, Filiaci, Gratton, & Fantini, 2000; Jasdzewski et al., 2002; Toronov et al., 2000).

NIRS appears to offer sensitivity and temporal resolution comparable to fMRI, spatial resolution comparable to and potentially better than MEG (at least for signals within a few centimeters of the surface), and quantitative precision of blood oxygenation comparable to PET at a cost in the range of EEG systems. Researchers can expect to see rapid development of both the underlying technologies and applications of NIRS for both clinical and cognitive neuroscience applications in the future.

### EROS

In addition to the well-established sensitivity of NIRS to hemodynamic factors varying on the scale of seconds, it is possible to measure signals (both amplitude and phase) that vary much more rapidly. This includes both *in vitro* and *in vivo* animal studies (Frostig, 1994;

Frostig et al., 1990; Grinvald, Lieke, Frostig, Gilbert, & Wiesel, 1986; Malonek & Grinvald, 1996; Rector, Rogers, Schwaber, Harper, & George, 2001) and noninvasive studies in humans (Gratton et al., 1994). These fast signals have been observed in response to a wide range of stimuli and cognitive events (Gratton & Fabiani, 1998) and are known as EROS.

Several hypotheses have been suggested for the biophysical mechanism underlying these fast responses. Changes in scattering, rather than absorption, appear to be the dominant cause. Scattering may be affected by cell size, which in turn is a function of membrane potential and the movement of hydrated ions into and out of the cells (Cohen, 1972; Hill & Keynes, 1949; MacVicar & Hochman, 1991). It has also been suggested that the orientation of membrane proteins may change with membrane potential and in turn alter the optical properties of the cell surface (Stepnoski et al., 1991).

Gabriele Gratton and his colleagues have reported a series of studies designed to explore the strengths and weaknesses of EROS. In 1995, Gratton and his colleagues reported detecting and localizing fast optical signals in response to both stimulation of different visual quadrants (Gratton, Corballis, et al., 1995) and finger tapping (Gratton, Fabiani, et al., 1995). Subsequent studies have demonstrated the sensitivity of EROS to manipulations of attention (Gratton, 1997) and memory (Gratton, Fabiani, Goodman-Wood, & Desoto, 1998). Recently, Rinne et al. (1999) showed that EROS can spatially discriminate the auditory mismatch negativity response from other auditory response components. A combined EROS/fMRI study of responses to visual stimuli presented at various eccentricities in the visual field demonstrates the accuracy of EROS estimates of response location in depth (Gratton, Sarno, Maclin, Corballis, & Fabiani, 2000).

The fact that EROS and NIRS measurements can be made simultaneously with the same instrument allows the direct comparison of neuronal and hemodynamic activation. Gratton, Goodman-Wood, and Fabiani (1999) compared the amplitude of EROS responses to visual gratings flashed at various frequencies with the magnitude of the simultaneously recorded NIRS. They found the NIRS magnitude to be proportional to the integral of the EROS amplitude. This combination of measures is the only way to simultaneously obtain neuronal and hemodynamic information from essentially the same volume of tissue, and it is likely to provide an important tool for studying the relation of neural and hemodynamic activity.

## PHYSIOLOGY: METABOLISM AND BLOOD FLOW

There are at least two major open neurophysiological questions that bear directly on the interpretation of cognitive neuroimaging data in healthy subjects: (a) What is the relation between neural activity and energy metabolism, and (b) what is the mechanism that couples blood flow to metabolism?

### Metabolism

Magistretti and Pellerin (1999) reviewed the metabolism issues. They described how converging lines of evidence suggest that astrocytes actively extract glucose from capillaries and reduce it to lactose, which is then actively transferred to neurons, where it may be the primary energy source for signaling related activity. This process appears to be regulated by glutamate, which, when released by neurons, is actively taken up by astrocytes, where it initiates glycolysis. Magistretti and Pellerin suggested that this model is consistent with the variable degree of coupling between glucose uptake and oxygen consumption as well as with transient peaks in lactate concentration. After clarification of several details—particularly the rates of each stage and the nature and capacities of any storage of substrates—this model may very well provide a quantitative description of cerebral energy metabolism, at least in the healthy brain.

### Blood Flow

The regulation of CBF is a far more complex issue (see Sanders, 1995, for an introduction). There are two competing classes of theories of CBF regulation: (a) metabolic (or humoral) theories and (b) neuronal theories. Sandor (1999) reviewed the history of the debate on the role of nervous versus humoral control of local CBF.

The metabolic hypothesis was first clearly espoused over 100 years ago by Roy and Sherrington (1890). It posits that a metabolic end product (typically $CO_2$ or lactate) diffuses from active neurons to local vessel walls, where it directly affects vessel diameter and blood flow. The humoral version of this theory substitutes any of a wide variety of nonmetabolic moieties but continues to rely on diffusion and direct action on blood vessels. These theories share at least two common weaknesses: (a) the magnitude of vessel reaction to putative CBF regulators is small, and (b) the preponderant site of CBF regulation appears to be in the precapillary arterioles, upstream from the active neurons.

Although it is well known that parenchymal blood vessels are richly innervated, the precise function of this innervation remains a subject of active research. There are more than a dozen recognized pathways for sympathetic and parasympathetic, trigeminovascular, and sensory innervation of cerebral blood vessels. Stimulation of the sympathetic nerve reduces CBF by 5%–10%, whereas parasympathetic stimulation has the opposite effect. Although these reactions are considerably smaller than reactions in other organs, it is generally believed that these systems play primarily a protective role in responding the extreme changes in blood pressure (Busija, 1996). Within the normal range, control of CBF is clearly local, as evidenced by the success of hemodynamically based cognitive neuroimaging. Although the details of possible neural mechanisms controlling CBF are likely to differ among regions of the brain, it is becoming clearer that neurovascular control plays a significant, if not dominant, role in the regulation of CBF (Lovick, Brown, & Key, 1999).

### Hemodynamic Dysregulation

If researchers' understanding of the mechanisms and parameters of the regulation of cerebral metabolism and blood in healthy subjects is still incomplete, their understanding of these issues in disease, in the very young, and in the elderly is very rudimentary. The normal relation between oxygen utilization and blood flow is known to be disrupted in epilepsy (Bruehl, Hagemann, & Witte, 1998), in migraine (Bednarczyk, Remler, Weikart, Nelson, & Reed, 1998), in elderly subjects (D'Esposito, Zarahn, Aguirre, & Rypma, 1999), and in stroke (Back, 1998). Indeed, in a study of the combined effect of increased brain topical K+ concentration and reduction of the nitric oxide in rats, Dreier et al. (1998) found that a disturbed coupling of metabolism and CBF can even cause ischemia.

A primary question in the diagnosis and management of stroke concerns the *penumbra*, or region of tissue whose hemodynamic supply has been acutely disrupted but whose neurons are in a delicate balance between recovery and further deterioration (Astrup, Siesjo, & Symon, 1981; Ginsberg, Belayev, Zhao, Huh, & Busto, 1999). Knowledge of the physiological state of the penumbra has, and continues to, evolve considerably (Back, 1998).

Clinical concepts of the penumbra and its role in recovery from stroke also continue to evolve (Kaufmann et al., 1999; Neubauer & James, 1998) and more precise quantitative data are becoming available. For example, in a group of 19 stroke patients, Marchal et al. (1999) used PET to determine putative thresholds for irreversible tissue damage as the lower limit of the 95% confidence interval calculated from all voxels within ultimately noninfarcted brain parenchyma ipsilateral to the insult. Voxels below these thresholds occurred significantly more frequently in the final infarct region than in the noninfarcted parenchyma for CBF and cerebral metabolic rate of oxygen ($CMRO_2$). These findings demonstrate the usefulness of PET-based CBF and $CMRO_2$ thresholds for probabilistic mapping of irreversible tissue damage within the 5- to 18-hr interval after stroke onset.

## Multimodal Studies of Neuronal Activity, Blood Flow, and Metabolism

Studies using multiple independent measures of neuronal, metabolic, and hemodynamic aspects of cerebral function are becoming increasingly common. The majority of these studies have been performed in patients with a variety of neurological disorders; relatively few have systematically investigated the relation of measures in healthy subjects. To fill this gap, Leuchter, Uijtdehaage, Cook, and Mandelkern (1999) conducted a combined EEG/PET study of 6 healthy subjects at rest and performing a simple motor task. They found EEG cordance (Leuchter, Cook, & Lachenbruch, 1994) of low frequency (4–8 Hz) and high frequency (20+ Hz) to be positively correlated with perfusion, whereas a band from 6 to 10 Hz was negatively correlated.

Hoshi, Kosaka, Xie, Kohri, and Tamura (1998) reported a strong correlation between EEG peak frequency and regional CBF measured with NIRS in resting subjects. They suggested that spontaneous variations in neural activity are reflected in continuous fluctuations in local cerebral hemodynamic parameters. Sadato et al. (1998) compared PET-measured CBF and EEG alpha power in healthy subjects and found negative correlations in the visual (striate) cortex and positive correlations in limbic areas. This illustrates both the regional variability of EEG–CBF coupling and the possible utility of EEG in studies of emotion. Villringer et al. (1997) compared PET–CBF and NIRS estimates of oxy-Hb, deoxy-Hb and total-Hb hemoglobin in 5 healthy subjects during rest and during a Stroop task. They found a significant correlation between total-Hb and CBF at a depth of 9 mm, confirming the validity of the NIRS estimates.

Litscher (1998) described an elaborate "multifunctional helmet for noninvasive neuromonitoring." This helmet includes six "active" EEG electrodes, two robotically positioned transcranial Doppler probes, and an

NIRS probe for transcranial cerebral oximetry. This system allows the simultaneous mapping of cerebral arteries, quantification of arterial blood flow, brainstem auditory evoked potentials, somatosensory evoked potentials, EEG, and cerebral oxygenation in a clinical environment. The apparent success of this prototype system suggests that such multimodal imaging will become more common and routine in the near future.

## CONCLUSION

Determination of the optimal strategy for the acute management of stroke patients is a difficult problem and remains controversial. Most current forms of therapy are designed to reduce complications of a recent stroke or prevent recurrences. The ability to topographically assess the physiological health of cerebral tissue in patients with ischemic disease will be useful in deciding the type, timing, and aggressiveness of therapeutic and preventative interventions. Such an ability will also be valuable for the assessment of experimental treatments and in understanding the fundamental basis of ischemic cell death and recovery. Assessment of both the amount of the cerebral cortex destroyed in a stroke and the remaining functionality of the adjacent cortex is currently difficult, if not impossible. MRI and CT show the size and location of necrotic tissue but give no information on the functionality of adjacent more normal appearing tissue. PET and single-photon emission CT give information regarding the level of blood flow to the tissue and glucose or oxygen consumption by the tissue but only indirectly yield information about its function. EEG, MEG, and evoked responses yield information about neurologic function but are difficult to localize unambiguously. NIRS and EROS offer information about blood flow and neuronal activity, respectively, and can be collected simultaneously with the same equipment. Improvements in both the technology and interpretation of optical data will make these techniques a valuable tool for the study and diagnosis of cerebral ischemic disease.

## REFERENCES

Aminoff, M. J. (1986). *Electrodiagnosis in clinical neurology*. New York: Churchill Livingstone.
Astrup, J., Siesjo, B. K., & Symon, L. (1981). Thresholds in cerebral ischemia—The ischemic penumbra. *Stroke, 12,* 723–725.
Back, T. (1998). Pathophysiology of the ischemic penumbra—Revision of a concept. *Cellular & Molecular Neurobiology, 18,* 621–638.
Bednarczyk, E. M., Remler, B., Weikart, C., Nelson, A. D., & Reed, R. C. (1998). Global cerebral blood flow, blood volume, and oxygen metabolism in patients with migraine headache. *Neurology, 50,* 1736–1740.

Beer, A. (1851). Versuch die absorbtions-verhältnisse des cordierites für rothes licht zu bestimmen (An attempt to determine the absorbtion coefficients of cordierites for near-red light). *Annalen der Physik und Chemie, 84*, 37–44.

Bonhoeffer, T., & Grinvald, A. (1996). Optical imaging based on intrinsic signals. In A. W. Toga & J. C. Mazziotta (Eds.), *Brain mapping: The methods* (pp. 55–97). San Diego, CA: Academic.

Boynton, G. M., Engel, S. A., Glover, G. H., & Heeger, D. J. (1996). Linear systems analysis of functional magnetic resonance imaging in human V1. *Journal of Neuroscience, 16*, 4207–4221.

Bruehl, C., Hagemann, G., & Witte, O. W. (1998). Uncoupling of blood flow and metabolism in focal epilepsy. *Epilepsia, 39*, 1235–1242.

Buckner, R. L., Bandettini, P. A., Savoy, R. L., Petersen, S. E., Raichle, M. E., & Rosen, B. R. (1996). Detection of cortical activation during averaged single trials of a cognitive task using functional magnetic resonance imaging. *Proceedings of the National Academy of Sciences of the USA, 93*, 14878–14883.

Busija, D. W. (1996). Nervous control of the cerebral circulation. In T. Bennett & S. M. Gardiner (Eds.), *Nervous control of blood vessels: The autonomic nervous system* (Vol. 8, pp. 177–205). UK: Harwood.

Chapman, R. M., Romani, G. L., Barbanera, S., Leoni, R., Modena, I., Ricci, G. B., & Campitelli, F. (1983). SQUID instrumentation and the relative covariance method for magnetic 3D localization of pathological cerebral sources. *Il Nuovo Cimento, 2, 38*, 549–554.

Cohen, L. B. (1972). Changes in neuron structure during action potential propagation and synaptic transmission. *Physiological Review, 53*, 373–417.

Conturo, T. E., Lori, N. F., Cull, T. S., Akbudak, E., Snyder, A. Z., Shimony, J. S., Mckinstry, R. C., Burton, H., & Raichle, M. E. (1999). Tracking neuronal fiber pathways in the living human brain. *Proceedings of the National Academy of Sciences, USA, 96*, 10422–10427.

Cooper, C. E., & Springett, R. (1997). Measurement of cytochrome oxidase and mitochondrial energetics by near-infrared spectroscopy. *Philosophical Transactions of the Royal Society of London Series B: Biological Sciences, 352*, 669–676.

Cope, M., Delpy, D. T., Reynolds, E. O., Wray, S., Wyatt, J., & van der Zee, P. (1988). Methods of quantitating cerebral near infrared spectroscopy data. *Advances in Experimental Medicine and Biology, 222*, 183–189.

Cui, W., Kumar, C., & Chance, B. (1991). Experimental study of migration depth for the photons measured at sample surface. *Proceedings of the International Society for Optical Engineering, 1431*, 180–191.

Danen, R. M., Wang, Y., Li, X. D., Thayer, W. S., & Yodh, A. G. (1998). Regional imager for low-resolution functional imaging of the brain with diffusing near-infrared light. *Photochemistry and Photobiology, 67*, 33–40.

Delpy, D. T., & Cope, M. (1997). Quantification in tissue near-infrared spectroscopy. *Philosophical Transactions of the Royal Society of London, Series B, 352*, 649–659.

Delpy, D. T., Cope, M., van der Zee, P., Arridge, S. R., Wray, S., & Wyatt, J. S. (1988). Estimation of optical path length through tissue from direct time of flight measurement. *Physics in Medicine and Biology, 33*, 1433–1442.

D'Esposito, M., Zarahn, E., & Aguirre, G. K. (1999). Event-related functional MRI: Implications for cognitive psychology. *Psychological Bulletin, 125*, 155–64.

D'Esposito, M., Zarahn, E., Aguirre, G. K., & Rypma, B. (1999). The effect of normal aging on the coupling of neural activity to the hemodynamic response. *NeuroImage, 10*, 6–14.

Dreier, J. P., Korner, K., Ebert, N., Gorner, A., Rubin, I., Back, T., Lindauer, U., Wolf, T., Villringer, A., Einhaupl, K. M., Lauritzen, M., & Dirnagl, U. (1998). Nitric oxide scavenging by hemoglobin or nitric oxide synthase by N-nitro-L-arginine induces cortical spreading ischemia when $K+$ is increased in the subarachnoid space. *Journal of Cerebral Blood Flow & Metabolism, 18*, 978–990.

Dujovny, M., Misra, M., & Widman, R. (1998). Cerebral oximetry—Techniques. *Neurological Research, 20*, S5–S12.

Duncan, A., Meek, J. H., Clemence, M., Elwell, C. E., Fallon, P., Tyszczuk, L., Cope, M., & Delpy, D. T. (1996). Measurement of cranial optical path length as a function of age using phase resolved near infrared spectroscopy. *Pediatric Research, 39*, 889–894.

Durduran, T., Culver, J. P., Holboke, M. J., Li, X. D., Zubkov, L., Chance, B., Pattanayak, D. N., & Yodh, A. G. (1999). Algorithms for 3D localization and imaging using near-field diffraction tomography with diffuse light. *Optics Express, 4,* 247–262.

Fallgatter, A. J., Muller, T. J., & Strik, W. K. (1998). Prefrontal hypooxygenation during language processing assessed with near-infrared spectroscopy. *Neuropsychobiology, 37,* 215–218.

Fallgatter, A. J., & Strik, W. K. (1998). Frontal brain activation during the Wisconsin Card Sorting Test assessed with two-channel near-infrared spectroscopy. *European Archives of Psychiatry and Clinical Neuroscience, 248,* 231–239.

Fierro, B., La Bua, V., Oliveri, M., Daniele, O., & Brighina, F. (1999). Prognostic value of somatosensory evoked potentials in stroke. *Electromyography and Clinical Neurophysiology, 39,* 155–160.

Firbank, M., Elwell, C. E., Cooper, C. E., & Delpy, D. T. (1998). Experimental and theoretical comparison of NIR spectroscopy of cerebral hemoglobin changes. *Journal of Applied Physiology, 85,* 1915–1921.

Firbank, M., Hiraoka, M., Essenpries, M., & Delpy, D. T. (1993). Measurement of the optical properties of the skull in the wavelength range 650–950 nm. *Physics in Medicine and Biology, 38,* 503–510.

Firbank, M., Okada, E., & Delpy, D. T. (1998). A theoretical study of the signal contribution of regions of the adult head to near-infrared spectroscopy studies of visual evoked responses. *Neuroimage, 8,* 69–78.

Fishkin, J. B., Fantini, S., van de Ven, M. J., & Gratton, E. (1996). Gigahertz photon density waves in a turbid medium: Theory and experiments. *Physical Reviews, E, 53,* 183–189.

Fishkin, J. B., & Gratton, E. (1993). Propagation of photon-density waves in strongly scattering media containing an absorbing semi-infinite plane bounded by a straight edge. *Journal of the Optical Society of America, 10,* 127–140.

Fox, P. T., Raichle, M. E., Mintun, M. A., & Dence, C. (1988, July). Nonoxidative glucose consumption during focal physiologic neural activity. *Science, 241,* 462–464.

Frackowiak, S. J. R., Lenzi, G.-L., Jones, T., & Heather, J. D. (1980). Quantitative measurement of regional cerebral blood flow and oxygen metabolism in man using 15O and positron emission tomography: Theory, procedure and normal values. *Journal of Computer Assisted Tomography, 4,* 727–736.

Franceschini, M. A., Toronov, V., Filiaci, L., Gratton, E., & Fantini, S. (2000). On-line optical imaging of the human brain with 100 ms. temporal resolution. *Optics Express, 6,* 49–57.

Frostig, R. D. (1994). What does *in vivo* optical imaging tell us about the primary visual cortex in primates? In A. Peters & K. S. Rockland (Eds.), *Cerebral cortex* (Vol. 10, pp. 331–358). New York: Plenum.

Frostig, R. D., Lieke, E. E., Ts'o, D. Y., & Grinvald, A. (1990). Cortical functional architecture and local coupling between neuronal activity and the microcirculation revealed by *in vivo* high-resolution optical imaging of intrinsic signals. *Proceedings of the National Academy of Sciences, 87,* 6082–6086.

Gallen, C. C., Hampson, S., & Bloom, F. E. (1990). Alteration of neuromagnetic alpha reactivity in stroke. *Neurology, 40,* 190.

Gallen, C. C., Schwartz, B., Pantev, C., Hampson, S., Sobel, D., Hirschkoff, E., Rieke, K., Otis, S., & Bloom, F. (1992). *Detection and localization of delta frequency activity in human stroke.* In M. Hoke, S. N. Erne, Y. C. Okada, & G. L. Romani (Eds.), Biomagnetism—Clinical Aspects (pp. 301–305). Amsterdam, Elsevier Science Publishers.

Germon, T. J., Evans, P. D., Manara, A. R., Barnett, N. J., Wall, P., & Nelson, R. J. (1998). Sensitivity of near infrared spectroscopy to cerebral and extra-cerebral oxygenation changes is determined by emitter–detector separation. *Journal of Clinical Monitoring and Computing, 14,* 353–360.

Germon, T. J., Young, A. E., Manara, A. R., & Nelson, R. J. (1995). Extracerebral absorption of near infrared light influences the detection of increased cerebral oxygenation monitored by near infrared spectroscopy. *Journal of Neurology, Neurosurgery and Psychiatry, 58,* 477–479.

Giltvedt, J., Sira, A., & Helme, P. (1984). Pulsed multifrequency photoplethysmography. *Medical and Biological Engineering and Computing, 22,* 212–215.

Ginsberg, M. D., Belayev, L., Zhao, W., Huh, P. W., & Busto, R. (1999). The acute ischemic penumbra: Topography, life span, and therapeutic response. *Acta Neurochirurgica Supplementum, 73,* 45–50.

Ginsberg, M. D., & Bogousslavsky, J. (1998). *Cerebrovascular disease: Pathophysiology, diagnosis and management*. Malden, MA: Blackwell Science.

Gratton, G. (1997). Attention and probability effects in the human occipital cortex: An optical imaging study. *NeuroReport, 8*, 1749–1753.

Gratton, G., Corballis, P. M., Cho, E., Fabiani, M., & Hood, D. C. (1995). Shades of gray matter: Non-invasive optical images of human brain responses during visual stimulation. *Psychophysiology, 32*, 505–509.

Gratton, G., & Fabiani, M. (1998). Dynamic brain imaging: Event-related optical signal (EROS) measures of the time course and localization of cognitive related activity. *Psychonomic Bulletin and Review, 5*, 535–563.

Gratton, G., Fabiani, M., Friedman, D., Franceschini, M. A., Fantini, S., Corballis, P. M., & Gratton, E. (1995). Rapid changes of optical parameters in the human brain during a tapping task. *Journal of Cognitive Neuroscience, 7*, 446–456.

Gratton, G., Fabiani, M., Goodman-Wood, M. R., & Desoto, M. C. (1998). Memory-driven processing in human medial occipital cortex: An event-related optical signal (EROS) study. *Psychophysiology, 35*, 348–351.

Gratton, G., Goodman-Wood, M., & Fabiani, M. (1999, March). *Comparison of neuronal and hemodynamic responses: An optical imaging study.* Paper presented at the annual meeting of the Cognitive Neuroscience Society, Washington, DC.

Gratton, G., Maier, N. J. S., Fabiani, M., Mantulin, W. W., & Gratton, E. (1994). Feasibility of intracranial near-infrared optical scanning. *Psychophysiology, 31*, 211–215.

Gratton, G., Sarno, A. J., Maclin, E., Corballis, P. M., & Fabiani, M. (2000). Toward non-invasive 3-D imaging of the time course of cortical activity: Investigation of the depth of the event-related optical signal (EROS). *NeuroImage, 11*, 491–504.

Grinvald, A., Lieke, E., Frostig, R. D., Gilbert, C. D., & Wiesel, T. N. (1986). Functional architecture of cortex revealed by optical imaging of intrinsic signals. *Nature, 324*, 361–364.

Harris, D. N. F., Cowans, F. M., Wertheim, D. A., & Hamid, S. (1994). NIRS in adults—Effects of increasing optode separation. *Advances in Experimental Medicine and Biology, 345*, 837–841.

Heekeren, H. R., Kohl, M., Obrig, H., Wenzel, R., von Pannwitz, W., Matcher, S. J., Dirnagl, U., Cooper, C. E., & Villringer, A. (1999). Noninvasive assessment of changes in cytochrome-c oxidase oxidation in human subjects during visual stimulation. *Journal of Cerebral Blood Flow and Metabolism, 19*, 592–603.

Heiss, W.-D. (1998). Application of positron emission tomography to the study of cerebral ischemia. In M. D. Ginsberg & J. Bogousslavsky (Eds.), *Cerebrovascular disease: Pathophysiology, diagnosis and management* (pp. 761–772). Malden, MA: Blackwell Science.

Hill, D. K., & Keynes, R. D. (1949). Opacity changes in stimulated nerve. *Journal of Physiology, 108*, 278–281.

Hirth, C., Obrig, H., Valdueza, J., Dirnagl, U., & Villringer, A. (1997). Simultaneous assessment of cerebral oxygenation and hemodynamics during a motor task: A combined near infrared and transcranial Doppler sonography study. *Advances in Experimental Medicine and Biology, 411*, 461–469.

Hock, C., Villringer, K., Muller-Spahn, F., Wenzel, R., Heekeren, H., Schuh-Hofer, S., Hofmann, M., Minoshima, S., Schwaiger, M., Dirnagl, U., & Villringer, A. (1997). Decrease in parietal cerebral hemoglobin oxygenation during performance of a verbal fluency task in patients with Alzheimer's disease monitored by means of near-infrared spectroscopy (NIRS)—Correlation with simultaneous rCBF–PET measurements. *Brain Research, 755*, 293–303.

Hoge, R. D., Atkinson, J., Gill, B., Crelier, G. R., Marrett, S., & Pike, G. B. (1999). Linear coupling between cerebral blood flow and oxygen consumption in activated human cortex. *Proceedings of the National Academy of Sciences USA, 96*, 9403–9408.

Hoshi, Y., Kosaka, S., Xie, Y., Kohri, S., & Tamura, M. (1998). Relationship between fluctuations in the cerebral hemoglobin oxygenation state and neuronal activity under resting conditions in man. *Neuroscience Letters, 245*, 147–150.

Hoshi, Y., & Tamura, M. (1993). Dynamic multichannel near-infrared optical imaging of human brain activity. *Journal of Applied Physiology, 75*, 1842–1846.

Howseman, A. M., Thomas, D. L., Pell, G. S., Williams, S. R., & Ordidge, R. J. (1999). Rapid T2* mapping using interleaved echo planar imaging. *Magnetic Resonance in Medicine, 41*, 368–374.

Jasdzewski, G., Strangman, G., Wagner, J., Kwong, K., Boas, D., & Poldrack, R. (2002, April). *Now you see it, now you don't: The initial dip as measured using near-infrared spectroscopy and event-re-*

*lated paradigms.* Paper presented at the 9th annual meeting of the Cognitive Neuroscience Society, San Francisco.

Jobsis, F. F. (1977). Noninvasive, infrared monitoring of cerebral and myocardial oxygen sufficiency and circulatory parameters. *Science, 198,* 1264–1267.

Kappelle, L. J., van Huffelen, A. C., & van Gijn, J. (1990). Is the EEG really normal in lacunar stroke? *Journal of Neurology, Neurosurgery, and Psychiatry, 53,* 63–66.

Kaufman, L., Curtis, S., Wang, J. Z., & Williamson, S. J. (1991). Changes in cortical activity when subjects scan memory for tones. *Electroencephalography and Clinical Neurophysiology, 82,* 266–284.

Kaufmann, A. M., Firlik, A. D., Fukui, M. B., Wechsler, L. R., Jungries, C. A., & Yonas, H. (1999). Ischemic core and penumbra in human stroke. *Stroke, 30,* 93–99.

Kitamura, J., Iwai, R., Tsumura, K., Ono, J., & Terashi, A. (1998). Electroencephalography and prognosis in stroke patients. *Journal of the Nippon Medical School, 65,* 28–33.

Knight, R. T., & Nakada, T. (1998). Cortico–limbic circuits and novelty: A review of EEG and blood flow. *Reviews in the Neurosciences, 9,* 57–70.

Kurth, C. D., & Thayer, W. S. (1999). A multiwavelength frequency-domain near-infrared cerebral oximeter. *Physics in Medicine and Biology, 44,* 727–740.

Kwong, K. (1995). Functional magnetic resonance imaging with echo planar imaging. *Magnetic Resonance Quarterly, 11,* 1–20.

Kwong, K., Belliveau, J. W., Chesler, D. A., Goldberg, I. E., Weisskoff, R. M., Poncelet, B. P., Kennedy, D. N., Hoppel, B. E., Cohen, M. S., Turner, R., Cheng, H.-M., Brady, T. J., & Rosen, B. R. (1992). Dynamic magnetic resonance imaging of human brain activity during primary sensory stimulation. *Proceedings of the National Academy of Sciences, 89,* 5675–5679.

Labar, D. R., Fisch, B. J., Pedley, T. A., Fink, M. E., & Solomon, R. A. (1991). Quantitative EEG monitoring for patients with subarachnoid hemorrhage. *Electroencephalography and Clinical Neurophysiology, 78,* 325–332.

Lauterbur, P. C. (1973). Image formation by induced local interactions: Examples employing nuclear magnetic resonance. *Nature, 242,* 190–191.

Leuchter, A. F., Cook, I. A., & Lachenbruch, P. A. (1994). Assessment of Cerebral Perfusion Using Quantitative EEG Cordance. *Psychiatry Research Neuroimaging, 55*(3), 141.

Leuchter, A. F., Uijtdehaage, S. H., Cook, I. A., & Mandelkern, M. (1999). Relationship between brain electrical activity and cortical perfusion in normal subjects. *Psychiatry Research, 90,* 125–140.

Lichty, W., Sakatani, K., Lin, F., Sun, P., Ding, H., & Wang, F. (1999). Near-infrared spectroscopic investigations of oxygenation changes related to brain activation. *SPIE, 3863,* 197–201.

Litscher, G. (1998). A multifunctional helmet for noninvasive neuromonitoring. *Journal of Neurosurgical Anesthesiology, 10,* 116–119.

Logothetis, N. K., Pauls, J., Augath, M., Trinath, T., & Oeltermann, A. (2001). Neurophysiological investigation of the basis of the fMRI signal. *Nature, 412,* 150–157.

Lovick, T. A., Brown, L. A., & Key, B. J. (1999). Neurovascular relationships in hippocampal slices: Physiological and anatomical studies of mechanisms underlying flow–metabolism coupling in intraparenchymal microvessels. *Neuroscience, 92,* 47–60.

Macdonell, R. A. L., Donnan, G. A., Bladin, P. F., Berkovic, S. F., & Wriedt, C. H. R. (1988). The electroencephalogram and acute ischemic stroke: Distinguishing cortical from lacunar infarction. *Arch Neurol, 45,* 520–524.

Maclin, E. L., Robinson, S. E., Knight, J. E., & Paulson, K. (1992, October). *Magnetoencephalographic identification of extrastriate visual areas in man.* Paper presented at the 22nd annual meeting of the Society for Neuroscience, Anaheim, CA.

Maclin, E., Rose, D., Knight, J., Orrison, W., & Davis, L. (1994). Somatosensory evoked magnetic fields in patients with stroke. *Electroencephalography and Clinical Neurophysiology, 91,* 468–475.

Maclin, E. L., Rose, D. F., & Paulson, K. (1991, August). *Functional mapping of occipital lesions: Correlation of perceptual deficits, electrophysiological sources and MRI lesions.* Paper presented at the 8th International Conference on Biomagnetism, Munster, FRG.

MacVicar, B. A., & Hochman, D. (1991). Imaging of synaptically evoked intrinsic optical signals in hippocampal slices. *Journal Neuroscience, 11,* 1458–1469.

Madsen, P. L., & Secher, N. H. (1999). Near-infrared oximetry of the brain. *Progress in Neurobiology, 58,* 541–560.

Magistretti, P. J., & Pellerin, L. (1999). Cellular mechanisms of brain energy metabolism and their relevance to functional brain imaging. *Philosophical Transactions of the Royal Society of London Series B: Biological Sciences, 354*, 1155–1163.

Malonek, D., & Grinvald, A. (1996, April). Interactions between electrical activity and cortical microcirculation revealed by imaging spectroscopy: Implications for functional brain mapping. *Science, 272*, 551–554.

Marchal, G., Benali, K., Iglesias, S., Viader, F., Derlon, J. M., & Baron, J. C. (1999). Voxel-based mapping of irreversible ischaemic damage with PET in acute stroke. *Brain, 122*, 2387–2400.

Miezin, F. M., Maccotta, L., Ollinger, J. M., Petersen, S. E., & Buckner, R. L. (2000). Characterizing the hemodynamic response: Effects of presentation rate, sampling procedure, and the possibility of ordering brain activity based on relative timing. *NeuroImage, 11*.

Millikan, G. A. (1942). Oximeter, instrument for measuring continuously oxygen saturation of arterial blood in man. *Rev, Sci. Instrum., 13*, 434.

Murri, L., Gori, S., Massetani, R., Bonanni, E., Marcella, F., & Milani, S. (1998). Evaluation of acute ischemic stroke using quantitative EEG: A comparison with conventional EEG and CT scan. *Neurophysiologie Clinique, 28*, 249–257.

Neubauer, R. A., & James, P. (1998). Cerebral oxygenation and the recoverable brain. *Neurological Research, 20*, S33–S536.

Obrig, H., Wolf, T., Doge, C., Hulsing, J. J., Dirnagl, U., & Villringer, A. (1996). Cerebral oxygenation changes during motor and somatosensory stimulation in humans, as measured by near-infrared spectroscopy. *Advances in Experimental Medicine and Biology, 388*, 219–224.

Ogawa, S., Lee, T. M., Kay, A. R., & Tank, D. W. (1990). Brain magnetic resonance imaging with contrast dependent on blood oxygenation. *Proceedings of the National Academy of Sciences, 87*, 9868–9872.

Oishi, M., & Mochizuki, Y. (1998). Correlation between contingent negative variation and regional cerebral blood flow. *Clinical Electroencephalography, 29*, 124–127.

Okada, E., Firbank, M., Schweiger, M., Arridge, S. R., Cope, M., & Delpy, D. T. (1997). Theoretical and experimental investigation of near-infrared light propagation in a model of the adult head. *Applied Optics, 36*, 21–31.

Pereon, Y., Aubertin, P., & Guiheneuc, P. (1995). Prognostic significance of electrophysiological investigations in stroke patients: Somatosensory and motor evoked potentials and sympathetic skin response. *Clinical Neurophysiology, 25*, 146–157.

Posner, M. I., & Raichle, M. E. (1994). *Images of mind*. New York: Freeman.

Posner, M. I., & Raichle, M. E. (1998). The neuroimaging of human brain function. *Proceedings of the National Academy of Sciences USA, 95*, 763–764.

Pritchard, W. (1998). Cognitive event-related potential correlates of schizophrenia. *Psychological Bulletin, 100*, 44–66.

Raichle, M. E. (1998). Behind the scenes of functional brain imaging: A historical and physiological perspective. *Proceedings of the National Academy of Sciences USA, 95*, 765–772.

Rector, D. M., Rogers, R. F., Schwaber, J. S., Harper, R. M., & George, J. S. (2001). Scattered-light imaging *in vivo* tracks fast and slow processes of neurophysiological activation. *NeuroImage, 14*, 977–994.

Richter, W. (1999). High temporal resolution functional magnetic resonance imaging at very-high-field. *Topics in Magnetic Resonance Imaging, 10*, 51–62.

Rinne, T., Gratton, G., Fabiani, M., Cowan, N., Maclin, E., Stinard, A., Sinkkonen, J., Alho, K., & Naatanen, R. (1999). Scalp-recorded optical signals make sound processing in the auditory cortex visible. *NeuroImage, 10*, 620–624.

Roy, C. S., & Sherrington, C. S. (1890). On the regulation of the blood supply of the brain. *Journal of Physiology, 11*, 85–108.

Rugg, M. D. (1998). Convergent approaches to electrophysiological and hemodynamic investigations of memory. *Human Brain Mapping, 6*, 394–398.

Sadato, N., Nakamura, S., Oohashi, T., Nishina, E., Fuwamoto, Y., Waki, A., & Yonekura, Y. (1998). Neural networks for generation and suppression of alpha rhythm: A PET study. *Neuroreport, 9*, 893–897.

Sakatani, K., Lichty, W., Xie, Y., Li, S., & Zuo, H. (1999). Effects of aging on language activated cerebral blood oxygenation changes of the left prefrontal cortex: Near infrared spectroscopy study. *Journal of Stroke and Cerebrovascular Diseases, 8*, 398–403.

Sanders, J. A. (1995). Functional magnetic resonance imaging. In W. W. Orrison Jr. (Ed.), *Functional brain imaging* (pp. 239–326). St. Louis, MO: Mosby.

Sandor, P. (1999). Nervous control of the cerebrovascular system: Doubts and facts. *Neurochemistry International, 35,* 237–259.

Schwarzbauer, C., & Heinke, W. (1999). Investigating the dependence of BOLD contrast on oxidative metabolism. *Magnetic Resonance in Medicine, 41,* 537–543.

Stejskal, L., & Sobota, J. (1985). Somatosensory evoked potentials in patients with occlusions of cerebral arteries. *Electroencephalography and Clinical Neurophysiology, 61,* 482–490.

Stepnoski, R. A., La Porta, A., Raccuia-Behling, F., Blonder, G. E., Slusher, R. E., & Kleinfeld, D. (1991). Noninvasive detection of changes in membrane potential in cultured neurons by light scattering. *Proceedings of the National Academy of Sciences, 88,* 9382–9386.

Toronov, V., Franceschini, M. A., Wolf, M., Michalos, A., Filiaci, L., & Gratton, E. (2000). Near-infrared study of fluctuations in cerebral hemodynamics during rest and motor stimulation: Temporal analysis and spatial mapping. *Medical Physics, 27,* 801–815.

Toronov, V., Webb, A., Choi, J. H., Wolf, M., Michalos, A., Gratton, E., & Hueber, D. (2001). Investigation of human brain dynamics by simultaneous near-infrared spectroscopy and functional magnetic resonance imaging. *Medical Physics, 28,* 521–527.

Totaro, R., Barattelli, G., Quaresima, V., Carolei, A., & Ferrari, M. (1998). Evaluation of potential factors affecting the measurement of cerebrovascular reactivity by near-infrared spectroscopy. *Clinical Science, 95,* 497–504.

Toyoda, K., Ibayashi, S., Yamamoto, T., Kuwabara, Y., & Fujishima, M. (1998). Auditory evoked neuromagnetic response in cerebrovascular diseases: A preliminary study. *Journal of Neurology, Neurosurgery and Psychiatry, 64,* 777–84.

Turner, R., LeBihan, D., Moonen, C. T. W., Despres, D., & Frank, J. (1991). Echo-planar time course of cat brain oxygenation changes. *Magnetic Resonance in Medicine, 22,* 159–166.

van der Zee, P., Arridge, S. R., Cope, M., & Delpy, D. T. (1990). The effect of optode positioning on optical pathlength in near infrared spectroscopy of brain. *Advances in Experimental Medicine and Biology, 277,* 79–84.

van der Zee, P., Essenpries, M., & Delpy, D. T. (1993). Optical properties of brain tissues. *Proceedings of the International Society for Optical Engineering, 1888,* 454–465.

Vieth, J. B. (1990). Magnetoencephalography in the study of stroke (cerebrovascular accident). In S. Sato (Ed.), *Advances in neurology* (Vol. 54, pp. 261–269). New York: Raven.

Vieth, J., Sack, G., Kober, H., Grummich, P., Schneider, S., Abraham-Fuchs, K., Haerer, W., Friedrich, S., & Moeger, A. (1991, August). *The efficacy of the dipole-density-plot (DDP) compared to the dipole pathway technique in multichannel MEG.* Paper presented at the 8th International Conference on Biomagnetism, Münster, Germany.

Vieth, J., Sack, G., Schueler, P., Grummich, P., & Schneider, S. (1989). Ischemic and epileptic lesions measured by AC- and DC-MEG. In S. J. Williamson, M. Hoke, G. Stroink, & M. Kotani (Eds.), *Advances in biomagnetism* (pp. 307–310). New York: Plenum.

Villringer, A., & Chance, B. (1997). Non-invasive optical spectroscopy and imaging of human brain function. *Trends in Neurosciences, 20,* 435–442.

Villringer, A., & Dirnagl, U. (1995). Coupling of brain activity and cerebral blood flow: Basis of functional neuroimaging. *Cerebrovascular and Brain Metabolism Reviews, 7,* 240–276.

Villringer, K., Minoshima, S., Hock, C., Obrig, H., Ziegler, S., Dirnagl, U., Schwaiger, M., & Villringer, A. (1997). Assessment of local brain activation. A simultaneous PET and near-infrared spectroscopy study. *Advances in Experimental Medicine and Biology, 413,* 149–153.

Warach, S. D., & Schlaug, G. (1998). Diffusion-weighted and perfusion magnetic resonance imaging in cerebral ischemia. In M. D. Ginsberg & J. Bogousslavsky (Eds.), *Cerebrovascular disease: Pathophysiology, diagnosis and management* (pp. 780–792). Malden, MA: Blackwell Science.

Watanabe, E., Maki, A., Kawaguchi, F., Takashiro, K., Yamashita, Y., Koizumi, H., & Mayanagi, Y. (1998). Non-invasive assessment of language dominance with near-infrared spectroscopic mapping. *Neuroscience Letters, 256,* 49–52.

Wray, S., Cope, M., Delpy, D. T., Wyatt, J. S., & Reynolds, E. O. (1988). Characterization of the near infrared absorption spectra of cytochrome and haemoglobin for the non-invasive monitoring of cerebral oxygenation. *Biochimica et Biophysica Acta, 933,* 184–192.

# 12

## High-Frequency Oscillations From the Human Somatosensory Cortex: The Interneuron Hypothesis

Isao Hashimoto
*Kanazawa Institute of Technology*

High-frequency oscillations (300–900 Hz) from the human somatosensory cortex have been the subject of great interest for the last 10 years. This is because physiological characteristics of the oscillations are so much different from the previously known lower frequency somatosensory evoked responses, such as N20, P25, and P27 components, to median nerve stimulation. In this chapter I present a short review of previous studies on somatosensory evoked high-frequency oscillations. I then describe the presence of tangential and radial dipoles for the high-frequency oscillations superimposed on N20 and P25 components, respectively. I also described briefly data on the detection of high-frequency oscillations to posterior tibial and digital nerve stimulation. These findings demonstrate that high-frequency oscillations are generated not only from area 3b but also from area 1 of the primary somatosensory cortex. Furthermore, high-frequency oscillations are not specific to median nerve stimulation but represent activity common to stimulation of any nerve. Developmental changes of the high-frequency oscillations or changes by an aging process are also presented. High-frequency oscillations are now used as a tool for functional diagnosis of neurological diseases such as Parkinson's disease, multiple system atrophy, and myoclonus epilepsy. Reciprocal modulation of high-frequency oscillations and the underlying N20 primary response by a wake–sleep cycle and by interference stimulation is a robust phenomenon. On the basis of the reciprocity between the 2 activities in the somatosensory cortex, I hypothesize that the high-frequency oscillations represent activity of fast-spiking GABAergic inhibitory interneurons in the somatosensory cortex, because it has been established that N20 is generated by ensemble excitatory postsynaptic potentials (EPSPs). Further evidence for the distinct generators for the 2 components is provided by the difference in the orientation of the dipoles calculated at the same time slices.

With recent advances in high spatial and temporal resolution magnetoencephalographic (MEG) and electroencephalographic (EEG) systems, it is now feasible to study in detail the dynamics of brain activity non-invasively. This has led to a remarkable resurgence of interest in high-frequency oscillations from the human somatosensory cortex. Until recently, it has been traditionally considered that MEG and EEG reflect population excitatory postsynaptic potentials (EPSPs) of the pyramidal neurons. Recent studies indicate that the high-frequency component of MEG and EEG signals represents action potentials of the thalamocortical projection fibers (Curio et al., 1994; Gobbele, Buchner, & Curio, 1998). Furthermore, it is also possible that somatosensory evoked high-frequency oscillations represent activity of fast-spiking GABAergic inhibitory interneurons controlling the output of pyramidal cells in the cortex (Hashimoto, Mashiko, & Imada, 1996). These possibilities to observe activity not only from the thalamocortical afferent fibers but also from cortical interneurons widen the type of signals that can be measured with MEG and EEG and expand their applications in basic and clinical neuroscience. This will have a particular impact on somatosensory neurophysiology, because thalamocortical axons projecting to the cortex, and interneurons in different layers of the cortex, constitute two of the three important neural elements in cortical microcircuitry.

## EARLY STUDIES OF HIGH-FREQUENCY OSCILLATIONS

Previous somatosensory evoked potential studies have revealed several brief wavelets superimposed on the ascending slope of the N20 primary response after stimulation of the median nerve (Abbruzzese, Favale, Leandri, & Ratto, 1978; Cracco & Cracco, 1976; Eisen, Roberts, Low, & Laurence, 1984; Maccabee, Pinkhasow, & Cracco, 1983). Because these wavelets are of much higher frequencies (>300 Hz) compared with the N20 component (30–50 Hz), it is natural that these high-frequency oscillations are considered to represent a different generator substrate from that of the N20, which itself is generated by population EPSPs of the pyramidal cells in area 3b of the somatosensory cortex. To further the notion of a distinct generator for the high-frequency oscillations, Yamada et al. (1988) and Emerson, Sgro, Pedley, and Hauser (1988) have found that high-frequency oscillations change dramatically during a wake–sleep cycle despite the remarkable stability of the underlying N20. In addition, Yamada et al. showed that amplitude of the high-frequency oscillations decreased markedly from waking to increasingly deepening sleep stages but recovered partially in REM sleep. They also found that the amplitudes of subcortically generated P14 and subsequent N15 remained almost the same throughout a wake–sleep cycle. From differential recovery curves for individual high-frequency peaks, Emori et al. (1991) speculated that the oscillations are generated within a cortical polysynaptic network and that at least one synapse is interposed between the neighboring peaks.

Curio et al. (1994) first reported magnetic recordings of high-frequency oscillations superimposed on the N20m (the magnetic counterpart of the electric N20) and, on the basis of a relatively constant amplitude ratio of high-frequency oscillations to N20m across the sensor arrays, suggested a similar field distribution for the two components. They speculated that the high-frequency signals are of heterogeneous origins with contributions from presynaptic action potentials as well as postsynaptic potentials of different populations of cortical neurons. As discussed earlier, there have been a number of speculations as to the generator(s) of the high-frequency oscillations, ranging from the thalamus (Eisen et al., 1984), to thalamocortical radiation (Gobbele et al., 1998; Maccabee et al., 1983; McLaughlin & Kelly, 1993; Yamada et al., 1988), to the cortex (Curio et al., 1994; Curio et al., 1997; Emori et al., 1991; Hashimoto et al., 1999; Hashimoto et al., 1996; Maccabee et al., 1983; Ozaki et al., 1998; Sakuma & Hashimoto, 1999; Sakuma, Sekihara, & Hashimoto, 1999). Thus, precise anatomic locations of the generators for high-frequency oscillations remain undetermined. In this respect, recent recordings of high-frequency oscillations from the surface of the human somatosensory cortex are important, because it has been established that the oscillations are really generated from area 3b (Kojima et al., 2001; Maegaki et al., 2000). However, physiological mechanisms of the high-frequency oscillations have been the subject of considerable controversy (Curio et al., 1994; Curio et al., 1997; Curio, 2000; Gobbele et al., 1998; Hashimoto, 2000, 2001; Hashimoto et al., 1999; Hashimoto et al., 2000; Hashimoto et al., 1996; Ozaki et al., 2001).

## ARE HIGH-FREQUENCY OSCILLATIONS AN ARTIFACT
## DUE TO HIGH-PASS FILTERING?

High-frequency oscillations are isolated from low-frequency signals with the use of high-pass filtering (>300 Hz). Since the first detection of the high-frequency oscillations there has been a persistent argument that they are simply an artifact due to high-pass filtering. This artifact hypothesis has not been supported on the basis of rigorous experiments on the one hand or simulations on the other. However, it is important to rule out the erroneous interpretation before discussing underlying anatomical or physiological mechanisms of the high-frequency oscillations.

There is much physiological evidence in favor of genuine cortical activity for the high-frequency oscillations and against the artifact hypothesis. First, high-frequency oscillations after high-pass filtering can be detected clearly as small notches superimposed on wide-band recorded somatosensory evoked potentials (Mochizuki et al., 1999; Nakano & Hashimoto, 2000; Yamada et al., 1988) and fields (Curio et al., 1994; Hashimoto et al., 1996; Ozaki et al., 2001). Second, different frequency analysis methods, including a fast-Fourier transform (Curio et al., 1994; Hashimoto et al., 1996; Nakano & Hashimoto, 1999a), a maximum-entropy method (Ozaki et al., 1998; Ozaki et al., 1999), and a time–frequency domain multiple signal classification algorism (Sakuma et al., 1999) have demonstrated unanimously a peak between 300 Hz and 750 Hz. Third, the amplitude of high-frequency oscillations decreased selectively during sleep while the underlying N20 (Emerson et al., 1988; Halboni et al., 2000; Yamada et al., 1988) and N20m (Hashimoto et al., 1996) remained unchanged or increased. Fourth, interference stimulation increased the number of high-frequency oscillation peaks, while N20m decreased its amplitude (Hashimoto et al., 1999). These reciprocal behaviors of high-frequency oscillations and the N20(m) under certain conditions strongly argue against the artifact hypothesis. Fifth, there is a population of fast-spiking interneurons in the somatosensory cortex that responds to synaptic volleys with a high-frequency burst of spikes more than 600 Hz with a high precision of timing (Rasmusson, 1996; Swadlow, Beloozerova, & Sirota, 1998). Furthermore, Jones et al. (2000) demonstrated that the fast-spiking inhibitory interneurons in area 3b in the rat respond to vibrissae stimulation with bursts of action potentials that closely approximate the periodicity of the surface-recorded high-frequency field potential oscillations. Sixth, direct recordings of somatosensory evoked potentials from the human primary somatosensory cortex disclosed localized high-frequency oscillations with a phase reversal across the central sulcus (Kojima et al., 2001; Maegaki et al., 2000). Seventh, a recent electrophysiological study in monkeys demonstrated that the high-frequency oscillations are directly recorded from areas 3b and 1, showing a phase reversal between the superficial and deeper layers (Shimazu et al., 2000). It is therefore concluded that high-frequency oscillations are not an artifact produced by high-pass filtering but reflect activity of a population of neurons in the somatosensory cortex.

## HIGH-FREQUENCY OSCILLATIONS CAN BE RECORDED TO STIMULATION OF OTHER NERVES THAN THE MEDIAN NERVE

Many studies have revealed that high-frequency oscillations in the range of 300–900 Hz have been shown to concur with the N20 primary response of the somatosensory cortex after median nerve stimulation (Abbruzzese et al., 1978; Cracco & Cracco, 1976; Curio et al., 1994; Eisen et al., 1984; Emori et al., 1991; Gobbele et al., 1998; Hashimoto et al., 1999; Hashimoto et al., 1996; Maccabee et al., 1983; Nakano & Hashimoto, 1999b, 2000; Ozaki et al., 1998; Ozaki et al., 1999; Ozaki et al., 2001; Yamada et al., 1988). Curio et al. (1997) succeeded in recording high-frequency oscillations to ulnar nerve stimulation after a "massive" averaging of 9,000 responses. For leg nerve stimulation there was only one report of high-frequency oscillations for common peroneal nerve stimulation (Eisen et al., 1984). In recent studies, my colleagues and I have been able to detect high-frequency oscillations both electrically (Nakano & Hashimoto, 1999a, 1999c) and magnetically (Sakuma & Hashimoto, 1999; Sakuma et al., 1999) for posterior tibial nerve stimulation. Similar to the high-frequency oscillations to median nerve stimulation, those evoked by posterior tibial nerve stimulation start approximately at the same time as or later than the onset of the primary cortical response (P37) and end in the middle of the second slope. In addition, the duration and number of peaks for the oscillation bursts evoked by the two different nerves are very similar. Recently, Tanosaki et al. (2001) recorded high-frequency oscillations to stimulation of the thumb and middle finger. The results suggest that high-frequency oscillations superimposed on the primary somatosensory response after stimulation of the median, ulnar, and digital nerves of the upper extremity, and the common peroneal and posterior tibial nerve of the lower limb, reflect a neural mechanism common to the somatosensory cortex. Figure 12.1

shows N20m and high-frequency oscillations after stimulation of the median nerve. Figure 12.2a and b illustrate P37m and high-frequency oscillations to the posterior tibial nerve stimulation. Also shown, in Fig. 12.2c, is the spectrogram computed from a time–frequency domain multiple-signal classification algorithm (Sakuma et al., 1999).

## HIGH-FREQUENCY OSCILLATIONS HAVE TANGENTIAL AND RADIAL DIPOLE COMPONENTS

MEG recordings are biased toward superficial and tangential sources in the brain (i.e., MEG is blind to radial sources). For this reason, previous studies on high-frequency oscillations have focused only on the tangential dipolar components (Curio et al., 1994; Curio et al., 1997; Hashimoto et al., 1999; Hashimoto et al., 1996; Sakuma & Hashimoto, 1999; Sakuma et al., 1999). To examine whether a radial component is present in high-frequency oscillations, Ozaki et al. (1998) recorded somatosensory evoked potentials after median nerve stimulation with a wide bandpass

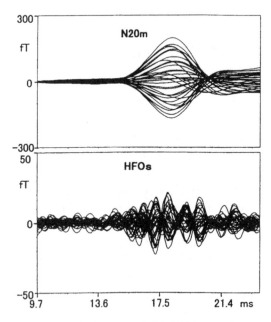

FIG. 12.1.  Somatosensory evoked magnetic fields (SEFs) to median nerve stimulation. The upper trace shows low-pass filtered (0.1–300 Hz) and the lower trace shows high-pass filtered (300–900 Hz) SEFs. Thirty-seven waveforms are superimposed to illustrate the polarity-reversed N20m deflections. The N20m primary response is superimposed by high-frequency oscillations.

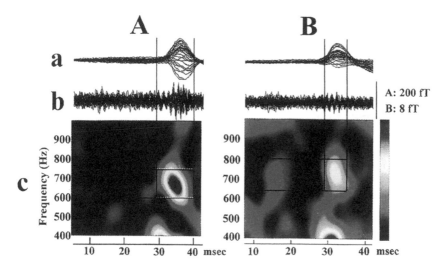

FIG. 12.2.    Panel A: wide-band recorded somatosensory evoked magnetic fields (SEFs) following posterior tibial nerve stimulation. Thirty-seven waveforms are superimposed to illustrate the polarity-reversed P37m deflections (a). High-frequency oscillations after digital filtering (500–800 Hz) of the wide-band SEFs in (a) are roughly coincident with the P37m (b). Averaged spectrogram for the frequency range above 400 Hz obtained from the magnetoencephalography data is shown in (c). A rectangle with a dotted line is the target region for the high-frequency oscillations. Panel B: a typical result from another subject showing a clear isolated region in the time–frequency spectrogram, although the equivalent current dipole of high-frequency oscillations could not be estimated with the single moving dipole model because of a low signal-to-noise ratio with a low correlation value (.74). From "Neural Source Estimation From a Time-Frequency Component of Somatic Evoked High-Frequency Magnetic Oscillations to Posterior Tibial Nerve Stimulation" by K. Sakuma, K. Sekihara, and I. Hashimoto, 1999, *Clinical Neurophysiology, 110,* p. 1587. Copyright 1999 by Elsevier Science. Reprinted by permission.

(0.5–2000 Hz). From multiple electrode arrays over the contralateral fronto–parietal scalp, they obtained a parietal N20 and a frontal P20, and a central P22 corresponding to P25 in the nomenclature of Allison et al. (1989). After digital bandpass filtering (300–1000 Hz), high-frequency oscillations consisting of five to eight peaks were discriminated from the P14 far field in all cases. The peaks showed a phase reversal between the frontal and parietal regions coincident with the underlying N20–P20 (see Fig. 12.3). In addition, a single high-frequency oscillation peak with a maximum at the central region was present in subjects with a high-amplitude central P22 in original wide-band recordings. Furthermore, this high-frequency component showed no phase reversal over the scalp, suggesting that this peak was generated by a radial dipole. These results indi-

**A**

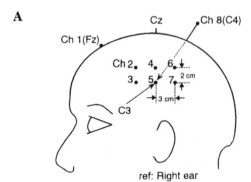

**B**

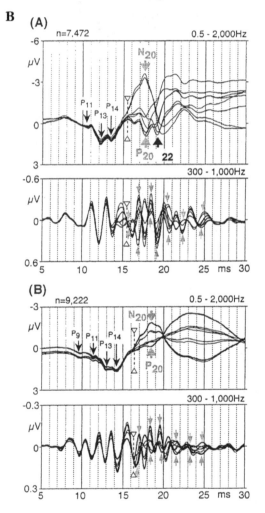

FIG. 12.3. Panel A: the position of the eight electrodes over the scalp. Channel 1 (Ch 1), Fz; Ch 2, 3 cm anterior and 2 cm medial to C3; Ch 3, 3 cm anterior to C3; Ch 4, 2 cm medial to C3; Ch 5, C3; Ch 6, 3 cm posterior and 2 cm medial to C3; Ch 7, 3 cm posterior to C3; Ch 8, C4. Panel B: the wide-band recorded somatosensory evoked potentials (SEPs; upper part) and digitally high-pass filtered SEPs (lower part) to right median nerve stimulation. Following the high-frequency components of P9, P11, P13, and P14 far fields, cortical oscillations start at the onset of the N20–P20 response (open triangle and dotted line). Phase reversal of the high-frequency oscillations is clearly shown (small gray arrows). At around 19 msec, when the central P22 potential is dominant in wide-band recordings, the high-frequency oscillation peak shows phase alignment (black arrow). From "High-Frequency Oscillations in Early Cortical Somatosensory Evoked Potentials" by I. Ozaki et al., 1998, *Electroencephalography and Clinical Neurophysiology, 108,* pp. 537–538. Copyright 1998 by Elsevier Science. Reprinted by permission.

cate that high-frequency oscillations are superimposed not only on the tangential N20-P20 but also on the radial P22 potential and are generated from both tangential (area 3b) and radial (area 1) current sources. In support of the somatosensory evoked potential study, Shimazu et al. (2000) found that in monkeys high-frequency oscillations directly recorded from area 3b and area 1 inverted polarity between the superficial and deeper layers, suggesting that the oscillations are generated in the primary somatosensory cortex.

## MODULATION OF HIGH-FREQUENCY OSCILLATIONS BY A WAKE–SLEEP CYCLE

Figure 12.4 illustrates wide-band records of somatosensory evoked fields obtained during wakefulness (Panel A) and during sleep (Panel B) from the same subject. The N20m showed a longer mean peak latency during sleep, but this difference (0.6 msec) did not reach significance. However, the mean N20m peak amplitude was significantly larger during sleep by approximately 10% (Hashimoto et al., 1996). Strong high-frequency oscillations present during waking (Panel C) were reduced in amplitude or no longer detected from the background noise during sleep (Panel D). This is in line with somatosensory evoked potential studies conducted by Yamada et al. (1988), Emerson et al. (1988), and Halboni et al. (2000) during a wake–sleep cycle.

## MODULATION OF HIGH-FREQUENCY OSCILLATIONS BY TACTILE INTERFERENCE

It is well established that the N20 primary response is attenuated by simultaneous tactile stimulation of the hand (S. J. Jones & Power, 1984; Kakigi et al., 1996) or by finger movements of the hand (Kakigi et al., 1995; Rossini et al., 1999; Schnitzler et al., 1995; Tanosaki, Kimura, et al., 2002a) ipsilateral to electrical median nerve stimulation.

For an interference session, continuous brushing of the palm and fingers of the electrostimulated hand was performed by the experimenter using a coarse cloth (Hashimoto et al., 1999). For a control session, the stimuli were applied to the subject without the concurrent brushing. Wide-band (0.1–1200 Hz) recorded responses were digitally low-pass (<300 Hz) and high-pass (>300 Hz) filtered. Figure 12.5 shows a typical N20m response and high-frequency oscillations for a control session and an interference session. The equivalent current dipole (ECD) localiza-

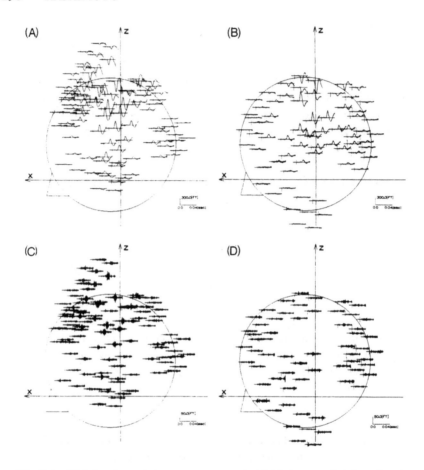

FIG. 12.4.    Wide-band recorded somatosensory evoked fields during wakefulness (Panel A) and sleep (Panel B). High-frequency oscillations during waking (Panel C) and sleep (Panel D) after the high-pass filtering (300–900 Hz) of the original data presented in Panels A and B, respectively. Note the remarkable reduction in amplitude of high-frequency oscillations during sleep. From "Somatic Evoked High-Frequency Magnetic Oscillations Reflect Activity of Inhibitory Interneurons in the Human Somatosensory Cortex" by I. Hashimoto, T. Mashiko, and T. Imada, 1996, *Electroencephalography and Clinical Neurophysiology, 100,* p. 196. Copyright 1996 by Elsevier Science. Reprinted by permission.

tions of the high-frequency peaks and the underlying N20m were close to each other. The mean N20m amplitude was 463 fT and 368 fT for the control and interference conditions, and the difference between the two was significant ($p < .005$). The amplitude ratios of N20m with and without interference stimulation (interference/control) ranged from 59% to 97%, with a mean of 79%. The number of high-frequency oscillation

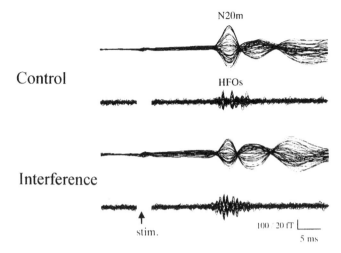

FIG. 12.5.   Modulation of median nerve N20m and high-frequency oscillations by con-current brushing of the ipsilateral palm. Control condition: low-pass filtered (0.1–300 Hz) and high-pass filtered (300–900 Hz) somatosensory evoked fields (SEFs) without brushing of the palm. Interference condition: corresponding SEFs with brushing. Note the reduction of the N20m amplitude and the increase in the number of peaks in high-fre-quency oscillations during brushing of the palm. The calibration is 100 fT for N20m and 20 fT for the high-frequency oscillations. From "Reciprocal Modulation of Somato-sensory Evoked N20m Primary Response and High-Frequency Oscillations by Interfer-ence Stimulation" by I. Hashimoto et al., 1999, *Clinical Neurophysiology, 110,* p. 1447. Copyright 1999 by Elsevier Science. Reprinted by permission.

peaks had a mean of 6.5 for the control condition and 8.1 for the interfer-ence condition. This increase in the number of peaks for interference stimulation was significant ($p < .05$); however, there was no difference in amplitude between the control and interference conditions. In accor-dance with earlier studies, N20m amplitude decreased dramatically dur-ing concurrent brushing of the palm and fingers (S. J. Jones & Power, 1984; Kakigi et al., 1996). Conversely, high-frequency oscillations in-creased in the number of peaks. The results clearly showed that the in-verse relation between N20m and high-frequency oscillations is present during interference stimulation.

## ENHANCED HIGH-FREQUENCY OSCILLATIONS
## FOR THUMB STIMULATION

Manipulation of objects by fine coordination of digit movements is one of the crucial functions that makes us humans distinct from nonhuman pri-mates. This requires accurate and fine control of hand movements, called *precision grasping.* It is widely accepted that the human thumb plays an important role in precision grasping and that its morphology has achieved prominent evolution compared with those of nonhuman primates (Susman, 1994). In fact, the structure of the human thumb has evolved for precision grasping and tool behavior. Compared with apes, the human thumb has three additional muscles for its rotatory, three-dimensional movements: (a) a flexor pollicis longus muscle, (b) a first volar interosseous muscle of Henle, and (c) a deep head of flexor pollicis brevis muscle. Thus, it is possible that somatosensory information from the thumb is processed adaptably for fine motor control. For example, the human thumb has the largest representation among digits in area 3b (Penfield & Boldrey, 1937; Sutherling, Levesque, & Baumgartner, 1992). Therefore, it seems reasonable to anticipate that N20m amplitude for the thumb would be higher than those for the other digits. However, this is not always the case (Okada, Tanenbaum, Williamson, & Kaufman, 1984; Suk, Ribary, Cappell, Yamamoto, & Llinas, 1991; Synek, 1986), and little attention has been paid to this obvious discrepancy so far. Therefore, my colleagues and I address the issue by examining the relation between N20m and high-frequency oscillations after thumb and middle-finger stimulation (Tanosaki et al., 2001).

The ECD location for N20m and high-frequency oscillations after thumb stimulation was lower than that for middle-finger stimulation, as expected. Figure 12.6 shows typical waveforms for 1 subject. The N20m amplitude did not show a significant difference between the thumb and middle finger. In contrast, the maximum and total amplitude of high-frequency oscillations for the thumb were significantly higher than those for the middle finger. Furthermore, the number of high-frequency oscillations for the thumb was significantly greater than that for the middle finger. Together with the finding that the N20m after thumb stimulation is disproportionately small in spite of its reported larger representational area, enhanced high-frequency oscillations for the thumb can be interpreted as an inverse relation between the two components. As I discuss in more detail later, I speculate that the enhanced high-frequency oscillations play an important role for fine-tuning of somatosensory information from the thumb.

## RECIPROCAL RELATION BETWEEN HIGH-FREQUENCY OSCILLATIONS AND N20M

Magnetophysiologic features of high-frequency oscillations and the underlying N20m can be summarized as follows. First, the equivalent di-

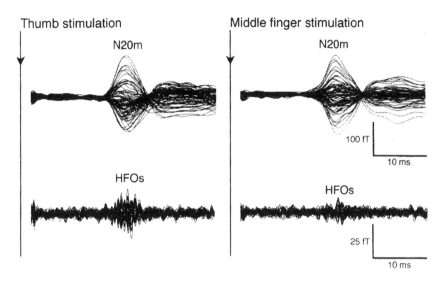

FIG. 12.6. Low-pass (3–300 Hz) and high-pass (300–900 Hz) filtered somatosensory evoked fields after stimulation of the thumb and middle finger. Waveforms recorded from 25 channels around the sensorimotor hand area contralateral to the stimulation side are superimposed. Note the greater number of peaks and higher amplitude for high-frequency oscillations after thumb than after stimulation of the middle finger. From "Specific Somatosensory Processing in Somatosensory Area 3b for Human Thumb: A Neuromagnetic Study" by M. Tanosaki et al., 2001, *Clinical Neurophysiology, 112,* p. 1518. Copyright 2001 by Elsevier Science. Reprinted by permission.

poles for the high-frequency peaks and the underlying N20m are overlapped temporally and colocalized spatially within area 3b. Second, the high-frequency oscillations have the main signal energy at 500–800 Hz and are distinct from the N20m, which has its principal signal energy at 30–50 Hz. Third, the high-frequency oscillations attenuate or disappear, whereas the underlying N20m increases its amplitude during sleep (Hashimoto et al., 1996). Fourth, the high-frequency oscillations increase in number of peaks, whereas the N20m decreases its amplitude for tactile interference stimulation (Hashimoto et al., 1999). Fifth, high-frequency oscillations are higher in maximum and total amplitude and in number of peaks, whereas the N20m is invariant for thumb stimulation as compared with middle finger stimulation (Tanosaki et al., 2001). Thus, it is clear that a reciprocal relation is present between the high-frequency oscillations and the N20m during a wake–sleep cycle, for interference stimulation, and for thumb and middle finger stimulation. The inverse relation between the high-frequency oscillations and the N20m representing ensemble EPSPs of the pyramidal neurons in area 3b (Allison et al., 1989) leads me to assume that some inhibitory mechanisms are involved in the generation of high-frequency oscillations. I argue that activity of fast-spiking inhibitory interneurons provides the basis for high-frequency oscillations. In the following sections I briefly describe anatomical and physiological features of inhibitory interneurons disclosed in animal experiments.

## ANATOMY OF CORTICAL INHIBITORY INTERNEURONS

The interneurons of layer 4 and pyramidal cells have both been shown to be the recipients of the direct thalamic synapses (E. G. Jones, 1975; White, 1986). Anatomic studies of monkey sensorimotor areas showed that there are several different types of interneurons, and the majority of them are nonspiny, GABAergic inhibitory interneurons (E. G. Jones, 1975). These interneurons receive thalamic axon synapses and have their own axon terminations focused on the cell somata, proximal dendrites, and initial segments of the pyramidal cells (DeFelipe, Conley, & Jones, 1986; E. G. Jones, 1993). Furthermore, the patterns of connectivity of many GABAergic interneurons are bidirectional, and the vertical axonal projections between the deep and superficial layers are particularly strong, whereas the horizontal projections are less prominent (E. G. Jones, 1993).

These synaptic connections suggest that GABA-mediated inhibition plays a powerful role in shaping the physiologic response profiles of pyramidal neurons. In addition, the parallel vertical and horizontal arrangement of the axonal arbors of the interneurons provides the anatomic basis for spatial summation of the axonal activity of individual neurons. Thus, synchronous activity of a population of GABAergic interneurons in area 3b with axonal arbors oriented tangentially to the scalp, by summing individual intracellular currents spatiotemporally, may produce magnetic fields strong enough to be detectable outside the head. I address this possibility further in a later section by comparing the orientation of the dipoles for the high-frequency oscillations and the N20m.

## PHYSIOLOGY OF CORTICAL INHIBITORY INTERNEURONS

An electrophysiologic characteristic of inhibitory interneurons in the somatosensory cortex is a high-frequency spike burst (200–1000 Hz) in response to synaptic volleys (Steriade, 1978; Swadlow, 1989, 1995; Swadlow et al., 1998). Second, the interneurons increase their activity during wakefulness (Livingstone & Hubel, 1981) and decrease their activity during sleep (Evarts, 1964; Moruzzi, 1966).

The functional roles of the inhibitory interneurons can be summarized as follows. First, the GABAergic inhibitory postsynaptic potentials ( IPSPs) play an important role in controlling the excitability and responsiveness in the pyramidal neurons (McCormick, 1989; Swadlow et al., 1998). Iontophoretic application of the GABA$_A$ antagonist bicuculline, in the somatosensory cortex, leads to an enlargement of the receptive fields of pyramidal cells (Dykes, Landry, Metherate, & Hicks, 1984; Tremere, Hicks, & Rasmusson, 2001), whereas enhanced inhibition leads to an enhanced response selectivity (Livingstone & Hubel, 1981). Second, cortical interneurons are activated by acetylcholine and serotonin on arousal, which causes enhancement of inhibition of downstream glutamatergic pyramidal cell activity (Steriade, Jones, & Llinás, 1990). Thus, with the interneurons controlling the pyramidal neurons by feed-forward inhibition, this inhibitory mechanism underlies an accurate discrimination of incoming sensory information (Steriade et al., 1990).

## INTERNEURON HYPOTHESIS
## FOR THE HIGH-FREQUENCY OSCILLATIONS

It is now well established that the N20m is generated within the apical dendrites of the pyramidal cells in area 3b (Allison et al., 1989). Area 3b in the posterior bank of the central sulcus receives skin afferent inputs (Nelson, Sur, Felleman, & Kaas, 1980) and gives rise to tangential current sources of both N20m and high-frequency oscillations (Curio et al., 1994; Hashimoto et al., 1999; Hashimoto et al., 1996). As discussed earlier, an electrophysiologic feature of inhibitory interneurons in the somatosensory cortex is a high-frequency spike burst up to 1000 Hz without adaptation in response to synaptic volleys. Therefore, the interneurons are considered to be extremely resistant to the refractoriness produced by continuous stimulation of the skin. It is surprising that the interference stimulation even increased the number of high-frequency peaks. The result suggests facilitatory effects of interference stimulation on GABAergic inhibitory interneurons by tonic excitation, leading to a response enhancement to the coherent afferent volley elicited by median nerve stimulation. Thus, with the interneurons controlling the pyramidal cells by feed-forward inhibition, this enhanced inhibitory mechanism underlies a remarkable reduction of the N20m during interference stimulation (Hashimoto et al., 1999). Therefore, I conclude that the attenuation of the N20m results from relative refractoriness of the pyramidal cells produced directly by the interference stimulation as well as the enhanced feed-forward inhibition from the interneurons.

During sleep, the interneurons decrease their activity (Evarts, 1964; Moruzzi, 1966), resulting in disinhibition of the downstream pyramidal cells. Thus, an amplitude reduction of high-frequency oscillations is associated with an increase in the N20m during sleep and vice versa during wakefulness (Hashimoto et al., 1996).

Although the thumb has a larger representation in area 3b than the middle finger does, the N20m is of the same amplitude for both digits (Tanosaki et al., 2001). This implies that the N20m after thumb stimulation is disproportionately small in amplitude. On the other hand, high-frequency oscillations are higher in amplitude and in number of peaks for thumb than for middle finger stimulation. I speculate that the enhanced high-frequency oscillations after thumb stimulation might facilitate primary somatosensory processing, which in turn provides the motor cortex finely tuned somatosensory information for fine motor control of the thumb. From these convergent lines of evidence it may be concluded that the high-frequency oscillations represent the activity of GABAergic inhibitory interneurons in layer 4 in area 3b of the primary somatosensory cortex, which receives monosynaptic excitatory input from the thalamus. Second, the underlying N20m represents activity of pyramidal neurons in the somatosensory cortex that receive monosynaptic excitatory input from the thalamus as well as the feed-forward inhibition from the interneurons (Hashimoto et al., 1999; Hashimoto et al., 1996; Tanosaki et al., 2001).

## SYNCHRONICITY OF CORTICAL INHIBITORY INTERNEURONS

High-frequency signals in somatosensory evoked potentials and fields have been ascribed to presynaptic action potentials and fields on the basis of their high-frequency spectral energy, which is common to peripheral nerve compound activity and subcortical white matter activity (Curio et al., 1994; Gobbele et al., 1998; Hashimoto, 1984; Hashimoto et al., 1994; Hashimoto et al., 1995; Hashimoto, Odaka, Gatayama, & Yokoyama, 1991; Katayama & Tsubokawa, 1987; Maccabee et al., 1983; McLaughlin & Kelly, 1993). It was recently suggested, on the basis of a mapping study of somatosensory evoked potentials over the scalp using a dense array of surface electrodes, and using a spatiotemporal analysis method, that the early part of high-frequency oscillations arises from an initial segment of the thalamocortical projection fibers (Gobbele et al., 1998). However, the decrease or total abolition of the high-frequency oscillations during sleep, despite an enhanced N20m (Hashimoto et al., 1996) or stable N20 (Yamada et al., 1988) reflecting ensemble EPSPs of the pyramidal neurons, would argue against the primary contribution of the thalamo-cortical afferent activity to the high-frequency oscillations.

A question naturally arises as to how averaged and summated activity of the somatosensory cortex has such a high-frequency component between 300 and 900 Hz in view of an inherent biological jitter in the activity of the central nervous system. In other words, a critical issue for the detection of averaged and summed activity of high-frequency oscillations is timing precision of the underlying individual neural activity. In awake rabbits, it has been demonstrated that the inhibitory interneurons of layer 4 in the primary somatosensory area respond to a brief airpuff stimulus on the trigeminal area with a high-frequency burst (>600 Hz) of three or more spikes (Swadlow, 1995; Swadlow et al., 1998). Individual interneurons are considered to receive a highly convergent input from a large population of thalamic afferent fibers, and many of the thalamic afferent fibers entering the cortex diverge to synapse on many interneurons in layer 4. This rich convergence and divergence of the thalamic afferents onto layer 4 interneurons can be characterized by high sensitivity and high temporal resolution. Furthermore, Rasmusson (1996) demonstrated in animal experiments that the inhibitory interneurons of layer 4 responded to electrical stimulation of the ventrobasal thalamus with an extremely small latency variation (SD = 0.04 msec). It has recently been demonstrated, using dual intracellular recordings, that electrotonic coupling by gap–junction acts to promote the synchronous firing of local networks of fast-spiking interneurons in the neocortex (Galarreta & Hestrin, 1999; Gibson, Beierlein, & Connors, 1999). Thus, it is possible that the mass response as an envelope of individual unit activities has a sharp temporal profile with a high-frequency component.

These findings suggest that the averaged activity of inhibitory interneurons can be recorded as high-frequency oscillations. In fact, simultaneous surface field potential recordings and intracellular recordings from fast-spiking interneurons from rat area 3b to vibrissa stimulation showed that the bursts of action potentials from the interneurons closely approximated the periodicity of the surface recorded high-frequency oscillations (M. S. Jones, MacDonald, Choi, Dudek, & Barth, 2000). The close association of stimulus-evoked activity in fast-spiking cells with the surface oscillations suggests that the fast-spiking interneurons are the generators of these oscillations. Morphological cell types for the fast-spiking cells are basket cells and chandelier cells with axonal arborizations near thick dendrites, somata, and initial segments (Kawaguchi & Kubota, 1997).

M. S. Jones et al. (2000) conjectured that the surface extracellular oscillations reflect fast IPSPs in the apical dendrites of target pyramidal cells rather than the activity of fast-spiking cells themselves. Because they did not record the activity of thalamocortical afferents in the experiment, the possible contribution of presynaptic activity of terminal arbors of thalamocortical afferents or even of their initial segments in the thalamus cannot be ruled out (Curio et al., 1994; Gobbele et al., 1998; Peterson, Schroeder, & Arezzo, 1995; Shimazu et al., 2000). Thus, this is an open question for future studies.

## FAST IPSPS OF PYRAMIDAL NEURONS VERSUS ACTION POTENTIALS OF FAST-SPIKING INTERNEURONS

Previous studies on humans and animals have identified three possible candidates for the generation of high-frequency oscillations: (a) fast IPSPs in the apical dendrites of pyramidal cells, (b) axonal activity of fast-spiking interneurons, and (c) action potentials conducted along the thalamocortical projection fibers. One simple way to test these possibilities is to compare the orientation of the ECD for high-frequency oscillations with that for the underlying N20m, because it has been established that the N20m is produced by EPSPs in the apical dendrites of the pyramidal cell population in area 3b (Allison et al., 1989; Hashimoto et al., 1996). The fast-IPSP hypothesis dictates that the dipole orientation for high-frequency oscillations should be just the same as that for the N20m, because the IPSPs and EPSPs are produced within the same apical dendrites of pyramidal neurons. Ozaki et al. (2001) and Ozaki and Hashimoto (2001) have found that the orientation of high-frequency oscillations shows more divergent pattern than that of the N20m (see Fig. 12.7A) and that there is a wide distribution in the angles formed by pairs of dipoles for the two components calculated at the same time slices (Fig. 12.7B). The mean difference in the angles formed by 114 pairs of ECD vectors obtained from 14 subjects was about 18°. The result seems to be contradictory to the fast-IPSP hypothesis of M. S. Jones et al. (2000), because according to their hypothesis the mean angle should be 0°. On the other hand, this angle favors the other hypothesis of axonal activity of

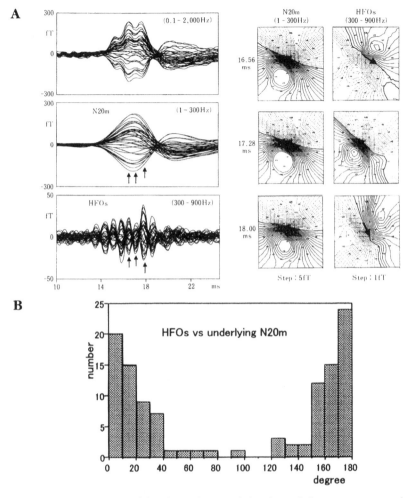

FIG. 12.7. Panel A: the left column shows wide-band recorded somatosensory evoked fields (SEFs, top row), low-pass (middle row) and high-pass (bottom row) filtered SEFs to right median nerve stimulation. Arrows indicate three high-frequency oscillation peaks (bottom row) and corresponding time slices in low-pass filtered N20m (middle row) where equivalent current dipole (ECD) vectors were calculated. The center and right columns show pairs of isofield maps with dipole directions superimposed for the N20m and high-frequency oscillation peaks at the three time slices indicated in the left column. Note the differences in dipole orientation between the two components. The orientation for a high-frequency oscillation peak is almost orthogonal to that for the N20m (bottom pair). From "High-Frequency Oscillations in Primary Somatosensory Cortex" by I. Ozaki and I. Hashimoto, 2001, *Clinical Electroencephalography, 43,* p. 675. Copyright 2001 by Nagai Shoten. Reprinted by permission. Panel B: distribution of the angles formed by 114 pairs of ECD vectors between N20m and high-frequency oscillations. The mean difference in the angles was about 18°. From "Dipole Orientation Differs Between High Frequency Oscillations and N20m Current Sources in Human Somatosensory Evoked Magnetic Fields to Median Nerve Stimulation" by I. Ozaki et al., 2001, *Neuroscience Letters, 310,* p. 43. Copyright 2001 by Elsevier Science. Reprinted by permission.

fast-spiking interneurons (Hashimoto et al., 1996). When fast-spiking interneurons oriented in vertical and horizontal axonal directions burst simultaneously, the vertical and horizontal currents result in a single ECD with an oblique direction against the apical dendrites of pyramidal neurons. I speculate that high-frequency oscillations represent the axonal activity of combined vertically and horizontally oriented fast-spiking interneurons in area 3b of the somatosensory cortex.

## HORIZONTAL FIBERS MEDIATE MONOSYNAPTIC EXCITATION OF PYRAMIDAL CELL POPULATION IN AREA 3B

The N20 primary response to median nerve stimulation has long been considered as a fixed tangential ECD in area 3b (Allison et al., 1989). However, our recent MEG studies provide evidence against this long-standing notion of a fixed source and give some insight into an early somatosensory processing mediated by horizontal fibers (Hashimoto et al., 2000; Hashimoto, Kimura, Iguchi, Takino, & Sekihara, 2001; Kimura & Hashimoto, 2001).

After filtering with a low-pass filter with a cutoff frequency of 300 Hz, low-amplitude high-frequency oscillations (HFOs) were removed from the N20m. I focused on ECD locations from 1.2 msec before and 1.2 msec after the peak, because the signal-to-noise ratio was sufficiently good during this period. The ECD moved sequentially toward the anterior, lateral, and inferior direction for a distance of 8.7 mm at a propagation velocity of 3.6 m/sec. Overlaying the successive ECD locations onto the MRI confirmed that the ECD movement was parallel to the surface of the posterior bank of the central sulcus at the 3b hand area and orthogonal to the direction of ECD orientation

It may be argued that the ECD movement detected in the study just described simply reflects the sequential activation of thalamocortical afferents from the ring, middle, and index fingers to the thumb, all innervated by the median nerve (Hashimoto et al., 2000, 2001). Therefore, Kimura and Hashimoto (2001) examined the ECD movement for stimulation of a single index finger after averaging 10,000 epochs. Localizations of ECDs were calculated for a period of 2.4 msec around the N20m peak (see Fig. 12.8A), as in the previous studies (Hashimoto et al., 2000; Hashimoto et al., 2001). The ECD moved toward the lateral and inferior direction with a mean distance of 8.4 mm, very similar to the findings following median nerve stimulation (see Fig. 12.8B). The results suggest that the distance of N20m ECD movement is independent of the size of projected cortical area.

Orthogonal to the direction of depolarization shift along the apical dendrites, the pyramidal cells whose somata are located in layer 3 are suc-

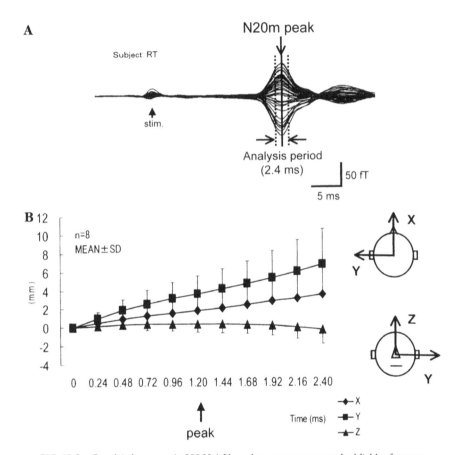

FIG. 12.8.   Panel A: low-pass (<300 Hz) filtered somatosensory evoked fields after averaging 10,000 epochs. The solid line shows the peak latency of the N20m, and the latency range between the two dotted lines indicates an equivalent current dipole (ECD) analysis period of 2.4 msec. Panel B: normalized movement (in millimeters) of the N20m ECD along $x$, $y$, and $z$ coordinates. The movement of the ECD is toward the anterior ($x$), lateral ($y$), and inferior ($z$) directions. The abscissa denotes the latency (in milliseconds) from a 1.2-msec pre-N20m peak that is set to zero. The ordinate indicates the distance (in millimeters) from the initial ECD location at a 1.2-msec pre-N20m peak. From "Source of Somatosensory Primary Cortical Evoked Magnetic Fields (N20m) Elicited by Index Finger Stimulation Moves Toward Mediolateral Direction in Area 3b in Man" by T. Kimura and I. Hashimoto, *Neuroscience Letters, 299,* p. 62. Copyright 2001 by Elsevier Science. Reprinted by permission.

cessively activated by the impulse transmitted through horizontal fibers (E. G. Jones, 1993; Langdon & Sur, 1990). Indeed, the horizontal intracortical collaterals of pyramidal cell axons can extend for 6 mm or more and are the principal route for horizontal spread of excitation in the neocortex (DeFelipe et al., 1986; Gilbert & Wiesel, 1989; McGuire, Gilbert, Rivlin, & Wiesel, 1991). What are the physiological functions of this horizontal connection? Horizontal fibers in monkey striate cortex connect functionally similar columns by which information over a wide area of the cortex is integrated (Gilbert, 1992). In the primary auditory cortex the horizontal fibers are oriented dorsoventrally along the organization of isofrequency bands and link columns of similar properties (Ojima, Honda, & Jones, 1991). This suggests that the connection may subserve sound localization. It remains unknown, however, what kind of information is integrated by the horizontal fibers in somatosensory area 3b. The studies just discussed show that the movement of the N20m ECD represents the sequential mediolateral activation of pyramidal cells in area 3b. Second, horizontal intracortical collaterals of pyramidal cell axons running parallel to the cortical surface mediate this activation. Third, the findings suggest that the initial somatosensory information processing in area 3b can be monitored noninvasively.

Magnetic recordings have made it possible to visualize for the first time robust serial mediolateral activation in area 3b (Hashimoto et al., 2001, 2000; Kimura & Hashimoto, 2001). In other words, cortical somatosensory evoked potential recordings have failed to detect this activation pattern (Allison et al., 1989). Because area 3b lies relatively deep within the central sulcus, direct recordings of activity in area 3b are difficult to achieve with surface electrodes. On the other hand, MEG source localization is better in the direction orthogonal to the dipole orientation (Hari, Joutsiniemi, & Sarvas, 1988), and the movement of the source is orthogonal to the N20m ECD orientation.

## HORIZONTAL FIBERS MEDIATE DISYNAPTIC INHIBITION OF PYRAMIDAL CELL POPULATION IN AREA 3B

### In-Field and Surround Inhibition Within Area 3b

Tanosaki et al. (2002b) studied modification of the N20m following electric middle finger stimulation with tactile interference to the same and surrounding digits to explore the neural mechanisms for the soma-

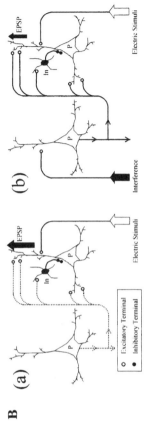

**A**

Rt middle finger stim.

Control

Interference

III

II + V

I + V

N20m, P30m, N40m, P60m

25 fT

10 ms/div

**B** (a)

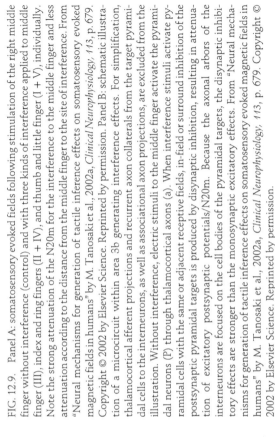

Excitatory Terminal
Inhibitory Terminal

EPSP

Electric Stimuli

(b)

EPSP

Electric Stimuli

Interference

FIG. 12.9. Panel A: somatosensory evoked fields following stimulation of the right middle finger without interference (control) and with three kinds of interference applied to middle finger (III), index and ring fingers (II + IV), and thumb and little finger (I + V), individually. Note the strong attenuation of the N20m for the interference to the middle finger and less attenuation according to the distance from the middle finger to the site of interference. From "Neural mechanisms for generation of tactile inference effects on somatosensory evoked magnetic fields in humans" by M. Tanosaki et al., 2002a, *Clinical Neurophysiology, 113*, p. 679. Copyright © 2002 by Elsevier Science. Reprinted by permission. Panel B: schematic illustration of a microcircuit within area 3b generating interference effects. For simplification, thalamocortical afferent projections and recurrent axon collaterals from the target pyramidal cells to the interneurons, as well as associational axon projections, are excluded from the illustration. Without interference, electric stimuli to the middle finger activate the pyramidal neurons (P) through thalamocortical axons (a). When interference stimuli activate pyramidal cells with the same or adjacent receptive fields, in-field or surround inhibition of the postsynaptic pyramidal targets is produced by disynaptic inhibition, resulting in attenuation of excitatory postsynaptic potentials/N20m. Because the axonal arbors of the interneurons are focused on the cell bodies of the pyramidal targets, the disynaptic inhibitory effects are stronger than the monosynaptic excitatory effects. From "Neural mechanisms for generation of tactile inference effects on somatosensory evoked magnetic fields in humans" by M. Tanosaki et al., 2002a, *Clinical Neurophysiology, 113*, p. 679. Copyright © 2002 by Elsevier Science. Reprinted by permission.

tosensory integration from multiple digits. During electric middle finger stimulation, concurrent tactile stimulation was applied to the middle finger (III), to the index and ring fingers (II + IV), and to the thumb and the little finger (I + V), individually (see Fig. 12.9a). The mean interference–control N20m amplitude ratios for the interference to III, to II + IV, and to I + V were 69%, 87%, and 93%, respectively. Thus, the attenuation of the N20m showed spatial gradients as a function of the distance from the middle finger to the site for the interference: the in-field inhibition (interference to the same finger [III]) was stronger than the adjacent-surround inhibition (interference to the adjacent digits [II + IV]), and the nonadjacent-surround inhibition was very weak.

When presynaptic pyramidal neurons generate axonal volleys by tactile stimulation they are transmitted horizontally along the intrinsic collaterals to the target postsynaptic pyramidal neurons and inhibitory interneurons. Thus, the activation of the intrinsic collaterals induces monosynaptic excitation and disynaptic inhibition (via inhibitory interneurons) to the target pyramidal neurons. In monkey somatosensory area 3b, the intrinsic horizontal collaterals of pyramidal neurons are widely distributed within cortical representations of the digits and interconnect them even if their representations are segregated (Burton & Fabri, 1995; Manger, Woods, Munoz, & Jones, 1997). In addition, the distribution of intrinsic collaterals has a spatial gradient: It is densest near the somata of the parent pyramidal cells and becomes sparse as a function of the distance from the soma. The spatial gradient of N20m attenuation suggests that the activation of intrinsic collaterals by tactile interference inhibits, on balance, the target pyramidal cells where the in-field inhibition is stronger than the surround inhibition. Although this study (Tanosaki et al., 2002b) focused only on modification of the N20m, in which high-frequency oscillations were not dealt with directly, I infer that enhanced activity of interneurons is the basis for the attenuated N20m as schematized in Fig. 12.9b (see also Figs. 12.5 and 12.10a).

## Activation of Area 3a by Voluntary Movements Inhibits Activity of Area 3b Through Horizontal Fibers

Voluntary movements of digits attenuate the N20m amplitude following median nerve stimulation (Kakigi et al., 1995; Rossini et al., 1999; Schnitzler et al., 1995). However, neural mechanisms of interaction between distinct submodalities in somatosensation remain to be elucidated. Somatosensory evoked magnetic fields following electric median

nerve stimulation were recorded with and without movement interference (Tanosaki et al., 2002a). During interference, the subject produced
repetitive opposing movements of the thumb with the index, middle and
ring fingers sequentially. Amplitudes of both N20m and high-frequency
oscillations were smaller in the movement condition (Fig. 12.10A). However, the attenuation was much greater for the N20m (67%) than for
high-frequency oscillations (85%). Thus, the ratio of decrement, computed by dividing 85% for high-frequency oscillations with 67% for
N20m, was 1.27, and was significantly higher than 1.0 ($p < .0005$), suggesting higher stability on the part of high-frequency oscillations than
the underlying N20m.

Area 3b, where the N20m is generated, mainly receives cutaneous afferent input, whereas area 3a receives inputs from muscle spindles and other
deep receptors (Kaas & Pons, 1988). Areas 3a and 3b are densely intercon-
nected by corticocortical axon collaterals of pyramidal neurons, and the connections are topographically organized (Burton & Fabri, 1995; DeFelipe et
al., 1986; Krubitzer & Kaas, 1990). These collaterals can provide monosynaptic excitatory and disynaptic inhibitory influences onto the postsynaptic pyramidal targets (Elhanany & White, 1990; McGuire et al., 1991;
Melchitzky, Sesack, Pucak, & Lewis, 1998; White & Keller, 1987). Attenuation of the N20m during movement is due to strong disynaptic inhibition
from the pyramidal neurons in area 3a through their corticocortical axon
collaterals toward the postsynaptic pyramidal targets in area 3b (see Fig.
12.10B). As the activity of the pyramidal targets is suppressed, the excitatory outputs onto the interneurons through recurrent axon collaterals decrease. This in turn decreases the enhanced activity of the interneurons
mediated by the corticocortical axon collaterals from area 3a. Attenuation of
high-frequency oscillations during movement is the net result of the converging influence on the interneurons from areas 3a and 3b.

## DEVELOPMENTAL CHANGES OF HIGH-FREQUENCY OSCILLATIONS

Although the effects of development on the N20 somatosensory evoked
potential component has been extensively studied (Allison, Hume, Wood,
& Goff, 1984; Desmedt, Brunko, & Debecker, 1976; Taylor & Fagan, 1988),
concurrent high-frequency oscillations have not been examined. Nakano
and Hashimoto (2000) recorded median nerve somatosensory evoked potentials from 15 healthy schoolchildren between ages 6 and 12 years. Fifteen healthy adult subjects aged between 19 and 32 years served as

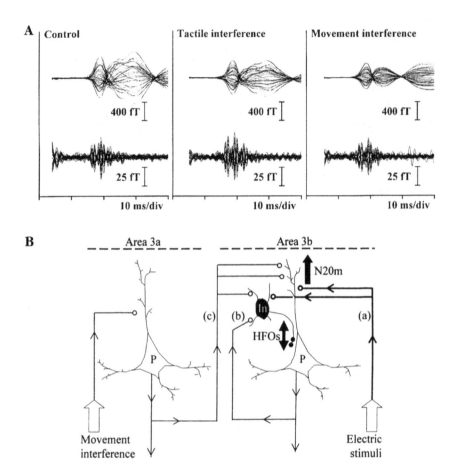

FIG. 12.10. Panel A: somatosensory evoked fields following right median nerve stimulation without interference (control) and with tactile and movement interferences. Note the attenuation of the N20m in tactile and movement interferences, in which the movement interference produces stronger attenuation. High-frequency oscillations are enhanced in the tactile interference and are attenuated in the movement interference. Attenuation is more prominent in the N20m than in high-frequency oscillations for movement interference. From "Movement interference attenuates somatosensory high-frequency oscilliations: Contribution of local axon collaterals of 3b pyramidal neurons" by M. Tanosaki et al., 2002a, *Clinical Neurophysiology, 113*, p. 999. Copyright © 2002 by Elsevier Science. Reprinted by permission. Panel B: schematic illustration of a microcircuit within areas 3a and 3b generating movement-interference effects. Electric stimuli to the median nerve activate the pyramidal neurons (P) and inhibitory interneurons through thalamocortical axons (a), which in turn generate N20m and high-frequency oscillations, respectively. Recurrent axon collaterals (b) of the pyramidal neurons in area 3b provide excitatory outputs onto the interneurons, which in turn inhibit the pyramidal neurons. Corticocortical axon collaterals of the pyramidal cells in area 3a provide excitatory synaptic outputs onto the pyramidal neurons and interneurons in area 3b. When movement-interference stimuli activate pyramidal cells in area 3a, the postsynaptic pyramidal targets in area 3b are disynaptically inhibited, resulting in attenuation of excitatory postsynaptic potentials (EPSPs)/N20m. *(continued on next page)*

controls. Wide-band somatosensory evoked potentials (a bandpass of 10–2000 Hz) were recorded from C3' (2 cm posterior to C3)–Fz derivation. Figure 12.11 shows the original wide-band, low-pass (<300 Hz) and high-pass (>300 Hz) filtered somatosensory evoked potentials from a typical adult subject (A) and a child (B). It is clear from the illustrations that high-frequency oscillations in the children are remarkably higher in amplitude, larger in number of peaks, and accordingly longer in the total burst duration than those of the adult subjects ($p < .0001$). Similarly, the amplitude of the N20 was also higher in children ($p < .05$). Besides, an amplitude ratio of high-frequency oscillations to the N20 was significantly larger in children ($p < .05$). This suggests that enhanced amplitude of high-frequency oscillations is not simply correlated with enhanced amplitude of the N20. The mechanisms for higher amplitude in high-frequency oscillations and the underlying N20 in children are still unresolved. One possibility is a thin skull and scalp in children, resulting in a lower resistance and a shorter distance between the cortex and the recording electrodes over the scalp. These physical characteristics alone can increase the amplitude of recorded cortical activity without any alterations in the cortical activity itself. There was no apparent inverse relation between high-frequency oscillations and the N20 in the developmental processes, because both high-frequency oscillations and N20 were enhanced in children. However, the amplitude ratio of high-frequency oscillations to the N20 was significantly larger in children, suggesting more enhanced activity of interneurons as compared with pyramidal neurons in area 3b. I speculate that cortical inhibitory mechanisms develop relatively earlier than the excitatory ones.

## MODULATION OF HIGH-FREQUENCY OSCILLATIONS BY AGING

The effects of aging on somatosensory evoked potentials after median nerve stimulation have been studied extensively (Desmedt & Cheron, 1980; Hume, Cant, Shaw, & Cowan, 1982; Luders, 1970; Shagass & Schwartz,

FIG. 12.10. *(continued)*   Because the axonal arbors of the interneurons are focused on the cell bodies of the pyramidal targets, the disynaptic inhibitory effects are stronger than the monosynaptic excitatory effects. Thus, decreased EPSPs reduce the activity of inhibitory interneurons, resulting in attenuation of high-frequency oscillations. From "Neural mechanisms for generation of tactile inference effects on somatosensory evoked magnetic fields in humans" by M. Tanosaki et al., 2002b, *Clinical Neurophysiology, 113*, p. 679. Copyright © 2002 by Elsevier Science. Reprinted by permission.

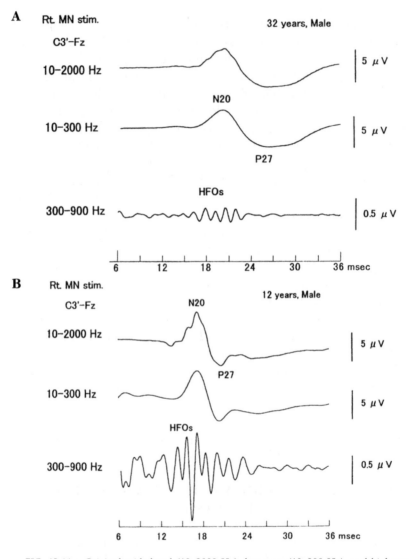

FIG. 12.11. Original wide-band (10–2000 Hz), low-pass (10–300 Hz), and high-pass (300–900 Hz) filtered somatosensory evoked potentials from C3'–Fz lead following median nerve stimulation in a normal adult subject (Panel A) and a child (Panel B). The high-pass traces show a short burst of high-frequency oscillations around N20 and P27, which can be recognized in the wide-band record as clear notches overlying the N20 response. Note the higher amplitudes and larger number of high-frequency oscillations in the child. From "Somatosensory Evoked High-Frequency Oscillations Are Enhanced in School Children" by S. Nakano and I. Hashimoto, 2000, *Neuroscience Letters, 291,* p. 114. Copyright 2000 by Elsevier Science. Reprinted by permission.

1965). In particular, the amplitude of the cortical primary response is well known to follow a $U$-shaped curve with aging such that it is high during adolescence, low during middle age, and high again in old age. However, the effects of aging on somatosensory evoked high-frequency oscillations after median nerve stimulation remain unknown. Fifteen normal subjects aged between 62 and 73 years were studied, and 15 normal young subjects aged between 19 and 32 years served as controls (Nakano & Hashimoto, 1999b).

Figure 12.12 shows the original wide-band (10–2000 Hz) recorded somatosensory evoked potentials, low-pass (<300 Hz) and high-pass (>300 Hz) filtered responses from a C3'–Fz lead in a typical young subject and a normal aged subject. The high-frequency oscillations started approximately at or after the onset of the primary cortical response (N20) and ended at the middle of the second slope in the young subject. In contrast, the high-frequency oscillations in the aged subject were clearly higher in amplitude and longer in total burst duration than those in the young subject. Specifically, the high-frequency oscillations between the N20 peak and the last peak of high-frequency oscillations were significantly higher in amplitude, longer in burst duration, and larger in area in the aged subjects than in the young subjects, whereas those between the onset of high-frequency oscillations and the N20 peak did not differ significantly. This suggests that the aging process affects differently the early and later parts of the high-frequency oscillations.

In agreement with previous reports, the N20 and P27 amplitudes have been shown to be higher in aged subjects (Desmedt & Cheron, 1980; Hume et al., 1982; Luders, 1970; Shagass & Schwartz, 1965). Given that the number of cortical neurons decreases with aging (Brody, 1955), it is surprising that the primary cortical potentials were enlarged in the aged subjects. Anatomically, pyramidal neurons in the cerebral cortex appear to show a greater reduction in their horizontal dendrites compared with apical dendrites (Scheibel, Lindsay, Tomiyasu, & Scheibel, 1975) and show hypertrophy of the apical dendrites with aging (Buell & Coleman, 1979). These morphologic changes in apical dendrites may produce a simplified and coherent flow of intracellular current generated by ensemble EPSPs, leading to an increased N20 amplitude. On the other hand, Kazis et al. (1983) speculated that a decrease in the cortical inhibitory mechanism leads to a predominance of the excitatory mechanism, which in turn produces higher amplitude in the primary cortical response in aged subjects. In the auditory system, P50m generated in the primary auditory cortex was larger in older subjects than in young subjects, and this

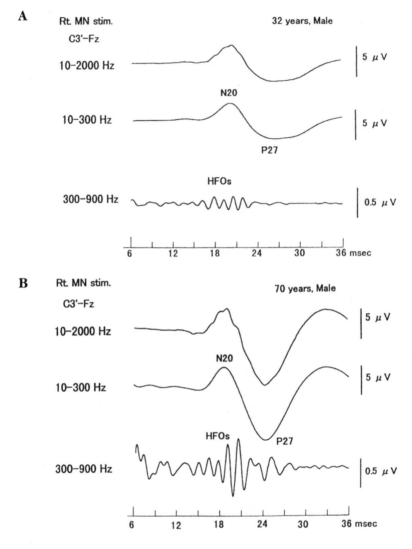

FIG. 12.12. Original wide-band (10–2000 Hz), low-pass (10–300Hz), and high-pass (300–900 Hz) filtered somatosensory evoked potentials from C3′–Fz lead following median nerve stimulation in a normal young (Panel A) and aged (Panel B) subject. Note the higher amplitudes in the later part of high-frequency oscillations in the aged subject. From "The Later Part of Human Somatic Evoked High-Frequency Oscillations Is Enhanced in Aged Subjects" by S. Nakano and I. Hashimoto, 1999, *Neuroscience Letters, 276,* p. 84. Copyright 1999 by Elsevier Science. Reprinted by permission.

enlargement was presumably caused by impaired inhibition of afferent inputs in the auditory cortex (Pekkonen et al., 1995).

Research indicates that the early part of high-frequency oscillations may be generated by inhibitory interneurons with a feed-forward inhibition to the pyramidal neurons in area 3b (Hashimoto et al., 1999; Hashimoto et al., 1996). The later part of high-frequency oscillations may be generated by inhibitory interneurons with a feedback inhibition to the pyramidal neurons. Provided that an enhanced N20 reflects a genuine increase in cortical activity and is not due to the morphologic changes in the apical dendrites, increased activity of pyramidal neurons will lead to increased activity of the postsynaptic inhibitory interneurons through recurrent axon collaterals. This results in higher amplitude of the later part of high-frequency oscillations. As a consequence, the increased activity of inhibitory interneurons should also inhibit the activity of pyramidal neurons by recurrent inhibition, resulting in a possible reduction in P27 amplitude. However, the P27 primary cortical response was increased in aged subjects. I speculate that the P27 response increment is due to a relative insensitivity of the pyramidal neurons to the feedback inhibitory input.

## HIGH-FREQUENCY OSCILLATIONS
## IN NEUROPATHOLOGICAL CONDITIONS

In regard to Parkinson's disease, Mochizuki et al. (1999) reported that the later part of high-frequency oscillations to median nerve stimulation was selectively enhanced, whereas the early part remained unchanged (see Fig. 12.13A). In myoclonus epilepsy, extremely enhanced high-frequency oscillations were superimposed on the peaks of P27 and N35 (see Fig. 12.13B). These ultra-late high-frequency oscillations are never observed in normal subjects. It is interesting that the early part of high-frequency oscillations in myoclonus epilepsy is not different from those of the normal controls. In a more recent study, high-frequency oscillations superimposed on the P37 primary response after stimulation of the posterior tibial nerve were shown to increase in amplitude threefold or more in Parkinson's disease and in multiple-system atrophy (Inoue, Hashimoto, & Nakamura, 2001). Noteworthy is that the underlying P37 was smaller than that of the normal controls. Thus, the mean amplitude ratios of high-frequency oscillations to the P37 were 0.028, 0.021, and 0.006 for multiple system atrophy, Parkinson's disease, and normal controls, respectively. The findings suggest that there exists a reciprocal relation be-

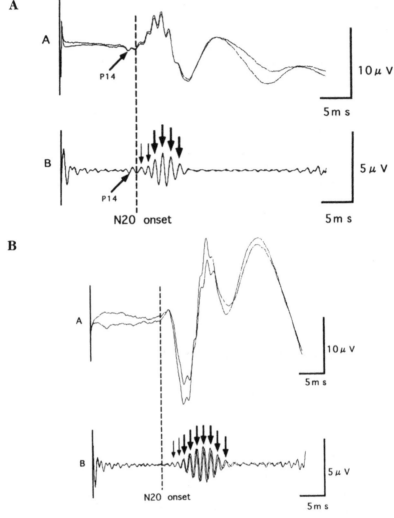

FIG. 12.13.   Panel A: somatosensory evoked potentials (SEPs) in a patient with Parkinson's disease. The upper trace shows original wide-band (0.5–3000 Hz) records and lower trace, high-pass (500–1000 Hz) filtered SEPs. Six high-frequency peaks, indicated by arrows, followed the P14 subcortical component, and later four peaks (indicated by large arrows) were abnormally enlarged. Panel B: SEPs in a patient with myoclonus epilepsy. The upper trace shows original wide-band and lower trace, high-pass filtered SEPs. Abnormally enlarged P27 (first downward deflection) and N35 (following upward deflection) were superimposed by nine high-frequency peaks in which later seven peaks were abnormally large. This ultra-late component of high-frequency oscillations is not observed in normal subjects. From "Somatosensory Evoked High-Frequency Oscillation in Parkinson's Disease and Myoclonus Epilepsy" by H. Mochizuki et al., 1999, *Journal of Clinical Neurophysiology, 110,* pp. 188–189. Copyright 1999 by Elsevier Science. Reprinted by permission.

tween high-frequency oscillations and the underlying P37 primary response in these diseases.

The study of high-frequency oscillations in various central nervous system diseases is in a stage of infancy. At present, neural mechanisms for an ultra-late component of the high-frequency oscillations observed in myoclonus epilepsy remain unknown. Further research on normal subjects and on patients with neurological diseases is needed to clarify the roles of the high-frequency oscillations in information processing.

## ACKNOWLEDGMENTS

I thank T. Fukushima, Y. Iguchi, T. Imada, K. Inoue, Y. Iwase, S. Kato, T. Kimura, T. Mashiko, S. Nakano, I. Ozaki, Y. Saito, K. Sakuma, K. Sekihara, A Suzuki, R. Takino, and M. Tanosaki for close collaboration, and G. Curio, Y. Okada, and H. Swadlow for insightful discussions.

## REFERENCES

Abbruzzese, M., Favale, E., Leandri, M., & Ratto, S. (1978). New subcomponents of the cerebral somatosensory evoked potential in man. *Acta Neurologica Scandinavica, 58,* 352–332.

Allison, T., Hume, A. L., Wood, C. C., & Goff, W. R. (1984). Developmental and aging changes in somatosensory, auditory and visual evoked potentials. *Electroencephalography and Clinical Neurophysiology, 58,* 14–24.

Allison, T., McCarthy, G., Wood, C. C., Darcey, T. M., Spencer, D. D., & Williamson, P. D. (1989). Human cortical potentials evoked by stimulation of the median nerve: I. Cytoarchitectonic areas generating short-latency activity. *Journal of Neurophysiology, 62,* 694–710.

Brody, H. (1955). Organization of cerebral cortex. *Journal of Comparative Neurology, 102,* 511–556.

Buell, S. J., & Coleman, P. D. (1979). Dendritic growth in the aged human brain and failure of growth in senile dementia. *Science, 206,* 854–856.

Burton, H., & Fabri, M. (1995). Ipsilateral connections of physiologically defined cutaneous representations in area 3b and 1 of macaque monkeys: Projections in the vicinity of the central sulcus. *Journal of Comparative Neurology, 355,* 508–538

Cracco, R. Q., & Cracco, J. B. (1976). Somatosensory evoked potential in man: Far-field potentials. *Electroencephalography and Clinical Neurophysiology, 41,* 460–466.

Curio, G. (2000). Linking 600-Hz "spikelike" EEG/MEG wavelets ("σ-burst") to cellular substrates. *Clinical Neurophysiology, 17,* 377–396.

Curio, G., Mackert, B.-M., Burghoff, M., Koetitz, R., Abraham-Fuchs, K., & Harer, W. (1994). Localization of evoked neuromagnetic 600 Hz activity in the cerebral somatosensory system. *Electroencephalography and Clinical Neurophysiology, 91,* 483–487.

Curio, G., Mackert, B.-M., Burghoff, M., Neumann, J., Nolte, G., Scherg, M., & Marx, P. (1997). Somatic source arrangement of 600 Hz oscillatory magnetic fields at the human primary somatosensory hand cortex. *Neuroscience Letters, 234,* 131–134.

DeFelipe, J., Conley, M., & Jones, E. G. (1986). Long-range focal collateralization of axons arising from corticocortical cells in monkey sensory–motor cortex. *Journal of Neuroscience, 6,* 3749–3766.

Desmedt, J. E., Brunko, E., & Debecker, J. (1976). Maturation of the somatosensory evoked potentials in normal infants and children, with special reference to the early N1 component. *Electroencephalography and Clinical Neurophysiology, 40,* 43–58.

Desmedt, J. E., & Cheron, G. (1980). Somatosensory evoked potentials in healthy octogenarians and in young adults: Wave forms, scalp topography and transit times of parietal and frontal components. *Electroencephalography and Clinical Neurophysiology, 50,* 404–425.

Dykes, R. W., Landry, P., Metherate, R., & Hicks, T. P. (1984). Functional role of GABA in cat primary somatosensory cortex: Shaping receptive fields of cortical neurons. *Journal of Neurophysiology, 52,* 1066–1093.

Eisen, A., Roberts, K., Low, M., & Laurence, P. (1984). Questions regarding the sequential neural generator theory of the somatosensory evoked potential raised by digital filtering. *Electroencephalography and Clinical Neurophysiology, 59,* 388–395.

Elhanany, E., & White, E. L. (1990). Intrinsic circuitry: Synapses involving the local axon collaterals of corticocortical projection neurons in the mouse primary somatosensory cortex. *Journal of Comparative Neurology, 291,* 43–54.

Emerson, R. G., Sgro, J. A., Pedley, T. A., & Hauser, A. (1988). State-dependent changes in the N20 component of median nerve somatosensory evoked potential. *Neurology, 38,* 64–68.

Emori, T., Yamada, T., Seki, Y., Yasuhara, A., Ando, K., Honda, Y., Leis, A. A., & Vachatimanont, P. (1991). Recovery functions of fast frequency potentials in the initial negative wave of median. *Electroencephalography and Clinical Neurophysiology, 78,* 116–123.

Evarts, E. V. (1964). Temporal patterns of discharge of pyramidal tract neurons during sleep and waking in the monkey. *Journal of Neurophysiology, 27,* 152–172.

Galarreta, M., & Hestrin, S. (1999). A network of fast-spiking cells in the neocortex connected by electrical synapses. *Nature, 402,* 72–75.

Gibson, J. R., Beierlein, M., & Connors, B. W. (1999). Two networks of electrically coupled inhibitory neurons in neocortex. *Nature, 402,* 75–79.

Gilbert, C. D. (1992). Horizontal integration and cortical dynamics. *Neuron, 9,* 1–13.

Gilbert, C. D., & Wiesel, T. N. (1989). Columnar specificity of intrinsic horizontal and corticocortical connections in cat visual cortex. *Journal of Neuroscience, 9,* 2432–2442.

Gobbele, R., Buchner, H., & Curio, G. (1998). High-frequency (600 Hz) SEP activities originating in the subcortical and cortical human somatosensory system. *Electroencephalography and Clinical Neurophysiology, 108,* 182–189.

Halboni, B., Kaminski, R., Gobbele, R., Zuchner, S., Waberski, T. D., Herrmann, C. S., Topper, R., & Buchner, H. (2000). Sleep stage dependent changes of the high-frequency part of the somatosensory evoked potentials at the thalamus and cortex. *Clinical Neurophysiology, 111,* 2277–2787.

Hari, R., Joutsiniemi, S.-L., & Sarvas, J. (1988). Spatial resolution of neuromagnetic records: Theoretical calculations in a spherical model. *Electroencephalography and Clinical Neurophysiology, 71,* 64–72.

Hashimoto, I. (1984). Somatosensory evoked potentials from the human brain-stem: Origins of short latency potentials. *Electroencephalography and Clinical Neurophysiology, 57,* 21–227.

Hashimoto, I. (2000). High-frequency oscillations of somatosensory evoked potentials and fields. *Clinical Neurophysiology, 17,* 309–320.

Hashimoto, I. (2001). Exploring the neural mechanisms of high-frequency oscillation (300–900 Hz) from the human somatosensory cortex. *NeuroReport, 12,* A7–A8.

Hashimoto, I., Kimura, T., Fukushima, T., Iguchi, Y., Saito, Y., Terasaki, O., & Sakuma, K. (1999). Reciprocal modulation of somatosensory evoked N20m primary response and high-frequency oscillations by interference stimulation. *Clinical Neurophysiology, 110,* 1445–1451.

Hashimoto, I., Kimura, T., Iguchi, Y., Takino, R., & Sekihara, K. (2001). Dynamic activation of distinct cytoarchitectonic areas of the human S1 cortex after median nerve stimulation. *NeuroReport, 12,* 1891–1897.

Hashimoto, I., Kimura, T., Sakuma, K., Iguchi, Y., Saito, Y., Terasaki, O., & Fukushima, T. (2000). Dynamic mediolateral activation of the pyramidal cell population in human somatosensory 3b area can be visualized by magnetic recordings. *Neuroscience Letters, 280,* 25–28.

Hashimoto, I., Mashiko, T., & Imada, T. (1996). Somatic evoked high-frequency magnetic oscillations reflect activity of inhibitory interneurons in the human somatosensory cortex. *Electroencephalography and Clinical Neurophysiology, 100,* 189–203.

Hashimoto, I., Mashiko, T., Mizuta, T., Imada, T., Iwase, Y., & Okazaki, H. (1994). Visualization of a moving quadrupole with magnetic measurements of peripheral nerve action fields. *Electroencephalography and Clinical Neurophysiology, 93,* 459–467.

Hashimoto, I., Mashiko, T., Mizuta, T., Imada, T., Iwase, Y., Okazaki, H., & Yoshikawa, K. (1995). Multichannel detection of magnetic compound action fields with stimulation of the index and little fingers. *Electroencephalography and Clinical Neurophysiology, 97,* 102–113.

Hashimoto, I., Odaka, K., Gatayama, T., & Yokoyama, S. (1991). Multichannel measurements of magnetic compound action fields of the median nerve in man. *Electroencephalography and Clinical Neurophysiology, 81,* 332–336.

Hume, A. L., Cant, B. R., Shaw, N. A., & Cowan, J. C. (1982). Central somatosensory conduction time from 10 to 79 years. *Electroencephalography and Clinical Neurophysiology, 54,* 49–54.

Inoue, K., Hashimoto, I., & Nakamura, S. (2001). High-frequency oscillations in human posterior tibial somatosensory evoked potentials are enhanced in patients with Parkinson's disease and multiple system atrophy. *Neuroscience Letters, 297,* 89–92.

Jones, E. G. (1975). Varieties and distribution of non-pyramidal cells in the somatic sensory cortex of the squirrel monkey. *Journal of Comparative Neurology, 160,* 205–268.

Jones, E. G. (1993). GABAergic neurons and their role in cortical plasticity in primates. *Cerebral Cortex, 3,* 361–372.

Jones, M. S., MacDonald, K. D., Choi, B., Dudek, F. E., & Barth, D. S. (2000). Intracellular correlates of fast (>200 Hz) electrical oscillations in rat somatosensory cortex. *Journal of Neurophysiology, 84,* 1505–1518.

Jones, S. J., & Power, C. N. (1984). Scalp topography of human somatosensory evoked potentials: The effect of interfering tactile stimulation applied to the hand. *Electroencephalography and Clinical Neurophysiology, 58,* 25–36.

Kaas, J. H., & Pons, T. P. (1988). The somatosensory system in primates. In D. H. Steklis & J. Erwin (Eds.), *Comparitive Primate Biology (Neurosciences, 4,* pp. 421–468). New York. Alan R. Liss.

Kakigi, R., Koyama, S., Hoshiyama, M., Kitamura, Y., Shimojo, M., Watanabe, S., & Nakamura, A. (1996). Effects of tactile interference stimulation on somatosensory evoked magnetic fields. *NeuroReport, 7,* 405–408.

Kakigi, R., Koyama, S., Hoshiyama, M., Watanabe, S., Shimojo, M., & Kitamura, Y. (1995). Gating of somatosensory evoked responses during active finger movements: Magnetoencephalographic studies. *Journal of Neural Science, 128,* 195–204.

Katayama, Y., & Tsubokawa, T. (1987). Somatosensory evoked potentials from the thalamic sensory relay nucleus (VPL) in humans: Correlations with short latency somatosensory evoked potentials recorded at the scalp. *Electroencephalography and Clinical Neurophysiology, 68,* 187–201.

Kawaguchi, Y., & Kubota, Y. (1997). GABAergic cell subtypes and their synaptic connections in rat frontal cortex. *Cerebral Cortex, 7,* 476–486.

Kazis, A., Vlaikidis, N., Pappa, P., Papanastasiou, J., Vlahveis, G., & Routsonis, K. (1983). Somatosensory and visual evoked potentials in human aging. *Electroencephalography and Clinical Neurophysiology, 23,* 49–59.

Kimura, T., & Hashimoto, I. (2001). Source of somatosensory primary cortical evoked magnetic fields (N20m) elicited by index finger stimulation moves toward mediolateral direction in area 3b in man. *Neuroscience Letters, 299,* 61–64.

Kojima ,Y., Uozumi, T., Akamatsu, N., Matsunaga, K., Urasaki, E., & Tsuji, S. (2001). Somatosensory evoked high frequency oscillations recorded from subdural electrodes. *Clinical Neurophysiology, 112,* 2261–2264.

Krubitzer, L. A., & Kaas, J. H. (1990). The organization and connections of somatosensory cortex in marmosets. *Journal of Neuroscience, 10,* 952–974.

Langdon, R. B., & Sur, M. (1990). Components of field potentials evoked by white matter stimulation in isolated slices of primary visual cortex: Spatial distribution and synaptic order. *Journal of Neurophysiology, 64,* 1484–1501.

Livingstone, M. S., & Hubel, D. H. (1981). Effects of sleep and arousal on the processing of visual information in the cat. *Nature, 291,* 554–561.

Luders, H. (1970). The effects of aging on the wave form of the somatosensory cortical evoked potential. *Electroencephalography and Clinical Neurophysiology, 29,* 450–460.

Maccabee, R J., Pinkhasow, E. I., & Cracco, R. J. (1983). Short-latency somatosensory evoked potentials to median nerve stimulation: Effect of low-frequency filter. *Electroencephalography and Clinical Neurophysiology, 55,* 34–44.

Maegaki, Y., Najm, I., Terada, K., Morris, H. H., Bingaman, W. E., Kohaya, N., Takenobu, A., Kadonaga, Y., & Luders, H. O. (2000). Somatosensory evoked high-frequency oscillations recorded directly from the human cerebral cortex. *Clinical Neurophysiology, 111,* 1916–1926.

Manger, P. R., Woods, T. M., Munoz, A., & Jones, E. G. (1997). Hand/face border as a limiting boundary in the body representation in monkey somatosensory cortex. *Journal of Neuroscience, 17,* 6338–6351.

McCormick, D. A. (1989). GABA as an inhibitory neurotransmitter in human cerebral cortex. *Journal of Neurophysiology, 62,* 1018–1027.

McGuire, B. A., Gilbert, C. D., Rivlin, P. K., & Wiesel, T. N. (1991). Targets of horizontal connections in macaque primary visual cortex. *Journal of Comparative Neurology, 305,* 370–392.

McLaughlin, D. F., & Kelly, E. F. (1993). Evoked potentials as indices of adaptation in the somatosensory system in humans: A review and prospectus. *Brain Research Reviews, 18,* 151–206.

Melchitzky, D. S., Sesack, S. R., Pucak, M. L., & Lewis, D. A. (1998). Synaptic targets of pyramidal neurons providing intrinsic horizontal connections in monkey prefrontal cortex. *Journal of Comparative Neurology, 390,* 211–224.

Mochizuki, H., Ugawa, Y., Machii, K., Terao, Y., Hanajima, R., Furubayashi, T., Uesugi, H., & Kanazawa, I. (1999). Somatosensory evoked high-frequency oscillation in Parkinson's disease and myoclonus epilepsy. *Clinical Neurophysiology, 110,* 185–191.

Moruzzi, G. (1966). The functional significance of sleep with particular regard to the brain mechanisms underlying consciousness. In J. C. Eccles (Ed.), *Brain and conscious experience* (pp. 345–379). New York: Springer-Verlag.

Nakano, S., & Hashimoto, I. (1999a). Comparison of somatosensory evoked high-frequency oscillations after posterior tibial and median nerve stimulation. *Clinical Neurophysiology, 110,* 1948–1952.

Nakano, S., & Hashimoto, I.(1999b). The later part of human somatic evoked high-frequency oscillations is enhanced in aged subjects. *Neuroscience Letters, 276,* 83–86.

Nakano, S., & Hashimoto, I. (1999)c. Somatosensory evoked high-frequency oscillations after posterior tibial nerve stimulation. In I. Hashimoto & R. Kakigi (Eds.), *Recent advances in human neurophysiology* (pp. 27–31). Amsterdam: Elsevier.

Nakano, S., & Hashimoto, I. (2000). Somatosensory evoked high-frequency oscillations are enhanced in school children. *Neuroscience Letters, 291,* 113–116.

Nelson, R. J., Sur, M., Felleman, D. J., & Kaas, J. H. (1980). Representations of the body surface in postcentral parietal cortex of *Macaca fascicularis. Journal of Comparative Neurology, 192,* 611–643.

Ojima, H., Honda, C. N., & Jones, E. G. (1991). Patterns of axon collateralization of identified supragranular pyramidal neurons in the cat auditory cortex. *Cerebral Cortex, 1,* 80–91.

Okada, Y. C., Tanenbaum, R., Williamson, S. J., & Kaufman, L. (1984). Somatotopic organization of the human somatosensory cortex revealed by neuromagnetic measurements. *Experimental Brain Research, 56,* 197–205.

Ozaki, I., & Hashimoto, I. (2001). High-frequency oscillations in primary somatosensory cortex (2). *Clinical Electroencephalography, 43,* 669–678.

Ozaki, I., Suzuki, C., Yaegashi, Y., Baba, M., Matsunaga, M., & Hashimoto, I. (1998). High-frequency oscillations in early cortical somatosensory evoked potentials. *Electroencephalography and Clinical Neurophysiology, 108,* 536–542.

Ozaki, I., Suzuki, C., Yaegashi, Y., Baba, M., Matsunaga, M., & Hashimoto, I. (1999). High-frequency oscillations in early cortical somatosensory EPs. In C. Barber, G. Celesia, I. Hashimoto, & R. Kakigi (Eds.), *Functional neuroscience: Evoked potentials and magnetic fields* (EEG Suppl., 49, pp. 52–55). Amsterdam: Elsevier Science.

Ozaki, I., Yaegashi, Y., Kimura, T., Baba, M., Matsunaga, M., & Hashimoto, I. (2001). Dipole orientation differs between high frequency oscillations and N20m current sources in human somatosensory evoked magnetic fields to median nerve stimulation. *Neuroscience Letters, 310,* 41–44.

Pekkonen, E., Huotilainen, M., Virtanen, J., Sinkkonen, J., Rinne, T., Ilmoniemi, R. J., & Naatanen, R. (1995). Age-related functional differences between auditory cortices: A whole-head MEG study. *NeuroReport, 6,* 1803–1806.

Penfield, W., & Boldrey, E. (1937). Somatic motor and sensory representation in the cerebral cortex of man as studied by electrical stimulation. *Brain, 60,* 387–443.

Peterson, N. N., Schroeder, D. E., & Arezzo, J. C. (1995). Neural generators of early cortical somatosensory evoked potentials in the awake monkey. *Electroencephalography and Clinical Neurophysiology, 96,* 248–260.

Rasmusson, D. D. (1996). Changes in the response properties of neurons in the ventroposterior lateral thalamic nucleus of the raccoon after peripheral deafferentation. *Journal of Neurophysiology, 75,* 2441–2450.

Rossini, P. M., Babiloni, C., Babiloni, F., Ambrosini, A., Onorati, P., Carducci, F., & Urbano, A. (1999). "Gating" of human short-latency somatosensory evoked cortical responses during execution of movement: A high resolution electroencephalographic study. *Brain Research, 843,* 161–170.

Sakuma, K., & Hashimoto, I. (1999). High-frequency magnetic oscillations evoked by posterior tibial nerve stimulation. *NeuroReport, 10,* 227–230.

Sakuma, K., Sekihara, K., & Hashimoto, I. (1999). Neural source estimation from a time–frequency component of somatic evoked high-frequency magnetic oscillations to posterior tibial nerve stimulation. *Clinical Neurophysiology, 110,* 1585–1588.

Scheibel, M. E., Lindsay, R. D., Tomiyasu, U., & Scheibel, A. B. (1975). Progressive dendritic changes in aging human cortex. *Experimental Neurology, 47,* 392–403.

Schnitzler, A., Witte, O. W., Cheyne, D., Haid, G., Vrba, J., & Freund, H. J. (1975). Modulation of somatosensory evoked magnetic fields by sensory and motor interferences. *NeuroReport, 6,* 1653–1658.

Shagass, C., & Schwartz, M. (1965, June). Age, personality and somatosensory cerebral evoked responses. *Science, 148,* 1359–1361.

Shimazu, H., Kaji, R., Tsujimoto, T., Ikeda, A., Kimura, J., & Shibasaki, H. (2000). High-frequency SEP components generated in the somatosensory cortex of the monkey. *NeuroReport, 11,* 2821–2826.

Steriade, M. (1978). Cortical long-axoned cells and putative interneurons during the sleep–waking cycle. *Behavioral and Brain Sciences, 3,* 465–514.

Steriade, M., Jones, E. G., & Llinás, R. (1990). *Thalamic oscillations and signaling.* New York: Wiley.

Suk, J., Ribary, U., Cappell, J., Yamamoto, T., & Llinas, R. (1991). Anatomical localization revealed by MEG recordings of the human somatosensory system. *Electroencephalography and Clinical Neurophysiology, 78,* 186–196.

Susman, R. L. (1994, September). Fossil evidence for early hominid tool use. *Science, 265,* 1570–1573.

Sutherling, W. W., Levesque, M. F., & Baumgartner, C. (1992). Cortical sensory representation of the human hand: Size of finger regions and nonoverlapping digit somatotopy. *Neurology, 42,* 1020–1028.

Swadlow, H. A. (1989). Efferent neurons and suspected interneurons in S-1 vibrissa cortex of awake rabbit: Receptive fields and axonal properties. *Journal of Neurophysiology, 62,* 288–308.

Swadlow, H. A. (1995). Influence of VPM afferents on putative inhibitory interneurons in SI of the awake rabbit: Evidence from cross-correlation, microstimulation, and latencies to peripheral sensory stimulation. *Journal of Neurophysiology, 73,* 1584–1599.

Swadlow, H. A., Beloozerova, I. N., & Sirota, M. G. (1998). Sharp, local synchrony among putative feed-forward inhibitory interneurons of rabbit somatosensory cortex. *Journal of Neurophysiology, 79,* 567–582.

Synek, V. M. (1986). Somatosensory evoked potentials after stimulation of digital nerves in upper limbs: Normative data. *Electroencephalography and Clinical Neurophysiology, 65,* 460–463.

Tanosaki, M., Hashimoto, I., Iguchi, Y., Kimura, T., Takino, R., Kurobe, Y., Haruta, Y., & Hoshi, Y. (2001). Specific somatosensory processing in somatosensory area 3b for human thumb: A neuromagnetic study. *Clinical Neurophysiology, 112,* 1516–1522.

Tanosaki, M., Kimura, T., Takino, R., Iguchi, Y., Suzuki, A., Kurobe, Y., Haruta, Y., Hoshi, Y., & Hashimoto, I. (2002a). Movement interference attenuates somatosensory high-frequency oscillations: Contribution of local axon collaterals of 3b pyramidal neurons. *Clinical Neurophysiology, 113,* 993–1000.

Tanosaki, M., Suzuki, A., Takino, R., Kimura, T., Iguchi, Y., Kurobe, Y., Haruta, Y., Hoshi, Y., & Hashimoto, I. (2002b). Neural mechanisms for generation of tactile interference effects on somatosensory evoked magnetic fields in humans. *Clinical Neurophysiology, 113,* 672–680.

Tanosaki, M., Suzuki, A., Kimura, T., Takino, R., Haruta, Y., Hoshi, Y., & Hashimoto, I. (2002c). Contribution of primary somatosensory area 3b to somatic cognition: A neuromagnetic study. *NeuroReport, 13,* 1519–1522.

Taylor, M. J., & Fagan, E. R. (1983). SEPs to median nerve stimulation: Normative data for paediatrics. *Electroencephalography and Clinical Neurophysiology, 71,* 323–330.

Tremere, L., Hicks, T. P., & Rasmusson, D. D. (2001). Expansion of receptive fields in raccoon somatosensory cortex *in vivo* by GABA$_A$ receptor antagonism: Implications for cortical reorganization. *Experimental Brain Research, 136,* 447–455.

White, E. L. (1986). Termination of thalamic afferents in the cerebral cortex. In E. G. Jones, & A. Peters (Eds.), *Cerebral cortex: Vol 5. Sensory–motor areas and aspects of cortical connectivity* (pp. 271–290). New York: Plenum .

White, E. L., & Keller, A. (1987). Intrinsic circuitry involving the local axon collaterals of corticothalamic projection cells in mouse SmI cortex. *Journal of Comparative Neurology, 262,* 13–26.

Yamada, T., Kameyama, S., Fuchigami, Y., Nakazumi, Y., Dickins, Q. S., & Kimura, J. (1988). Changes of short latency somatosensory evoked potential in sleep. *Electroencephalography and Clinical Neurophysiology, 70,* 126–136.

# 13

## Measuring Sensory Memory: Magnetoencephalography Habituation and Psychophysics

Zhong-Lin Lu
*University of Southern California*

George Sperling
*University of California, Irvine*

Vision and audition each have several levels of sensory memory, and constructing experiments to selectively measure one or another of these memories has been an elusive goal. In this chapter we consider one apparently successful example: Z.-L. Lu, S. J. Williamson, and L. Kaufman (1992b), who measured the retention of the precise loudness of a tone in a very short term auditory memory. The psychophysically measured immediate memory for tonal loudness decayed in a period of a few seconds (depending on the observer) to the average loudness of recently heard tones (which was maintained in a higher level short-term auditory sensory memory). A critical component of this experiment was the establishment of a well-defined higher level sensory-memory representation so that the decay of the very short term memory trace could be observed without contamination. In their habituation paradigm, the same tonal stimulus was repeatedly presented with a fixed interval between presentations, and the magnetoencephalography (MEG) response was recorded. The longer the interval between successive presentations, the greater the response. The recovery of response amplitude from prior stimulation reflects continuing activation and therefore offers physiological access to memory duration. MEG recordings of habituation to the stimuli in the loudness experiments revealed two sites in temporal cortex: (a) a primary A1 site that reflects the tonal memory studied psychophysically and (b) another auditory memory site in the nearby auditory association cortex. By replicating the psychophysical conditions precisely in habituation, and by separating the two N1 MEG components, for each subject both the psychophysically measured memory for loudness and the memory inferred from habituation of A1 were found to decay with an identical time constant. Between subjects, the lifetime (time constant of the decay) of memory for loudness varied from 0.8 to 3 sec. In addition, an example of the decay of very short term visual memory (iconic memory) is given in which the psychophysically measured lifetime and the electroencephalographic (EEG) lifetime determined in a habituation experiment seem to agree quite closely. MEG is preferred to EEG because of its superior ability to isolate and localize sources, and MEG is preferred to functional magnetic resonance imaging (fMRI) because of its temporal resolution. MEG is an ideal tool for studying sensory memory.

## MEMORY REGISTERS

*Sensory memory* refers to the initial, modality-specific neural representation of sensory stimuli. Sensory memory is often contrasted with *short-term memory* and *working memory* (which are assumed to be less modality specific than sensory memory), and all of these are distinct from *long-term memory*. In functional terms, sensory memory is comparable to a register in a computer. In a human or a computer, if one wants to know what the last auditory input was, one examines the auditory sensory register. On the other hand, accessing the contents of long-term memory in a computer requires two registers: (a) a *memory access* register, for the memory address of the particular contents, and (b) a *memory contents* register for the contents themselves. In human long-term memory, the address of the contents (memory access) is computed from *retrieval cues*, which may be partial contents, context, or related items. The brain mechanism by which the contents become available and useful is not understood.

The prevailing view of short- and long-term memory systems is that there are one or more modality-specific sensory registers in each sensory modality, plus a register or registers for short-term and/or working memory, plus functionally distinct long-term memory systems (i.e., for episodic, semantic, procedural, and perhaps other forms of long-term memory).

## LEVELS OF MEMORY AND PROCESSING

The conceptualization of sensory memories as registers is almost certainly too simplistic. In biological sensory processing there is a considerable amount of memory—perhaps more aptly called *retention*—that is inherent in the processing itself, and this memory may differ for different stimuli at every stage of processing. For example, visual sensory memory exists in the receptors and bipolar cells of the retina as an afterimage. These cells do not constitute a register in the usual meaning of the word, but they can retain a representation of the input image long after it has been removed. The afterimage is a negative of the original stimulus that is perceived on subsequent stimulation. The original stimulus can itself persist in the retina as *persistence of sensation*.

An *afterimage* is sensory memory that is specific to the eye of stimulation. Stimulating the other eye may make it more difficult to extract the information, but it is relatively easy to demonstrate the eye specificity. A characteristic that has often been used to define visual sensory memory is that a subsequent stimulus overwrites the memory. To the extent that subsequent stimuli in the same eye are more effective at overwriting memory contents than stimuli in the other eye, the memory is maintained in neurons prior to binocular combination. In the literature there is a clear distinction between (retinal) afterimages and perhaps non-retinal retention mechanisms, which are eye specific, on the one hand, and visual sensory memory (Sperling, 1960; called *iconic memory* by Neisser, 1967), which is not eye specific, on the other hand.

*Repetition detection* (or simply *recognition memory*) is a paradigm that reveals memory that survives being overwritten. Repetition detection probes short-term visual or auditory memories that store successive events concurrently. The modality specificity of visual sensory memory can be demonstrated in a variety of psychophysical tasks, such as memory for successively presented nonverbalizable nonsense shapes. Beyond visual sensory (iconic) and visual short-term memory, deriving the taxonomy of visual memory systems has not been possible by means of psychophysical tasks. The taxonomy of auditory sensory memory systems is probably even more complicated than that of visual sensory memory systems, because auditory signals are subjected to much more complicated processing prior to reaching auditory temporal cortex area A1 than are visual signals before reaching occipital cortex area V1.

## HABITUATION

In trying to sort through the complexities of sensory memory systems, it would be ideal if there were a method whereby each sensory and short-term memory system could be identified by (a) its brain location, (b) the time constant for which it retains information, and (c) the format (or encoding) of the information it retains. This is where Sam Williamson had a great insight. Habituation is an extremely powerful tool that offers a means of quickly providing the first two components of a sensory memory (location and time constant) and perhaps the third (encoding) as well.

Magnetoencephalography (MEG) is an ideal method for studying habituation, because it permits better spatial localization than electroencephalography (EEG) and because response amplitude in MEG is more directly related to neural activity than in functional magnetic resonance imagery (fMRI). The principle is as follows (Fig. 13.1). Presenting a stimulus repeatedly causes the MEG response to the stimulus to weaken. Presenting it at a slower rate gives the response more time to recover than in rapid presentations. The reference point is a stimulus sequence presented with an extremely long interval between successive presentations (stimulus onset asynchrony) that permits full recovery of the MEG response. At some critical, faster presentation rate the MEG response is reduced to only $1 - (1/e) = 0.63$ of its response to an extremely slow stimulus. The time between successive stimuli at this rate defines the *time constant* of recovery. In fact, the situation may be slightly more complicated in that recovery may not begin immediately after termination of a stimulus; there may be a *refractory period* before recovery begins. In general, therefore, there are two parameters to describe the temporal properties of habituation: (a) time constant and (b) refractory period. It is remarkable that in the examples offered by Williamson and in the other instances described in this chapter the recovery from habituation is of a simple form, exponentially limited growth, so that these two parameters are sufficient to describe the temporal dynamics.

Using flickering checkerboard stimuli and MEG recording, Uusitalo, Williamson, and Seppä (1996) were able to detect 10 brain locations with different recovery time constants. Each one of these brain locations represents a process with an inherent retention time, a process that could become a component of the overall retention time observed in a psychophysical memory experiment.

The observed retention time and resistance to interference in a psychophysical experiment will depend on whether a stimulus is re-

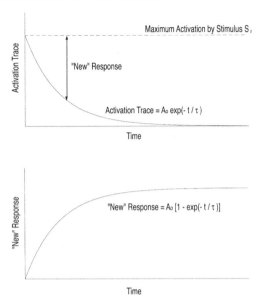

FIG. 13.1. The logic of the habituation paradigm: model relationship between activation trace and measured neuronal response from magnetoencephalography. When a stimulus $S_i$ is presented for the first time at time $t = 0$ it produces an activation trace, $A_o \exp(-t/\tau)$ for $t \geq 0$. When the stimulus is presented again after a time $t_1$, it again produces an internal activation of $A_o$. The new response $A_1$ observed externally is only the difference between the residual response $A_o\exp(-t/\tau)$ and $A_o$, that is, $A_1 = A_o (1- \exp(-t/\tau))[(-\exp((t-t_1)/\tau)], t \geq t_1$.

peated exactly or whether it is changed somewhat between "repetitions." Psychophysical tasks that use early sensory memories have shorter retention times than tasks in which more abstract comparisons suffice. So, a task that requires an observer to decide if two tones have exactly the same loudness will suffer when the interval between tones exceeds several seconds. A task that requires listeners to decide whether two tonal *sequences* (melodies) are identical can tolerate much longer delays between the two successive presentations, because it uses a higher level memory system. There are similar examples from visual tasks.

The corresponding habituation experiments seek to determine the relative effectiveness for habituation of an exact repetition compared with an altered repetition. We expect that habituation of higher brain centers that process visual stimuli would not be affected when successive stimuli alternate between a lowercase *a* and an uppercase *A* or when the spatial location of the letter *A* is jittered from presentation to presentation. Early brain processes would regard such semantically equivalent stimuli as being visually quite different and would adapt less in an alternating sequence than in a homogeneous sequence. Such alternating-feature sequences have been used in repetition-detection experiments to determine the level of processing of human visual repetition detection (e.g., Sperling, Wurst, & Lu, 1993). The possibility of using the same or very similar sequences to study habituation in MEG and in psychophysical performance in a detection or memory experiment offers an opportunity to correlate brain and behavior in the study of sensory processing and sensory memory.

As noted earlier, of all the paradigms used to study sensory memory, habituation paradigms are especially well adapted to MEG because of MEG's temporal resolution; the relatively direct relation of magnetic signal intensity to neural output; and because of the accuracy of brain localization relative to EEG. Another advantage of habituation paradigms is that there are psychophysical paradigms that can be related to habituation. Here we consider two instances in which habituation measured at brain locations was correlated with behavior to define the location and time constant of a sensory memory: (a) an auditory study to determine the brain location and time course of echoic memory for subtle differences in loudness and (b) a visual study of iconic memory (mostly under 1 sec) for arrays of sine-wave patches.

The auditory study of echoic memory is complete, and the main part has been published (Lu, Williamson, & Kaufman, 1992b); the visual study is still incomplete and unpublished (Yang, 1999). Although repetition detection in psychophysical visual studies and habituation in MEG might have been the ideal setting in which to correlate psychophysically derived sensory memory systems with sensory memory systems derived from MEG habituation, in fact one of the first successful correlations of a psychophysically determined sensory memory system with an MEG-determined system occurred in the auditory system.

## AUDITORY SENSORY MEMORY

### Very Short Term Memory for Tonal Loudness

Auditory sensory memory, also called *echoic memory* (Neisser, 1967), lasts about 2–5 sec (Glanzer & Cunitz, 1966; Treisman, 1964; Wickelgren, 1969) and is essential for integrating acoustic information presented sequentially over an appreciable period of time (Crowder, 1976). Prior to 1992, there was no physiological evidence regarding the locus of human auditory sensory memory, although psychophysical experiments

(Massaro, 1975) suggested a central rather than a peripheral site. Electrophysiological investigations (Weinberger, et al, 1990) of auditory memory functions in animals provide evidence that similar short-term memory functions are served by sensory areas of the cerebral cortex.

Lu, Williamson, and Kaufman (1992a, 1992b) exploited advantages of MEG to investigate retention of stimulus-related information within areas of the primary and association auditory cortices. They found that the lifetime of a cortical activation trace in the primary auditory cortex predicts the lifetime of behaviorally determined auditory sensory memory.

The lifetime of a cortical activation trace was obtained from measurements of the magnetic field pattern across the side of the head when the subject was presented with repeating tone stimuli. In responding to a tone, cortical areas set up activation patterns of synaptic activity that result in a weaker cortical response to a subsequent tone. In this way, sensory areas "remember" information just presented. When identical tones are presented at a fixed time interval, the response strengthens with longer intervals, in a way that permits a lifetime to be determined for the activation trace. The primary cortex has a relatively short lifetime—just a couple of seconds—but the activation trace in the association cortex persists for several seconds longer. Remarkably, by extrapolating back to an interstimulus interval of zero, it is possible to identify the time when the trace just begins to decay. For the association cortex it is the onset feature of the tone that counts. By contrast, for the primary cortex both the onset and the offset reset the trace. By extending such studies it should be possible to determine what aspects of sounds are preferentially processed by primary and association areas.

To establish psychological correlates of the lifetime of the activation traces in the auditory cortex, Lu et al. (1992b) set up a psychoacoustic experiment to study decay of loudness memory following the presentation of a pure sine wave tone. It is known from human behavioral studies carried out early in the twentieth century that a person's remembrance of the loudness of a tone decays exponentially with time to the mean loudness of recently heard tones; that is, a listener's memory of a particular tone is lost with time, and the listener is forced to rely on his or her memory of the mean loudness of all the tones recently heard (an effect known as the *central tendency;* Helson, 1964; Hollingworth, 1909, 1910; Ipsen, 1926; Lauenstein, 1933; Needham, 1935; Woodrow, 1933).

Lu et al. (1992b) showed that, for individual subjects, physiological lifetimes determined magnetically, and behavioral lifetimes determined from tone-matching studies, agree within an accuracy of better than 20%.

Memory lifetimes ranged from 0.8 to 3 sec for individuals who participated in this study. These results provide strong evidence that the primary auditory cortex serves auditory sensory memory, and the lifetime of that memory can be gauged by studies of neuronal activity in that area of the brain. We review this study later.

## Measuring Neural Activity in the Primary and Association Auditory Cortices

### *The N100 Component*

Technical advances in low-temperature physics have provided the essential instrumentation (MEG) for recording the magnetic field of the human brain. The N100 component, a major peak in the magnetic waveform of the evoked neuromagnetic response, normally occurs about 100 msec after the onset of a tone burst. Many aspects of the N100 component have been studied in both EEG and MEG over the past few decades. For example, from MEG research (Pantev et al., 1988) we know that neural sources of N100 in response to tone bursts of different frequencies lie in different locations within the primary auditory cortex (the so-called *tonotopic map*).

### *Separating Primary and Association Cortex Contributions to N100.* Before 1992, it had been speculated that activities from several brain regions contributed to the auditory N100, although there was no definitive evidence. Lu et al. (1992a) postulated that contributions to the N100 from other brain regions were obscured because the usual rates of tone burst presentation (about 1 per second) in previous studies were too fast to permit recovery of slower brain regions. Using a 6.0-sec interstimulus interval (ISI), they discovered a magnetic field pattern near the scalp (Fig. 13.2B) that is significantly different from the pattern using fast (ISI = 1.2 sec) presentation rates (Fig. 13.2A). Although it is possible to account for the observed field pattern at short ISIs with one neural source (in the primary auditory cortex), the field pattern at long ISIs indicates an additional neural source in association auditory cortex (see Fig. 13.3). These data showed that in addition to the neural contribution from the primary auditory cortex a neural source from auditory association cortex also contributed to the N100.

To distinguish the two sources that contribute to the early MEG response to a tonal burst, Lu et al. (1992a) designated the contribution from

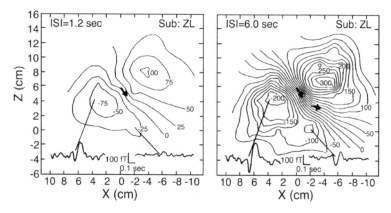

FIG. 13.2. Isofield contours for subject ZL characterizing the measured field pattern over the left hemisphere 100 msec following the onset of a tone burst stimulus. Arrows denote the direction of current dipole sources that account for each pattern, with their bases placed at the dipole's surface location. In the right panels, the upper arrow is the N100m source and the lower arrow is the L100m source. Insets illustrate response waveforms obtained at the indicated positions. Both waveforms also exhibit a 200-msec component. ISI = interstimulus interval. Reprinted from *Brain Research, 527,* Z.-L. Lu, S. J. Williamson, & L. Kaufman, Human auditory primary and association cortex having differing lifetimes for activation traces, pp. 236–241. Copyright © 1992, with permission from Elsevier Science.

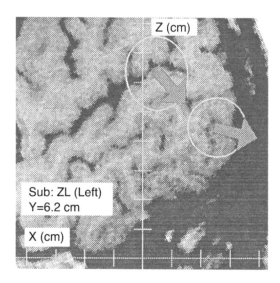

FIG. 13.3. Deduced locations for neuronal sources that are responsible for N100m (upper arrow) and L100m (second N100 source, lower arrow) on sagittal magnetic resonance images of the left hemispheres of 1 subject. Coordinates are expressed in the PPN system, with a distance of 1 cm between adjacent tics on the axes. The base of each arrow indicates the respective positions, with the ellipse indicating the estimated range of uncertainty (95% confidence level), and the direction of each arrow specifies the flow of intracellular current. The N100m source lies within the lateral sulcus, and the L100m source lies within 1 cm of the superior temporal sulcus. Reprinted from *Brain Research, 527,* Z.-L. Lu, S. J. Williamson, & L. Kaufman, Human auditory primary and association cortex having differing lifetimes for activation traces, pp. 236–241. Copyright © 1992, with permission from Elsevier Science.

327

the primary auditory cortex N100, and the contribution from the association auditory cortex L100.

### *Peripheral Refractory Effects Versus Central Habituation.*
It is also well known that the N100 component exhibits a *rate effect:* It is exceptionally sensitive to the rate at which the stimuli are repeated. Amplitudes diminish if stimuli are presented sufficiently soon after an identical preceding one (Celesia, 1976; Hari, Kaila, Katila, Tuomisto, & Varpula, 1982; Naatanen & Picton, 1987). However, it was not clear whether the rate effect arose from peripheral sense organs or from higher cortical regions.

Electrophysiological studies of the auditory system in cats conducted by Wickelgren (1968) and Weinberger et al. (1990) led to four criteria according to which a rate effect could be classified as a central process (habituation): (a) diminished response strength for shorter ISIs (see Fig. 13.4); (b) spontaneous recovery of full response strength after stimuli are withheld for a sufficiently long time (see Fig. 13.5); (c) enhanced response to a different stimulus (probe) which replaces the standard stimulus, thereby ensuring that the weak responses were not due to a state change (e.g., drowsiness; see Fig. 13.6); and (d) enhanced response to a standard stimulus if preceded by a deviant stimulus (dishabituation; see Fig. 13.7). Lu (1992) ob-

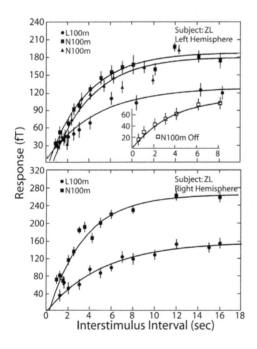

FIG. 13.4. Response amplitudes versus interstimulus interval over the left and right hemispheres for subject ZL, for tones of 0.5 sec (N100m: squares; L100m: circles), 1.2 sec (N100m: triangles), and 2 sec (N100m: inverted triangles) duration. Insets illustrate the dependence for the N100m offset response for tones of different duration indicated by the horizontal axis. Reprinted from *Brain Research, 527,* Z.-L. Lu, S. J. Williamson, & L. Kaufman, Human auditory primary and association cortex having differing lifetimes for activation traces, pp. 236–241. Copyright © 1992, with permission from Elsevier Science.

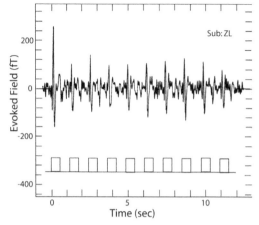

FIG. 13.5.   Average evoked magnetic field to trains of tones of the same frequency and intensity. One stimuli train is shown under the waveform. Sub = Subject.

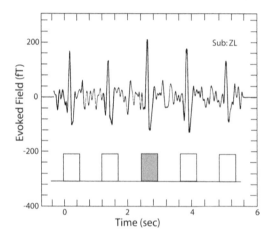

FIG. 13.6.   Recording of the probe response. The shadowed block represents the probe stimulus; the other four blocks denote the standard stimuli. Sub = Subject.

tained the first evidence that the N100 and L100 rate effects satisfy all the criteria from habituation and thereby reflect cortical processes.

## Modeling Neural Activity With Exponential Decay Functions

As noted earlier, one can separately measure magnetic fields arising from the primary and association auditory cortical areas. Figure 13.4 shows that response strengths increase systematically with increasing ISI for both cortical areas. Maximum responses are not attained until ISIs ex-

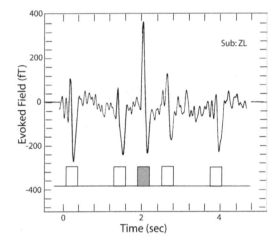

FIG. 13.7.   Recording of dishabituation. The shadowed block represents the probe stimulus (which is of a different temporal frequency); the other blocks denote standard stimuli. Sub = Subject.

ceed a few seconds, with the primary cortex approaching its asymptote sooner than the association cortex. Because of the similarity in the ISI trends, each set of data was fit with an exponential function. The solid curves in Fig. 13.4 are obtained with the function $A\,(1 - e^{-(t-t_0)/\tau})$, whose parameters are determined by a least-squares fit to the data. All the data are well fit by this expression ($\tau = 3.5$ sec for N100 and 5.1 sec for L100).

The following assumptions define a model of neural activation. (a) It is generally accepted that a stimulus produces a neural activation trace that decays after the stimulus is withdrawn (Fig. 13.1). We further propose (b) that neural activation decays exponentially and (c) that a subsequent identical stimulus resets the trace to its full strength. Thus, the observed response strength indicates how much the trace has decayed since the preceding stimulus. The assumptions provide a method for quantifying the strength of the neural activation trace in terms of the peak magnetic field strength that is observed from the responding populations of cortical neurons.

Within the framework of the preceding model (see Fig. 13.1), three parameters need to be estimated for empirical fits to data: $A, t_0, \tau$. The parameter $A$ determines the maximum response strength, $t_0$ denotes the time when the activation trace begins to decay, and $\tau$ specifies the lifetime of the decay. Lu et al. (1992a) found that $t_0$ for the primary auditory cortex is very close to the offset of the previous tone, indicating that the activation trace reflects the offset response to that tone. Indeed, it is well known that the offset of a tone evokes a response in the primary auditory cortex. It appears that the activation traces established by the onset and by the offset of a tone burst are very similar. In support of this notion, Lu et al. (1992a) showed that the offset response of a tone is habituated by the onset response to the same tone. A graph identical to those illustrated in Fig. 13.4 is obtained if the horizontal axis represents tone duration instead of ISI.

However, the situation is different in the association cortex: The value of $t_0$ matches the onset of the previous tone, not its offset. The response of association cortex consequently distinguishes between onset and offset in the sense that the offset of a tone does not establish a new activation trace or enhance the activation trace left by the onset. It may well be that the primary auditory cortex cannot "tell" the difference between the onset and offset of a tone, because the activation traces are so similar. However, both onset and offset are clearly distinguished from each other when one takes into account the additional information provided by association cortex. Because neuronal activity is nearly simultaneous in the two cortical areas, the need for higher centers in the brain to rely on the output of the two areas in such a way would seem to impose no temporal disadvantage.

## Lifetime of Neural Activation Predicts Duration of Echoic Memory

It is quite remarkable that the lifetimes obtained by fitting the exponential function to the MEG ISI data for the N100 component vary considerably across the 4 subjects who were studied in detail. The values are: $\tau = 0.8, 1.4, 1.6,$ and $3.4$ sec, a range that spans a factor of 4. Approximately the same lifetimes were found for habituation of another component, with 180-msec latency, suggesting that the lifetime is characteristic of the specific cortical area. It is also noteworthy that the lifetime best accounting for the ISI data for the magnetic field arising from the association cortex is longer by about 2 sec for each subject. These ranges of values suggest that the activation trace in the primary auditory cortex may well be associated with very short term echoic memory. Lu et al. (1992b) carried out behavioral studies on the same subjects to determine whether a correlation could be found for individual subjects between their MEG habituation time constants and the behaviorally measured duration of their echoic memories.

## Measuring Duration of Echoic Memory

Early in this century, Hollingworth (1910) discovered the central tendency: A few seconds after experiencing a stimulus, the judged magnitude of the stimulus approaches the mean magnitude of all the stimuli used in the experiment. Lu et al. (1992b) were able to exploit this tendency to measure the decay of very short term echoic memory. They used a two-alternative forced-choice paradigm for the same subjects who had been studied using MEG. A test tone was provided to one ear, and after a delay a probe tone was provided to the other ear (see Fig. 13.8). The subject responded by indicating whether the probe tone was louder or softer than the test tone.

The frequency of the probe was always the same as the test tone, but its intensity was randomly chosen with equal probabilities from one of two lists. One list had a mean loudness that, together with the test tone, is 2.9 dB lower than the loudness of the test tone, and the other list had a mean loudness that is 2.5 dB greater (see Fig. 13.9). Subjects were unable to determine which list was presented in a given session. The hypothesis was that, for short delays, the subject would judge the loudness of the probe tone relative to the test tone. However, for long delays the subject would have lost the very short term echoic memory of the test tone and make judgments based on a "longer term" memory representing the long-term mean loudness of all tones. A total of 6,000 trials were col-

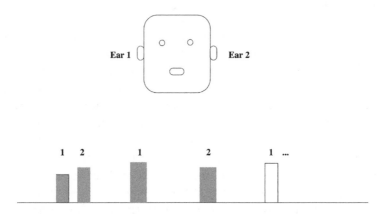

FIG. 13.8.    Loudness match paradigm. The loudness of test tone and the time between each pair of stimuli is fixed. Test and probe tones are of the same frequency and duration. For each pair of stimuli, the frequency is randomly chosen from 800, 900, and 1100 Hz with equal probability. The time delay between test and probe tones is randomly chosen from 0.5, 2.3, 4.3, 6.3, and 11.8 sec with equal probability.

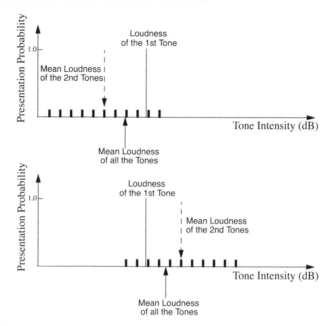

FIG. 13.9. Two histograms of probe tone loudness distributions. One list had a mean loudness that together with the test tone is 2.9 dB lower than the loudness of the test tone, and the other list has a mean loudness that is 2.5 dB greater. Only one list was used in a given experimental session.

lected for each subject. One of the challenges in carrying out studies of this kind is to determine how long it takes at the beginning of a session for the subject to acquire accurate judgment of the average loudness. In practice, several hundred of the initial trials were discarded without the subject's knowledge, so that stable results could be obtained.

Representative results for the decay of echoic memory are illustrated in Fig. 13.10. When the mean loudness of the probe tones is biased higher than that of the test, the subject's loudness judgments shift toward greater loudness as the delay between presentation of the test and probe increases. When the mean loudness of probe tones is lower than the test, the opposite trend is observed.

In MEG studies characterizing the dependence of N100 amplitude on ISI, an exponential function was used to achieve the data fit shown in Fig. 13.11. The behavioral measurements for the temporal dependence of remembered loudness are also well described by an exponential decay. A causal relation between the two phenomena would be suggested if the lifetimes of the two, behavioral and brain, were the same for each subject

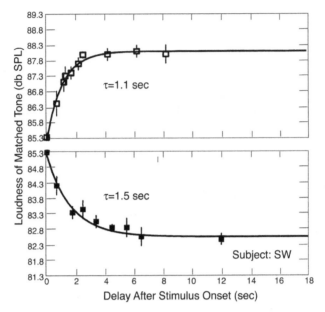

FIG. 13.10.   Remembered loudness of a tone as determined by a forced-choice match with a probe tone presented at various delays after the test tone. Data represented by the open symbols were obtained when the mean loudness of the test and probe tones was 2.5 dB greater than that of the test tone. Data represented by closed symbols were obtained with the mean loudness 2.9 dB lower. Error bars denote the standard deviation for each delay. Reprinted with permission from Lu, Z.-L., Williamson, S. J., & Kaufman, L. (1992). Physiological measurements predict the lifetime for human auditory memory of a tone. *Science, 258,* 1668–1670. Copyright © 1992 American Association for the Advancement of Science.

but differed between subjects. Figure 13.12, based on the data of 4 subjects, shows a correlation of .97 between the brain and behavioral echoic-memory lifetimes. The high correlation suggests that noninvasive measurements of the lifetime for cortical activation traces may provide an objective and meaningful characterization of sensory memory lifetime for individual subjects. This interpretation of the activation trace also provides a possible neural mechanism for very short term echoic memory.

## Other Auditory Sensory Memories

Cowan's (1995) review concluded that there are at least two forms of auditory sensory memory: (a) a very short-lived memory, such as the memory for tonal loudness just described, and (b) a second auditory sensory memory with a duration on the order of seconds.

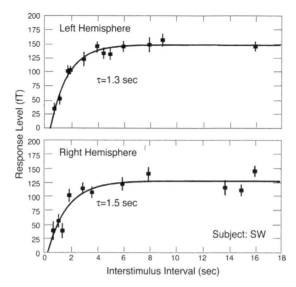

FIG. 13.11. Peak magnetic field strength near the scalp approximately 100 msec after the onset of a tone burst stimulus (the magnetic counterpart to the N100 component in the event-related potential) increases with interstimulus interval, as shown, in both hemispheres of Subject SW. The field sensor was placed over each hemisphere at a location where it monitors activity in the primary auditory cortex. Reprinted with permission from Lu, Z.-L., Williamson, S. J., & Kaufman, L. (1992). Physiological measurements predict the lifetime for human auditory memory of a tone. *Science, 258,* 1668–1670. Copyright © 1992 American Association for the Advancement of Science.

Indeed, it is not obvious that the next-higher auditory memory can be characterized by a time constant in seconds. It might be a limited-capacity memory based on retroactive interference in which new inputs push older material out of memory. In the absence of new auditory input (i.e., silence), periods of silence might themselves be recoded as memory events. This is a much more complex process than simple, exponential passive decay with time, although it may be difficult to distinguish from passive decay when new stimuli arrive at a constant rate. We consider here two instances of higher level auditory memory: one related to the loudness experiment and another that illustrates exponential decay based on retroactive interference and the kinds of significant complications that arise.

### Memory for the Mean Loudness of a Tonal Sequence

In the loudness experiment described earlier, the very short term auditory sensory memory decayed in a second or two to the average loudness

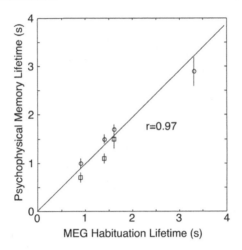

FIG. 13.12.   Agreement across 4 subjects between behavioral lifetimes for the decay of the loudness of a tone following its presentation and physiological lifetimes for the decay of the neuronal activation trace in the primary auditory cortex. Squares denote behavioral lifetimes measured in blocks when the mean loudness of the probe tones was higher that of the test tones, and circles denote the results when the mean loudness was lower. MEG = magnetoencephalography. Reprinted with permission from Lu, Z.-L., Williamson, S. J., & Kaufman, L. (1992). Physiological measurements predict the lifetime for human auditory memory of a tone. *Science, 258,* 1668–1670. Copyright © 1992 American Association for the Advancement of Science.

of the previous tonal sequence. Thus, the very same tone, after a 2- or 3-sec interval during which the very short term auditory memory trace decayed to insignificance, would be judged as louder following a sequence of loud tones and softer following a sequence of less intense tones. Obviously, the memory for the loudness of the previously heard tones in a test block is an auditory memory. In the context of tonal sequences, it has a time constant of many seconds. Using the memory for tonal sequence to establish the baseline to which the probe tones decayed was one of the critical design elements that made the measurement of very short term auditory memory decay so successful.

### Short-Term Phonemic Memory

**Exponentially Defined Capacity Limit.**   We describe here a simple model of an auditory memory (Sperling, 1968) that can be reasonably approximated as a memory for phonemes, and we indicate how it might be studied using MEG. This memory model explains the effect of acoustic similarity in short-term memory experiments (Conrad, 1963; Sperling

& Speelman, 1970): why sequences of similar-sounding letters (such as B, C, D, E, G, P, T, V, and Z) are remembered much less well than sequences of different sounding letters (such as A, B, F, O, Q, R, and Y).

The phonemic short-term memory model is illustrated in Fig. 13.13. Items enter memory and are stored in sequence. A spoken letter sequence "X, Y, Z" would enter memory as six phones: $1 = e$, $2 = ks$, $3 = w$, $4 = ii$, $5 = z$, $6 = ee$. Let $i$ be the index number of a phoneme, counting backward in time from the last phoneme heard. The probability of recalling the $i$th most recent phoneme is proportional to $e^{-i/\alpha}$, where $\alpha$ is the memory capacity (in phonemes). The brief silence that separates spoken letters is assumed to be stored without requiring additional space and without loss. A model with discrete, indexed phonemes is appropriate for an experimental procedure in which letters are distinct utterances (as opposed to continuous speech). The probability of correctly recalling a letter depends on which of its constituent phonemes are retrieved. If all constituent phones are retrieved, the letter is recalled correctly. If they are not, an informed guess is made on the basis of the phoneme (if any) that was retrieved. In a stimulus constructed

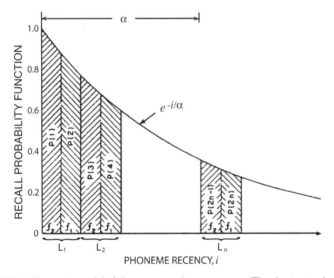

FIG. 13.13. Phonemic model of short-term auditory memory. The abscissa is phonemic recency; the most recent phoneme is numbered 1. The ordinate is the memory strength function; the area under the function describes the phoneme's strength in memory. As a simplification, recall probability (of a phoneme) is taken to be directly proportional to its memory strength. From "Phonemic model of short-term auditory memory," by G. Sperling, 1968, *Proceedings of the 76th Annual Convention of the American Psychological Association, 3*, p. 63. Copyright © 1968 by American Psychological Association.

out of an ideal acoustically unconfusable alphabet, retrieval of just one of a letter's two phonemes suffices for recall of that letter. In an acoustically confusable stimulus (B, T, V, P, Z, T) the phoneme *ee* is useless but nevertheless occupies space in memory. The initial consonant must be retrieved to recall the letter.

The simple phonemic model gives a good account of the acoustic-similarity phenomenon and of the relative difficulty of lists composed of different alphabets. It works especially well when the capacity of memory is tested by *partial reports* in which the listener reports only a subset of characters that is requested by a randomly selected poststimulus cue. The phonemic capacity of this short-term auditory sensory memory is relatively independent of presentation rate in the range of 1 to 4 items per second. This indicates that memory capacity is described in terms of number of phonemes rather than in units of time.

***Complications.***   When listeners have to make whole reports of the entire presented list, matters get more complicated because of subvocal rehearsal and because of *destructive readout*—a long response interferes more with the items still in memory than does a brief response. Matters get still more complicated when comparing memory for pseudodigits with real digits. Pseudodigits are carefully constructed nonsense syllables than have phonemic properties identical to real digits but are unfamiliar. Memory for pseudodigits is worse than memory for real digits. This indicates that a simple phonemic model of auditory short-term memory cannot give a full account of human performance, because familiarity, a much higher level process than echoic memory, plays a significant role.

The advantage of a reasonably good quantitative description of an auditory short-term memory is that it lends itself to MEG analysis by means of habituation paradigms. In this case, one would be presenting not repetitions of the same tone but repetitions of the same or similar phonemic sequences. If one could localize the phonemic memory illustrated in Fig. 13.13, would that memory use the same mechanisms as the memory for the mean loudness of the tonal sequences used to discover very short term auditory sensory memory? Indeed, to what extent does short-term memory for melodic sequences or for noise bursts share resources with short-term memory for phonemic sequences? These are precisely the sorts of questions that are extremely difficult to answer by means of psychophysics alone and that would benefit from collateral MEG brain-imaging data.

## VISUAL SENSORY MEMORY

### Visual Iconic Memory

Although this chapter deals primarily with auditory memory, it is useful to compare auditory with visual sensory memory. An unpublished experiment carried out by Sam Williamson's student Wei Yang (1999) is especially relevant. Yang measured the time course of the decay of visual very short term sensory memory (iconic memory) and compared it with the time course of recovery in a visual habituation procedure—a close parallel to Lu et al.'s (1992a) experiment, reviewed earlier.

### Stimuli and Results

Yang (1999) chose to measure iconic memory for a brief flash of 8 sine wave patches arrayed in an annular fashion around the fixation point (see Fig. 13.14). Each patch had one of four randomly chosen slants. At a variable interval $T$ after the presentation, a report cue (a pointer) appeared over the fixation point, and it directed the observer to report the slant of the pointed-to sine wave patch. The probability $p(T)$ of a correct report declined with increasing $T$. To a reasonable approximation, $p(T)$ decayed exponentially (with time constant $\alpha_\psi$) from an initial level of 91% (which represents memory for seven locations) to a value of 43% that represents a residual memory for about two locations. The average value of $\alpha_\psi$ was about 470 msec. A very interesting ancillary observation was that, with extensive practice, the value of $\alpha_\psi$ appeared to increase, doubling in some cases. Contrary to intuition, very short term visual memory for sine wave patches improves with practice.

For brain recording, Yang (1999) used a two-electrode EEG system of one reference electrode and one occipital placement. To measure recovery from habituation, Yang presented a stimulus consisting of eight sine wave patches (see Fig. 13.14) at various rates. Although there was a problem with noise level in the EEG recording that made determination of the habituation recovery time constant $\alpha_\phi$ somewhat problematic, Yang reported a high correlation between the time constant of iconic memory decay and the time constant of recovery from habituation. Remarkably, the habituation time constant measured by EEG appeared to increase with practice by the same amount as the time constant of the psychophysically measured decay of iconic memory, suggesting that, indeed, the same neurons were involved in psychophysical memory performance and in physiological habituation.

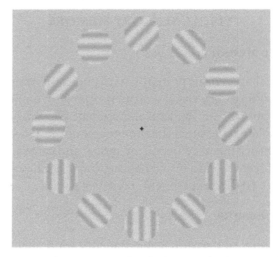

FIG. 13.14.   An array of sine wave patches displayed to the observer in Yang's (1999) psychophysical partial report and electroencephalography habituation procedures. The four orientations are horizontal, vertical, and 45° to the left and right of vertical. The background luminance is 20 cd/m$_2$. The contrast of the sine wave patches is 0.20.

## Complications

There are a number of problems not resolved in Yang's (1999) study. For example, although the stimuli to measure the psychophysical and physiological time constants were the same, the habituation was not slant specific (Yang, Kounios, & Bachman, 2000); the EEG recording method did not permit Yang to separate possibly different sources; and there was the EEG noise problem, to which we already alluded. Nevertheless, Yang's thesis represents a promising beginning and suggests that a combined psychophysical and MEG approach to measuring very short term visual sensory memory would very likely succeed.

### Higher Level Visual Sensory Memories and MEG

As in the determination of very short term auditory sensory memory, the asymptote to which the very short term visual memory decayed represents a form of longer duration visual sensory memory. In vision, even more than in audition, numerous paradigms have evolved to measure and characterize short-term visual memories (some of which we mentioned in the introductory paragraphs). Combining these paradigms with MEG (and EEG and fMRI) would seem to offer bountiful possibilities for the differentiation of the systems. Obviously, these methods of studying sensory memory have not been fully exploited.

## CONCLUSIONS

The sensory memory mechanism suggested by our studies is basically a strength model that has appeared in the psychology literature quite frequently (Loftus, Duncan, & Gehrig, 1992; Reeves & Sperling, 1986). Recent research applying the habituation methods to the human visual system found that each responding area of the brain habituates, indicating memory for past stimulation, and the lifetimes are organized in a hierarchy with lifetimes ranging from a few hundred milliseconds in the sensory areas to 10–30 sec in the parietal, temporal, and prefrontal areas (Uusitalo et al., 1996). The links between the psychological functions and the MEG response strengths of these cell populations remain to be established.

## REFERENCES

Celesia, G. G. (1976). Organization of auditory cortical areas in man. *Brain, 99,* 403–414.

Conrad, R. (1963). Acoustic confusions and memory span for words. *Nature, 197,* 1029–1030.

Cowan, N. (1995). *Attention and memory: An integrated framework.* New York: Oxford University Press.

Crowder, R. G. (1976). *Principles of learning and memory.* Hillsdale, NJ: Lawrence Erlbaum Associates.

Glanzer, M., & Cunitz, A. R. (1966). Two storage mechanisms in free recall. *Journal of Verbal Learning and Verbal Behavior, 5,* 351–360.

Hari, R., Kaila, K., Katila, T., Tuomisto, T., & Varpula, T. (1982). Interstimulus interval dependence of the auditory vertex response and its magnetic counterpart: Implications for their neural generation. *Electroencephalography and Clinical Neurophysiology, 54,* 561–569.

Helson, H. (1964). *Adaptation level theory: An experimental and systematic approach to behavior.* New York: Harper.

Hollingworth, H. L. (1909). *The inaccuracy of movement with special reference to constant errors.* New York: Science Press.

Hollingworth, H. L. (1910). The central tendency of judgment. *Journal of Philosophy, 7,* 461–468.

Ipsen, G. (1926). Über Gestaltauffassung. *Neue Psychologische Studien, 1,* 171–278.

Lauenstein, O. (1933). Ansatz an einer Physiologischen Theorie des Vergleichs und der Zeitfehler *Psychologische Forschung, 17,* 130–177.

Loftus, G. R., Duncan, J., & Gehrig, P. (1992). On the time course of perceptual information that results from a brief visual presentation. *Journal of Experimental Psychology: Human Perception and Performance, 18,* 530–549.

Lu, Z.-L. (1992). *Neuromagnetic investigation of sensory evoked and spontaneous activity of human cerebral cortex.* Unpublished doctoral dissertation, New York University.

Lu, Z.-L., Williamson, S. J., & Kaufman, L. (1992a). Human auditory primary and association cortex have differing lifetimes for activation traces. *Brain Research, 527,* 236–241.

Lu, Z.-L., Williamson, S. J., & Kaufman, L. (1992b, December). Physiological measurements predict the lifetime for human auditory memory of a tone. *Science, 258,* 1668–1670.

Massaro, D. W. (1975). *Experimental psychology and information processing.* Chicago: Rand McNally.

Naatanen, R., & Picton, T. (1987). The N1 wave of the human electric and magnetic response to sound. *Psychophysiology, 24,* 375–425.

Needham, J. G. (1935). The effect of the time interval upon the time-error at different intensive levels. *Journal of Experimental Psychology, 18,* 530–543.

Neisser, U. (1967). *Cognitive psychology.* New York: Appleton-Century-Crofts.

Pantev, C., Hoke, M., Lehnertz, K., Luntkenhoner, B., Anogianakis, G., & Wittkowski, W. (1988). Tonotopic organization of the human auditory cortex revealed by transient auditory evoked magnetic fields. *Electroencephalography and Clinical Neurophysiology, 69,* 160–170.

Reeves, A., & Sperling, G. (1986). Attention gating in short-term visual memory. *Psychological Review, 93,* 180–206.

Sperling, G. (1960). The information available in brief visual presentations. *Psychological Monographs, 74*(11, Whole No. 498).

Sperling, G. (1968). Phonemic model of short-term auditory memory. In *Proceedings of the 76th Annual Convention of the American Psychological Association* (Vol. 3, pp. 63–64). Washington, DC: American Psychological Association.

Sperling, G., & Speelman, R. G. (1970). Acoustic similarity and auditory short-term memory: Experiments and a model. In D. A. Norman (Ed.), *Models of human memory* (pp. 149–202). New York: Academic Press.

Sperling, G., Wurst, S. A., & Lu, Z.-L. (1993). Using repetition detection to define and localize the processes of selective attention. In D. E. Meyer & S. Kornblum (Eds.), *Attention and performance XIV: Synergies in experimental psychology, artificial intelligence, and cognitive neuroscience* (pp. 265–298). Cambridge, MA: MIT Press.

Treisman A. (1964). Monitoring and storage of irrelevant messages in selective attention. *Journal of Verbal Learning and Verbal Behavior, 3,* 449–459.

Uusitalo, M. A., Williamson, S. J., & Seppä, M. T. (1996). Dynamical organisation of the human visual system revealed by lifetimes of activation traces. *Neuroscience Letters, 213,* 149–152.

Weinberger, N. M., Ashe, J. H., Metherate, R., McKenna, T. M., Diamond, D. M., & Bakin, J. (1990). Retuning auditory cortex by learning: A preliminary model of receptive field plasticity. *Concepts in Neuroscience, 1,* 91–132.

Wickelgren, W. O. (1968). Effect of acoustic habituation on click-evoked responses in cats. *Journal of Neurophysiology, 31,* 777–785.

Wickelgren, W. A. (1969). Associative strength theory of recognition memory for pitch. *Journal of Mathematical Psychology, 6,* 13–61.

Woodrow, H. (1933). Weight discrimination with a varying standard. *Am. J. Psych., 45,* 391–416.

Yang, W. (1999). *Lifetime of human visual sensory memory: Properties and neural substrate.* Unpublished doctoral dissertation, New York University.

Yang, W., Kounios, J., & Bachman, P. (2000). Habituation of N1 component in visual evoked potential is specific to spatial location, but not to content of stimulus. *Journal of Cognitive Neuroscience* (Suppl.), 37–37.

# 14

# Clinical Applications of Brain Magnetic Source Imaging

Juergen B. Vieth
Helmut Kober
Oliver Ganslandt
Martin Möller
*University of Erlangen-Nürnberg*
Kyousuke Kamada
*University of Erlangen-Nürnberg*
*and Hokkaido University*

Brain lesions may influence their border zones anatomically and functionally. Magnetic source imaging (MSI) can give information on the function of these areas by localizing sources of evoked and spontaneous brain activity. The inherent multisource problem of MSI recordings can be handled by using spatial average techniques, the dipole density plot and the current density plot. In clinical routine the localizing of the somatosensory, motor cortex, and speech-related cortical areas is used for image-guided neurosurgery with neuronavigators. In subjects and patients, MSI results have been compared with the results of the functional magnetic resonance imaging (MRI). In the presurgical evaluation of epileptic patients the source localization of the spontaneous slow-wave activity can be an additional valuable tool by localizing the penumbra of the epileptogenic lesion, especially when the lesion is not visible in the MRI. In patients with multiple sclerosis it could be demonstrated that white matter lesions cause abnormal activity in adjacent neuronal areas. The penumbra associated with infarcts and transient ischemic attacks also can be localized. This was supported by comparisons of MSI results and those of the proton magnetic resonance spectroscopic imaging ($^1$H MRSI) of $N$-acetyl and lactate in patients with brain infarcts and tumors.

Brain lesions may alter the surrounding brain tissue structurally by moving or compressing it, by infiltration or edema, or by a mixture of these. In addition to the tumor area itself, the function of these border zones might also deteriorate. Electrophysiological signs of these functional deficits might be lesional activity (focal slow and fast waves) and epileptic activity (focal interictal spike or seizure activity) in the electroencephalogram (EEG) and the magnetoencephalogram (MEG). Therefore it is clinically of great interest to know the localization and the extent of focal sources of abnormal spontaneous activity in or around lesions.

However, it is clinically also very important to know the location and the extent of the evoked and event-related activity of functionally important areas around brain lesions, especially when the lesions should be removed surgically. Also, it is of clinical interest to know whether the electrophysiological part of the function is still normal and if a displacement of the functional area took place.

When these sources are to be localized, one must take into consideration that the electric (EEG) or magnetic fields (MEG) of brain activity originate not only from the sources of interest but also from those of the rest of the brain (background activity). Therefore, the so-called *multisource problem* must be handled in order to prevent misinterpretation of the signals. Thus, in this chapter we also give a short description of how this problem can be solved in magnetic source imaging (MSI). The main part of this chapter reports about clinical applications in neurosurgery and neurology with the present progress toward clinical relevance and acceptance. Multiple comparisons are presented of results of MSI with results of functional magnetic resonance imaging (fMRI) and with results of proton magnetic resonance spectroscopic imaging ($^1$H MRSI) of N-acetyl and lactate.

## METHOD

### MSI

#### *Biomagnetic Recording and Source Localization*

From 1990 to 1994, we used the 37-channel system (Krenikon®; Siemens, Erlangen, Germany; planar recording surface of 20 cm in diameter), and since 1995 we have used the 2 × 37 channel system (MAGNES II®; Biomagnetic Technologies Inc., now 4-D Neuroimaging; San Diego; curved recording surface with a 14-cm open diameter). The transfer of the coordinates from the head to the recording device and to the MRI data set was done with our surface fit (edge detection algorithm) of the electrically measured head surface (Isotrack™ 3D-digitizer, Polhemus Navigation Sciences, Colchester, Vermont) and the head surface that was reconstructed from the magnetic resonance images. With our procedure the error of the coordinate transfer is less than 2 mm. The advantages of our procedure are (a) the electrical scanning of the head surface is much easier to perform than using fiducial points, and (b) no MRI fiducial points are necessary at all. Thus, any three-dimensional MRI, or computer tomography, or positron emission tomography, or fMRI scan can be used to be fitted with the MEG sources or with each other (Kober, Grummich, & Vieth 1995).

We used the sphere as the MEG volume conductor model, because it is sufficient in most cases (Meijs, Bosch, Peters, & Lopes Da Silva, 1987; Zanow, 1997). Depending on the task, we used either the single current dipole model or a current distribution solution. To apply the single current dipole in a more adequate way, the localization procedure was done only on signal sections where one component predominantly describes the signal. The principal-components analysis selects these sections from the whole recording time (normally 10 min). Thus, typically only 1–2 % of the original signal will be used for the source localization, speeding it up substantially (Kober et al., 1992).

### MEG Multisource Problem

In order to reduce the background activity, we use in the first place the alpha blocking effect during the recording (eyes open). Additional measures can be applied, when the signal of interest is not in phase with that of other sources of the background activity and when it differs from the background by its focal nature, by its frequency band (slow or fast waves or epileptic activity), and by its time-locked appearance (evoked and event-related responses or epileptic activity).

For the dipole analysis we developed a kind of spatial averaging of the already-localized sources, to show the spatial distribution of the activity over the recording time. This is the *dipole density plot* (DDP), a three-dimensionally working convolution using a three-dimensional Gaussian envelope, that takes into account the localization uncertainty. Because the signal-to-noise ratio will be impaired when multiple sources are present, we found that the dipole methods are able to separate only up to two dominant dipole sources (Kober et al., 1992; Vieth, Kober, & Grummich, 1996; Vieth et al., 1992).

Our second approach—a current density proceeding—can be used when up to three dominant and extended sources are present. We adjusted for our needs a spatial filtering approach first described by Robinson and Rose (1992). In our proceeding, the current localization by spatial filtering (CLSF), the analyzing space (a sphere) consists of 7,000 voxels, which are adjusted in size and location to the area of interest. The individual current flow of each voxel is obtained at individual time instants by applying a spatial filter to the signals, which were measured at the surface of the skull (Grummich, Kober, & Vieth, 1992). As it is done as a part of the DDP a spatial averaging can also be applied on the CLSF, which we called the *current density plot* (CDP). The CDP shows the current intensity over the analyzing time, thus enhancing the separation of sources, which are active more or less continuously (Kamada, Kober, et al., 1998).

Our MSI evaluation process is illustrated in Fig. 14.1.

### *fMRI and Magnetic Resonance Spectroscopic Imaging*

For details of these comparing methods, see for fMRI Stippich et al. (1998); Nimsky et al. (1999); and Kober, Nimsky, et al. (2001); and for magnetic resonance spectroscopic imaging (MRS) ($^1$H MRSI) Kamada et al. (1997, 2001).

## RESULTS AND DISCUSSION

In previous years we have been able to develop clinical applications with different progress toward clinical usefulness, relevance, and acceptance. We validated these applications using structural lesions, when applicable.

### Evaluation With Structural Lesions

We tested the reliability of the DDP and the CDP with spontaneous focal activity of structural brain lesions (tumors, infarcts) and their border zones, up to June 2000, in 147 cases with focal slow-wave activity (2–6 Hz) and in 88 cases with fast-wave activity (12.5–30 Hz; Grummich et al., 1995). In patients with infarcts there was a tendency for fewer cases with fast activity than in patients with tumors. Nineteen cases of each group were additionally investigated using MRS. On the basis of our results, we found the accuracy to localize the associated sources of the abnormal brain activity to be considerably high when focal activity is present (Kamada et al., 2001; Kamada et al., 1997; Kober et al,. 1992; Vieth et al., 1996; Vieth et al., 1992) and we can be sure to localize at least the main portion of the area of the functionally impaired neuronal activity with or without visible structural lesions in the MRI.

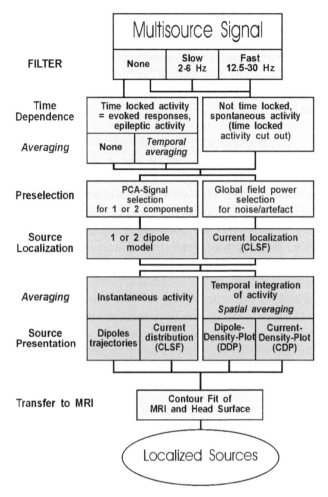

FIG. 14.1. Evaluation proceeding of the magnetic source imaging source localization in Erlangen. Data regarding signal processing and source localization are on light and dark gray background, respectively. The multisource signal (white background) can be processed according to the task: either as the raw (unfiltered) signal or as the signal in the 2–6 Hz (slow activity) or the 12.5–30 Hz (fast activity) band. The time-locked activity (evoked and event-related responses or epileptic activity) can either be temporally averaged or not. To prevent possible contamination of the filtered spontaneous activity, epileptic spike/wave activity can be eliminated. In the preselection phase either the principal-components analysis is used to select only signal sections that are predominantly described by only one (typically 1%–2% of the whole analyzing time only) or two components, or the global field power is used to give an indication of data sections that are contaminated by strong noise or artifacts, or both. The source localization can be either the application of the single- or two-dipole model or that of the current localization by spatial filtering (CLSF). The source presentation can be done either directly (trajectories) or as the result of a spatial averaging of the localization results over the whole analyzing time (isocontour lines), that is either the dipole density plot or the current density plot. The last step is the fit of the anatomical and the functional data before the localized sources (white background) are obtained.

We should stress here that our approaches (DDP and CLSF, including CDP) also could be used with EEG, provided that the EEG source localization has been done accurately enough.

## Normal Activity

The clinical application to determine the relation of tumors to the cortical somatosensory, motory, auditory and cortical speech areas was adapted and established in Erlangen by members of the Department of Experimental Neuropsychiatry with the goal of acceptance in the clinical environment. Now these approaches are routinely used by the Clinic of Neurosurgery in Erlangen for operation planning and intraoperative functional neuronavigation (Fahlbusch, Ganslandt, & Nimsky, 2000; Ganslandt et al., 1999). This image-guided neurosurgery is performed in a "twin operation room" with a Siemens Open-MRI (Magnetom Open) in one room and, in the other room, the movable operation table (to be moved into the Open-MRI), the Zeiss microscope neuronavigation system (MKM), and the additional Stealth pointer neuronavigation system (Steinmeier et al., 1998). Thus, an optimal degree of carefulness is possible during the operation, with special reference to important eloquent brain areas to have a minimum number of possible postoperational functional deficits.

## Somatosensory Evoked and Motor Event Related Responses

Gallen et al. (1993; Gallen et al., 1997) demonstrated first in neurosurgery the clinical usefulness of the somatosensory magnetic evoked responses. This technique was subsequently used by others: Fahlbusch et al. (2000); Ganslandt et al. (1999; Ganslandt et al., 1997; Ganslandt et al., 1996); Kamada et al. (1993); Morioka, Yamamoto, Katsuta, Fujii, and Fukui (1994); Nakasato et al. (1996); and Orrison et al. (1992). A coupling of MSI results to the neuronavigator was first described by Watanabe, Mayanagi, and Kaneko (1993). The interactive use of MSI in image-guided neurosurgery was reported first by Rezai et al. (1996).

Deecke, Weinberg, and Brickett (1982) reported first on a motor-related MEG activity of intention, the so-called *Bereitschaftsfeld*, in the supplementary motor area. Also later, the localization of directly motor-induced activity in the precentral gyrus was possible. More generally, Lewine and Orrison (1995) reported about this response. Our group developed for neurosurgical usage the localization of this cortical motor-induced activity. It was elicited by self-paced finger movements. The trigger signal was obtained from the rectified electromyogram of the corresponding muscles of the lower arm (Ganslandt et al., 1999; Kassubek et al., 1996; Kober, Nimsky, et al., 2001).

In Erlangen, we successfully localized (up to June 2001) in 157 patients with tumors around the central sulcus the somatosensory responses in 152 cases (97%) and the motor-associated cortical responses in 80 of 89 cases (90%). Thirty-two patients have not been operated on on the basis of the MSI findings (Ganslandt, Fahlbusch, Kober, Gralla, & Nimsky, 2002). In all patients the projection of the magnetic single-dipole localization on the brain surface of the postcentral gyrus coincided with the intraoperatively evoked phase reversal of the potentials measured at the surface of the cortex, which was elicited by electric finger stimulation (cf. Ganslandt et al., 2002; Ganslandt et al., 1999; Ganslandt et al., 1997; Ganslandt et al., 1996; Stippich et al., 1996). One hundred twenty-eight of 155 operated patients were operated on by using the functional neuronavigation.

Figure 14.2 shows an example of a patient with a left meningioma: the localization of the somatosensory evoked response in the postcentral gyrus combined with the display of the Stealth neuronavigator.

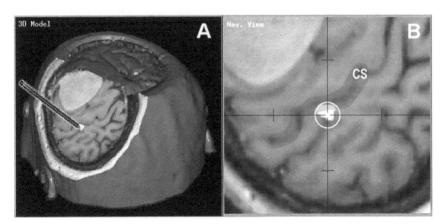

FIG. 14.2.    Single-dipole magnetic source imaging (MSI) source localization of the postcentral gyrus using the somatosensory evoked field (SEF) at 50 msec after the tactile stimulus of the right index finger (200 samples, averaged) of a 65-year-old female patient (wwa) with a left meningioma. Panel A: display of the Stealth neuronavigator showing in a tangential plane the tumor and the MSI SEF source and the intraoperatively used pointer instrument. Panel B: enlarged section of A; the central sulcus is shaded and marked by *CS* and the SEF source is marked by a white encircled spot (from Vieth et al. 1999 by courtesy of the organizers of NFSI '99, Zagreb 1999).

Figure 14.3 shows an example of a patient with a left astrocytoma: the localization of the motor-related responses and the somatosensory evoked responses in the pre- and postcentral gyrus, respectively.

### MSI and fMRI

Since 1991 (Belliveau et al., 1991), fMRI has been used to localize three dimensionally the local oxygenation level change elicited by evoked or event-related brain activity. The effect is called the *blood oxygenation level dependent contrast* (BOLD). There are some fundamental differences between MSI and fMRI that can cause misinterpretation of fMRI results:

1. The signal-to-noise ratio in MSI is much higher than in fMRI, so it can be more difficult in fMRI than in MSI to differentiate the findings of interest from artifacts.
2. In fMRI a baseline recording is always necessary; MSI does not need this reference. So, in cases where the baseline status is not present anymore (i.e., infarcts, tumors) fMRI is unable to give meaningful results. MSI just localizes sources of focal normal and abnormal brain activity.

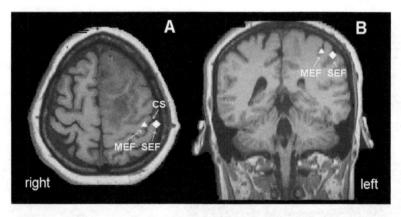

FIG. 14.3.    Single-dipole magnetic source imaging source localizations of the motor-related source (MEF) in the precentral and somatosensory evoked field (SEF) in the postcentral gyrus of a 39-year-old female patient (age) with a left astrocytoma. SEF and MEF dipole sources are marked, respectively. The central sulcus is marked by *CS* in Panel A. The SEF source was localized at 50 msec after the tactile stimulus of the index finger (200 samples, averaged). The MEF source was localized at 100 msec after the movement onset (trigger obtained from the rectified surface electromyogram) of self-paced brisk movements of the right index finger (100 samples, averaged) (from Vieth et al. 1999 by courtesy of the organizers of NFSI '99, Zagreb 1999).

3. In fMRI, the patient movement during the recording may produce new (artifact) sources (Hajnal et al. 1994). This problem has not yet been solved completely. If the patient's movements are small, the artifacts can be reduced by image-based detection of the movements (Friston, Williams, Howard, Frackowiak, & Turner, 1996; Josephs, Wang, Athwal, & Turner, 1999). In MSI, patient movement during the recording will cause only a blurring of the localization results.

4. In MSI, the neuronal areas will be localized. In fMRI, the drainage section and the venous branch show the oxygen level change (cf. Segebarth et al., 1994). Thus, interpretation of fMRI findings should be done with general caution (Segebarth et al., 1994). Until now, no procedure was published to get around this situation.

5. In fMRI, the time resolution depends on the diffusion time of oxyhemoglobin to the draining vessels, which is on the order of seconds. In MSI, the time resolution depends on the electric properties of the tissue and the recording equipment, so it is on the order of 1 msec or less.

In three comparative studies with 6 subjects (Stippich et al., 1996), 15 patients (Nimsky et al., 1999), and 34 patients (Kober, Nimsky, et al., 2001), it was demonstrated that the localization of evoked cortical responses obtained by MSI and fMRI typically is dislocated by approximately 1 cm as the consequence of the two different principles: (a) the measurement of the electric neuronal activity (MSI) and (b) the measurement of blood oxygenation changes in the venous branch following the neuronal activity (fMRI; cf. Segebarth et al., 1994).

Figure 14.4 shows an example of the comparison of the localization of the motor-related MSI response and the motor-related fMRI response.

### *Event-Related Speech Responses*

It also is possible to localize the cortical areas, which are activated by speech recognition (Simos, Breier, Zouridakis, & Papanicolaou, 1998). In our approach (Kamada, Kober, et al., 1998; Kober, Möller, et al., 2001), similar to the WADA test (Wada & Rasmussen, 1960), we activate recognition visually with written words and pictograms of monosyllabic concrete objects. The presentation is conducted via a glass fiber bundle from a television screen located outside the shielded room. If the recognized term is also spoken internally, then the area of the speech induction (Broca's area) can be activated and localized (Grummich, Kober, Vieth,

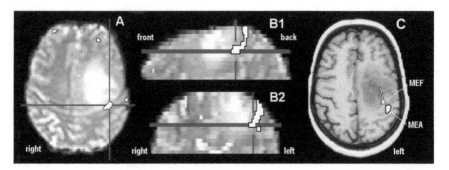

FIG. 14.4.  Localization of motor evoked activity (MEA) in functional magnetic resonance imaging (fMRI) in Panel A, Panel B Transverse Relaxation time constant (T2), and Panel C Longitudinal relaxation time constant (T1) and of the magnetic motor evoked field (MEF) in Panel C in a 32-year-old female patient (gdb) with a left astrocytoma suffering from a light motor deficit of the right hand. fMRI was measured using a T2*-weighted echo planar imaging (EPI) sequence. The recording consisted of three activation periods (iteratively clenching the right fist) and three baseline (rest) periods with 10 EPI volume data sets for each period. Functional activation maps were obtained by using the cross-correlation coefficient of the measured and expected activation at 0.7 or higher. Panel A: axial view; Panel B1: sagittal view; Panel B2: coronal view of the fMRI motor activity (MEA) blood oxygenation level dependent contrast effect; Panel C: axial view showing MEA and the magnetic source imaging single-dipole source localization (MEF). The MEF was localized 100 msec after the movement onset (trigger obtained from the rectified surface electromyogram) of self-paced brisk movements of the right index finger (100 samples, averaged). The MEF was localized on the edge of the tumor (light motor deficit of the right hand) in the precentral gyrus. The MEA was found in the central sulcus (venous drainage), which is especially visible in Panels B1 and B2 (from Vieth et al., 1999 by courtesy of the organizers of NFSI '99, Zagreb 1999).

Matschke, & Ganslandt, 1994). Meaningless pictograms also were presented to enhance the average of the speech-related signals by subtracting the signals of the meaningless presentation from the signals of the speech-related presentation (Kamada, Kober, et al., 1998; Kober, Möller et al., 2001).

In right-handed people the density of activity was highest in the posterior part of the left superior temporal gyrus (Wernicke's area) at around 350 msec (internal reading) and at around 500–600 msec (internal speaking) in the left inferior frontal gyrus (Broca's area) but also some at the same time in the superior temporal gyrus (Kamada, Kober, et al., 1998). This procedure also was used successfully to show differences of two differently written languages: (a) a phonetic oriented language (German) and (b) a language consisting of morphograms (*Kanji* characters of Japanese). The latter causes an additional late response (Kamada, Kober, et al., 1998). The nature of this response has yet to be clarified.

In Erlangen, 67 patients (57 right handed and 10 left handed) had brain tumors in the speech-related cortical areas. These areas were localized by using our averaging version of the CLSF, the CDP. The DDP, on the other hand, was not able to give clear enough results in almost all cases because of a too low signal-to-noise ratio.

Our approach was tested in 21 healthy subjects. Handedness was determined by the Edinburgh Handedness Inventory (Oldfield, 1971). Our approach allowed us to differ between the sensory and the motor speech areas (methods cf. Kamada, Kober, et al., 1998). Sixty-six of 68 patients suffered from transient or permanent speech disturbances. Only 2 patients suffered from an impairment. In 65 patients (95%) the sensory speech area could also be localized, and in 61 patients (90%) the motor speech area also could be localized (Ganslandt et al., 2002).

To determine the hemisphere with the larger activity, MEG recordings were done simultaneously on both sides. Our current density approach showed two to four times more activity on one side, sometimes up to eight times larger (laterality index). In all patients (right and left handed), higher activity was observed on the left side (Kober, Möller, et al., 2001). In 4 right-handed cases and in 1 left-handed patient the WADA test (Wada & Rasmussen, 1960) showed the speech dominance in the left hemisphere. Thus, the MSI results in these cases (higher CLSF speech intensity on the left side) were confirmed by the WADA test. An epicortical intraoperatively applied stimulation at Broca's area caused a speech arrest in 5 cases. Because of its invasiveness, the WADA test was restrictively applied according to clinical needs. Thus, this part of the WADA test might be supplemented or replaced by the MSI approach in the presurgical evaluation of patients. More comparing studies are necessary.

Up to now, 35 of the 67 patients had been operated on. Thirty had been operated on using the functional neuronavigation. Only 2 patients suffered from a postoperative deterioration of speech. Thirty-two patients have not been operated on on the basis of the MSI findings (Ganslandt et al., 2002; Kober, Möller, et al., 2001). Figure 14.5 shows an example of the localization of the speech areas and the somatosensory evoked responses in a patient with a left temporo–parietal glioma.

## Abnormal Activity

### Epileptogenic Lesion

One valuable application of localizing abnormal activity is in the field of the presurgical evaluation of epileptic patients: Normally, the epileptogenic

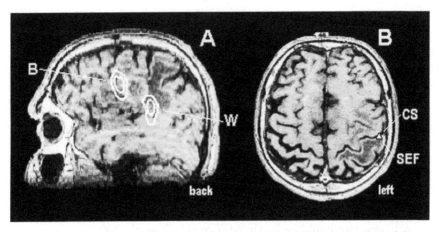

FIG. 14.5.   Speech-related magnetic source image source localizations in Panel A and the somatosensory evoked field (SEF) in Panel B of a 69-year-old male patient (jza) with a left temporo–parietal glioma. The speech responses were elicited by presenting pictograms of monosyllabic concrete objects for 800 msec on a television screen (conducted via a glass fiber bundle to the inside of the shielded room). Two hundred fifty samples were averaged and the current localization by spatial filtering (CLSF; current density) of the response determined. Isocontour lines show the intensity of the CLSF results. The task was to recognize the meaning of the object and to speak internally the word of the object. The first response was at 340 msec after the onset of the presentation in the posterior part of the left superior temporal gyrus (Wernicke's area), marked by W, and the second response was at 745 msec after the onset of the presentation in the left inferior frontal gyrus (Broca's area), marked by B. The SEF source (marked by SEF) was localized 50 msec after the tactile stimulus at the index finger (200 samples, averaged). The central sulcus is marked by CS. (From Vieth et al., 1999, by courtesy of the organizers of NFSI '99, Zagreb 1999.)

zone is removed to cure the epilepsy, but results with structural lesions show that the removal of the epileptogenic lesion (assumed to be the original cause of a seizure disorder) is also important for the clinical outcome (Awad, Rosenfeld, Ahl, Hahn, & Lüders, 1991; Cascino et al., 1992). On the other hand, the outcome of surgery of nonlesional focal neocortical epilepsy has a seizure-free rate of only 0%–20% (Kutsy, Farell, & Ojemann, 1999; Lee, Spencer, & Spencer, 2000; Zentner et al., 1996). Thus, the localization of the epileptogenic "lesion," the slow- (and fast-) wave focal activity associated with visible and without visible lesions, is of great interest. In addition, it is very easy to record the spontaneous interictal activity associated with epileptogenic lesions compared with the acquisition of spikes or even a seizure. Up to now, only two other groups and our group have demonstrated that the spontaneous slow-wave activity can be used to localize the epileptogenic lesion of focal epilepsies, which are associated either with or without structural lesions (Gallen et al., 1997; Lewine & Orrison, 1995; Vieth et al., 1994; Vieth, Kober, Kamada, & Ganslandt, 1998).

In our study with focal epilepsies, we had one group of epileptic patients with structural lesions as the reason for the epilepsy and another group without any visible structural lesions. In the first group we got in the border zone of the tumors a strong coincidence of the MSI localizations of the three different spontaneous interictal signal components: (a) epileptic spikes, (b) slow-wave activity, and (c) fast-wave activity. For signal enhancement, both the DDP and the CDP have been used. Occasionally, occurring spike/wave complexes have been discarded when spontaneous slow- and fast-wave activity was analyzed.

An example is shown in Fig. 14.6, which also gives an impression of a shell-like distribution of the slow- and fast-wave sources around the tumor. The same coincidence of the results in all six approaches also was found in the second group of epileptic patients, the ones with no visible structural lesion (Vieth et al., 1993; Vieth et al., 1994; Vieth et al, 1998).

Focal abnormal lesional activity has even been found to be associated with the (focal) Rolandic epilepsy of children (Kamada, Möller, et al., 1998). We demonstrated that even in these cases an epileptogenic lesion may be present with functional (psychopathological) deficits; in spite of

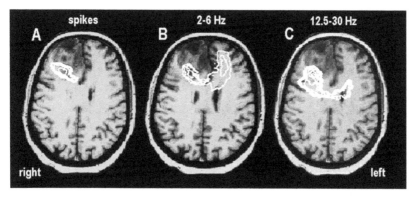

FIG. 14.6.   Magnetic source image source localization of focal abnormal spontaneous interictal activity in the border zone of a right frontal astrocytoma of a 67-year-old female patient (ida) with grand mal epileptic seizures. The averaging version of the current localization by spatial filtering, the current density plot, was used to localize the current density during the whole recording time of 10 min. Panel A: spikes; Panel B: slow- (2–6 Hz) and Panel C: fast- (12.5–30 Hz) wave activities. In Panels B and C, occurring spike/wave activity was eliminated out of the original signal to prevent contamination of the slow- and fast-wave spontaneous activity. The impression of a shell-like abnormal activity can be seen, especially in Panels B and C (from Vieth et al., 1999 by courtesy of the organizers of NFSI '99, Zagreb 1999).

that "per definitionem," no (visible structural) lesion is associated with this disease in the MRI. So the approach to localize the epileptogenic lesion seems to be a valuable additional complementary tool, especially in the presurgical evaluation of epilepsy patients, when no structural lesion is visible in the MRI. Thus, it is worthwhile to test in multicenter studies the value of our approach to localize the epileptogenic lesion compared with the localization of interictal spikes and that of the seizure-onset zone and the epileptogenic zone.

### White Matter Lesions

The sources of the MEG are mainly the longitudinally flowing currents inside the dendritic tree of neurons. These currents are generated at the synapses of the neurons by the postsynaptic potentials (Okada & Kyuhou, 1997). Therefore, it could be expected that lesions in the axonal section of the neurons (white matter) should have no significant contribution to the normal and abnormal electric activity of the brain. Multiple sclerosis (MS) is a disease that mainly destroys the myelin sheath of the neuronal fibers (axons). Therefore, in the MRI a contrast may appear in the white matter. We wanted to know if these fiber lesions produce abnormal activity at all and, if so, where it comes from.

In our study we included 8 patients with MS and a group of 8 healthy subjects serving as a baseline. The two groups received the same recording and evaluation protocol. The spatial dipole distribution was quantified and compared statistically between the groups. In all the MS patients the maximum of focal abnormal slow- and fast-wave activity was found in cortical (neuronal) areas adjacent to the fiber lesions, whereas in the healthy subjects no focal abnormal brain activity could be found (Kassubek, Sörös, Kober, Stippich, & Vieth, 1999). These results indicated that the interpretation of such MSI results should be done with care, because in the case of a fiber lesion and an additional—perhaps not visible—lesion in the gray matter it might be difficult to differentiate where the cause of the abnormal cortical activity is located: in the cortex itself or in the white matter. Additional information should clarify the answer.

### Cerebrovascular Accidents

Cerebrovascular accidents account for approximately one fourth of the total mortality and the bulk rate of disabled people. Therefore it would be of great value to have diagnostic measures for an early detection of prestages.

In our studies we have found that the MSI is able to localize not only the disturbed function around a structural brain lesion (infarct) but also that of an area with only functional—perhaps reversible—impairment. These can be *transient ischemic attacks* (TIAs), and infarcts that are too small to be detected by standard MRI resolution. Up to now, we have localized not only the pathological activity associated with brain infarcts in 23 patients but also the activity associated with the penumbra of TIAs (Kamada et al., 1997; Kober, Vieth, Stippich, Kassubek, & Hopfengärtner, 2000; Stippich, Kassubek, Kober, Sörös, & Vieth, 2000; Vieth et al., 1996; Vieth et al., 1992) in 21 cases.

Thus we have also been able to localize clinically silent reversible ischemic brain deficits in accordance with silent brain infarcts (Caplan, 1994). This finding is clinically important regardless of whether an extracranial stenosis of the internal carotid artery is to be assumed as symptomatic. In this case of a symptomatic stenosis, another indication for an endarterectomy can be assumed (Vieth et al., 1992). Very helpful for the idea of screening patients with an asymptomatic carotid stenosis in order to fetch such a silent reversible ischemic brain deficit is our finding that the abnormal activity of TIAs—caused by a symptomatic carotid stenosis—is lasting at least 4 weeks and never reached 10 weeks after the accident (Kober et al., 2000). The feasibility of localizing the penumbra of infarcts is also very important when new therapeutic approaches (i.e., neuroprotectors) are available that prevent neurons from being damaged irreversibly. More clinical studies should verify the value of these diagnostic tools.

### Brain Functions and Metabolism

More evidence that our approaches are able to localize abnormal activity of the penumbra comes from two other studies. We investigated one group of patients with brain infarcts and another one with tumors to compare the functional localization of the abnormal electric brain functions and the abnormal metabolic brain functions using the MSI and the proton MRS ($^1$H MRSI).

### Brain Infarcts

In the first study, we investigated 12 patients with a brain infarct and compared them with 12 normal cases. The goal was to study the MEG slow-wave DDP inside the infarct, in the border zone, and in normal tissue in relation to the MRS signal intensity of $N$-acetyl (NA; marker for normal function of the brain) and the lactate MRS signal intensity (an indicator of anaerobic metabolism). We found that the signal intensity of NA was significantly reduced in the regions with the highest slow-wave activity but was well correlated interindividually with the DDP of the quantified maximum of slow waves. Although lactate was mildly accumulated in these regions, the lactate level had no correlation with slow-wave magnetic activity. We could assume that preserved and metabolically active cortical tissue with remaining NA signal and the increased slow-wave activity under lactic acidosis (mild accumulation of lactate) could be one of the ischemic penumbra states. This study also shows that the slow-wave activity may well serve as a marker to localize the penumbra.

Figure 14.7 shows in a patient with a brain infarct the spatial distribution of the intensities of the abnormal slow waves, the lactate, and the NA activities.

Figure 14.8 shows an example of the same patient with the topographic development of the three activities (MSI, NA, lactate) along a line from normal to pathological tissue. It appears that all three distributions start with abnormal values relatively far away from the infarct, typically 3 cm or more. From the results of the study we can assume that the MEG quantified slow-wave sources give an indication of whether a

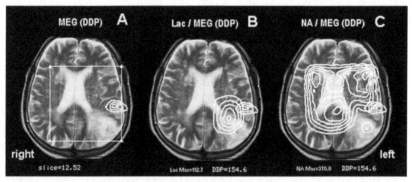

FIG. 14.7.    Dipole density plot magnetic source imaging source localization of focal abnormal spontaneous slow-wave (2–6 Hz) activity of a 60-year-old male patient (kfa) during the recording time of 10 min in the border zone of a left brain infarct in Panels A, B, and C. Additional overlay of a separately recorded proton magnetic resonance spectroscopic imaging ($^1$H MRSI) signals of lactate are presented in Panel B and of $N$-acetyl (NA) in Panel C. The field of view is 200 × 200 mm, marked in Panel A by a white line and seen in Panel C by the outer limit of the NA activity; 16 × 16 phase encoding; nominal in-plane resolution: 12.5 mm, point-resolved spectroscopy; repetition time (TR): 1,500 msec; echo time (TE): 135 and 270 msec. For details, see Kamada et al. (1997, 2001). (From Vieth et al., 1999 by courtesy of the organizers of NFSI '99, Zagreb 1999.)

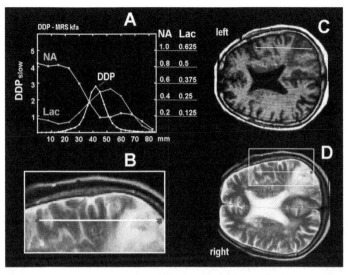

FIG. 14.8.   Intensity of abnormal spontaneous slow-wave (2–6 Hz) activity, lactate (Lac) $^1$H MRSI activity, and N-acetyl (NA) $^1$H MRSI activity of the same patient (kfa) as in Fig. 14.7 with a left brain infarct along a line drawn from normal tissue through the bulk of the brain infarct. The recording protocol is the same as in Fig. 14.7. Panel C: line seen in a T1 image; Panel D: line seen in a T2 image enclosed by a white rectangular line marking the enlarged area in Panel B. For comparison, the line in Panel B is in direct spatial relation to the three different activities in Panel A. A relatively distant start of the decrease of NA and the increase of Lac appears in the border zone of the infarct (3.5–4 cm apart from the visible limit of the infarct). Abnormal slow-wave activity also starts that far, coming to a peak 2 cm apart from the infarct limit. Then the slow-wave activity steadily decreases to zero until the limit of the infarct. The neurons beyond this limit are not able to produce even slow waves anymore or a sufficient intensity of them. For details see Kamada et al. (2001; Kamada et al., 1997). DDP = dipole density plot. (From Vieth et al. 1999 by courtesy of the organizers of NFSI '99, Zagreb 1999.)

penumbra is present and where it is located (Kamada et al., 1997). The clinical importance of this is to have a diagnostic tool to find areas of neurons where therapeutic measures (i.e., neuroprotectors) might prevent neurons from being damaged irreversibly.

### Brain Tumors

In the second study, 7 patients with common invasive and noninvasive brain tumors (i.e., astrocytic tumor and meningioma) were compared with a group of 10 healthy subjects. The recording protocol of MEG and $^1$H MRSI was in both groups the same as in the previous study. Increased slow- and fast-wave activities and spikes were observed in the neuronal area adjacent to the bulk of the tumor with a mild reduction of

NA and a slight accumulation of lactate. Lactate intensity was less pronounced than in the study with the infarcts.

The bulk of the tumors were magnetically silent. The extension of the tumor border zone seems to depend on the invasiveness of the tumor, but it seems to be smaller than that of the infarcts, typically about 2 cm.

Figure 14.9 shows an example of the intensity of the three activities along a line from tissue of the border zone of a tumor through the tumor and back to tissue outside the tumor again. We could assume also in this study that preserved and metabolically active cortical tissue in the border region of a tumor with a remaining NA signal and the increased slow-wave activity under lactic acidosis could be one of the ischemic pen-

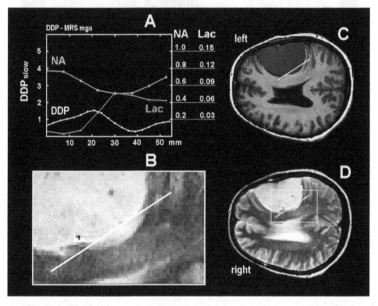

FIG. 14.9.    Intensity of abnormal spontaneous slow-wave (2–6 Hz) activity, lactate (Lac) [1]H MRSI activity, and N-acetyl (NA) [1]H MRSI activity of a 53-year-old female (mga) with a left meningioma along a line drawn from tissue in the border zone through one pole of the tumor and back to border zone tissue on the other side of the meningioma. The recording protocol is the same as in Figs. 14.7 and 14.8. Panel C: line seen in a T1 image; Panel D: line seen in a T2 image enclosed by a white rectangular line marking the enlarged area in Panel B, where the line is in direct spatial relation to the three different activities for comparison. Starting from tissue in the border zone, NA is decreasing to the tumor tissue and increasing to border zone tissue again. Lac is increasing mildly (compared with infarcts) from border zone tissue to the tumor tissue and does not reach the baseline on the other side of the tumor. The slow-wave activity has two peaks in both border zones of the tumor according to the assumption that only outside the meningioma are neurons capable of producing sufficient electric activity. For details, see Kamada et al. (2001; Kamada et al., 1997). DDP = dipole density plot (from Vieth et al. 1999 by courtesy of the organizers of NFSI 99, Zagreb 1999).

umbra states of tumors, too. This study also shows that the slow-wave activity might well serve as a marker to localize the penumbra of tumors. Thus, the clinical importance of the MSI may be the early detection or prestages of tumors and the follow-up investigation. Details are in Kamada et al. (2001; Kamada et al., 1997).

## CONCLUSION

In our studies we demonstrated that the localization of the function of eloquent cortical areas is well suited to be used as a valuable additional tool in functional image-guided neurosurgery. The localization of the epileptogenic lesion also is a very promising tool in the presurgical investigation of epileptic patients. The penumbras of TIAs, infarcts, and tumors can be localized. A possible screening for "asymptomatic TIAs" (clinically silent reversible neuronal deficit) might also be a promising tool in the prevention of strokes. In patients with infarcts, knowledge of the localization and the extent of the penumbra may serve as a basis to prevent the increase of irreversibly damaged tissue. In patients with tumors, localization of the border zone activity may serve as a tool of early detection or prestages of tumors. More clinical studies should verify the value of these promising tools.

## REFERENCES

Awad, I. A., Rosenfeld, J., Ahl, J., Hahn, J. F., & Lüders, H. (1991). Intractable epilepsy and structural lesions of the brain: Mapping, resection, strategies, and seizure outcome. *Epilepsia, 32,* 179–186.

Belliveau, J. W., Kennedy, D. N. Jr., McKinstry, R. C., Buchbinder, B. R., Weisskoff, R. M., Cohen, M. S., Vevea, J. M., Brady, T. J., & Rosen, B. R. (1991, November). Functional mapping of the human visual cortex by magnetic resonance imaging. *Science, 254,* 716–719.

Caplan, L. R. (1994). Silent brain infarcts. *Cerebrovascular Diseases, 4*(Suppl. 1), 32–40.

Cascino, G. D., Kelly, P. J., Sharbrough, F. W., Hulihan, J. F., Hirschorn, K. A., & Trenerry, M. R. (1992). Longterm followup of stereotactic lesionectomy in partial epilepsy: Predictive factors and electroencephalographic results. *Epilepsia, 33,* 639–644.

Deecke, L., Weinberg, P., & Brickett, P. (1982). Magnetic fields of the human brain accompanying voluntary movement: *Bereitschaftsmagnetfeld. Experimental Brain Research, 48,* 144–148.

Fahlbusch, R., Ganslandt, O., & Nimsky, C. (2000). Intraoperative imaging with open magnetic resonance imaging and neuronavigation. *Child's Nervous System, 16,* 829–831.

Friston, K. J., Williams, S. R., Howard, R., Frackowiak, S. R. J., & Turner, R. (1996). Movement-related effects in fMRI time series. *Magnetic Resonance in Medicine, 35,* 346–355.

Gallen, C. C., Sobel, D. F., Waltz, T., Aung, M., Copeland, B., Schwartz, B. J., Hirschkoff, E. C., & Bloom, F. E. (1993). Noninvasive presurgical neuromagnetic mapping of somatosensory cortex. *Neurosurgery, 33,* 260–268.

Gallen, C. C., Tecoma, E., Iragui, V., Sobel, D. F., Schwartz, B. J., & Bloom, F. E. (1997). Magnetic source imaging of abnormal low-frequency magnetic activity in presurgical evaluations of epilepsy. *Epilepsia, 38,* 452–460.

Ganslandt, O., Fahlbusch, R., Kober, H., Gralla, J., & Nimsky, C. (2002). On the utility of magnetoencephalography and functional neuronavigation in the planning and treatment of brain tumors. *Nervenarzt, 73,* 155–161.

Ganslandt, O., Fahlbusch, R., Nimsky, C., Kober, H., Möller, M., Steinmeier, R., Romstöck, J., & Vieth, J. (1999). Functional neuronavigation with magnetoencephalography: outcome in 50 patients with lesions around the motor cortex. *Journal of Neurosurgery, 91,* 73–79.

Ganslandt, O., Steinmeier, R., Kober, H., Vieth, J., Kassubek, J., Romstöck, J., Strauss, C., & Fahlbusch, R. (1997). Magnetic source imaging combined with image guided, frameless stereotaxy: A new method in surgery around the motor strip. *Neurosurgery, 41,* 621–627.

Ganslandt, O., Ulbricht, D., Kober, H., Vieth, J., Strauss, C., & Fahlbusch, R. (1996). SEF–MEG localization of somatosensory cortex as a method for presurgical assessment of functional brain area. *Electroencephalography and Clinical Neurophysiology, 46*(Suppl.), 209–213.

Grummich, P., Kober, H., & Vieth, J. (1992). Localization of the underlying currents of magnetic brain activity using spatial filtering. *Biomedical Engineering (Berlin), 37*(Suppl. 2), 158–159.

Grummich, P., Kober, H., Vieth, J., Matschke, J., & Ganslandt, O. (1994). Sensory speech area investigated by magnetoencephalography. *Biomedical Engineering (Berlin), 37*(Suppl.), 129–130.

Grummich, P., Vieth, J., Kober, H., Pongratz, H., Ulbricht, D., & Ganslandt, O. (1995). Localization of focal spontaneous beta wave activity associated with structural lesions in the brain. In C. Baumgartner, L. Deecke, G. Stroink, & S. J. Williamson (Eds.), *Biomagnetism: Fundamental research and clinical applications* (pp. 75–79). Amsterdam: Elsevier Science.

Hajnal, J. V., Myers, R., Oatridge, A., Schwieso, J. E., Young, I. R., & Bydders, G. M. (1994). Artifacts due to stimulus correlated motion in functional imaging of the brain. *Magnetic Resonance in Medicine, 31,* 283–291.

Josephs, O., Wang, J. J., Athwal, B. S., & Turner, R. (1999). Reduction of motion artifact in fMRI. *NeuroImage, 9*(Suppl.),

Kamada, K., Kober, H., Saguer, M., Möller, M., Kaltenhäuser, M., & Vieth, J. (1998). Responses to silent *kanji* reading of the native Japanese and German in task subtraction magnetoencephalography. *Cognitive Brain Research, 7,* 89–98.

Kamada, K., Möller, M., Saguer, M., Ganslandt, O. Kaltenhäuser, M., Kober, H., & Vieth, J. (2001). A combined study of tumor-related brain lesions using MEG and proton MR spectroscopic imaging. *Journal of Neurological Sciences, 186,* 13–21.

Kamada, K., Möller, M., Saguer, M., Kassubek, J., Kaltenhäuser, M., Kober, H., Überall, M., Lauffer, H., Wenzel, D., & Vieth, J. (1998). Localization analysis of neuronal activities in benign rolandic epilepsy using magnetoencephalography. *Journal of Neurological Sciences, 154,* 164–172.

Kamada, K., Saguer, M., Möller, M., Wicklow, K., Kaltenhäuser, M., Kober, H., & Vieth, J. (1997). Functional and metabolic analysis of cerebral ischemia using magnetoencephalography and proton magnetic resonance spectroscopy. *Annals of Neurology, 42,* 554–563.

Kamada, K., Takeuchi, F., Kuriki, S., Oshiro, O., Houkin, K., & Abe, H. (1993). Functional neurosurgical stimulation with brain surface magnetic resonance images and magnetoencephalography. *Neurosurgery, 33,* 269–273.

Kassubek, J., Sörös, P., Kober, H., Stippich, C., & Vieth, J. (1999). Focal slow and beta wave activity in patients with multiple sclerosis revealed by magnetoencephalography. *Brain Topography, 11,* 193–200.

Kassubek, J., Stippich, P., Sörös, P., Ganslandt, O., Kamada, K., Hopfengärtner, R., Kober, H., Steinmeier, R., & Vieth, J. B. (1996). A motor field source localization protocol using magnetoencephalography. *Biomedical Engineering (Berlin), 41*(Suppl. 1), 334–335.

Kober, H., Grummich, P., & Vieth, J. (1995). Fit of the digitized head surface with the surface reconstructed from MRI–tomography. In C. Baumgartner, L. Deecke, G. Stroink, & S. J. Williamson (Eds.), *Biomagnetism: Fundamental research and clinical applications* (pp 309–312). Amsterdam: Elsevier Science.

Kober, H., Möller, M., Nimsky, C., Vieth, J., Fahlbusch, R., & Ganslandt, O. (2001). New approach to localize speech relevant brain areas and hemispheric dominance using spatially filtered magnetoencephalography. *Human Brain Mapping, 14,* 236–250.

Kober, H., Nimsky, C., Möller, M., Hastreiter, P., Fahlbusch, R., & Ganslandt, O. (2001). Correlation of sensorimotor activation with functional magnetic resonance imaging and magnetoencephalography in presurgical functional imaging: A spatial analysis. *NeuroImage, 14,* 1214–1228.

Kober, H., Vieth, J., Grummich, P., Daun, A., Weise, E., & Pongratz, H. (1992). The factor analysis used to improve the dipole-density-plot (DDP) to localize focal concentrations of spontaneous magnetic brain activity. *Biomedical Engineering (Berlin), 37*(Suppl. 2), 164–165.

Kober, H., Vieth, J. B., Stippich, C., Kassubek, J. R., & Hopfengärtner, R. (2000). Time course of abnormal MEG activity associated with transient ischemic attacks. In C. J. Aine, Y. Okada, G. Stroink, S. J. Swithenby, & C. C. Wood (Eds.), *Biomag96: Proceedings of the Tenth International Conference on Biomagnetism* (pp 1033–1036). New York: Springer-Verlag.

Kutsy, R. L., Farell, D. F., & Ojemann, G. A. (1999). Ictal patterns of neocortical seizures monitored with intracranial electrodes: Correlation with surgical outcome. *Epilepsia, 40,* 257–260.

Lee, S. A., Spencer, D. D., & Spencer, S. S. (2000). Intracranial EEG seizure-onset patterns in neocortical epilepsy. *Epilepsia, 41,* 297–307.

Lewine, J. D., & Orrison, W. W. (1995). Magnetoencephalography and magnetic source imaging. In *Functional brain imaging* (pp. 369–417). St. Louis, MO: Mosby YearBook.

Meijs, J. W. H., Bosch, F. G. C., Peters, M. J., & Lopes Da Silva, F. H. (1987). On the magnetic field distribution generated by a dipolar current source situated in a realistically shaped compartment model of the head. *Electroencephalography and Clinical Neurophysiology, 66,* 268–298.

Morioka, T., Yamamoto, T., Katsuta, T., Fujii, K., & Fukui, M. (1994). Presurgical three dimensional magnetic source imaging of the somatosensory cortex in a patient with a peri-Rolandic lesion: Technical note. *Neurosurgery, 34,* 930–934.

Nakasato, N., Seki, K., Kawamura, T., Ohtomo, S., Kanno, A., Fujita, S., et al. (1996). Cortical mapping using an MRI-linked whole head MEG system and presurgical decision making. *Electroencephalography and Clinical Neurophysiology, 47*(Suppl.), 333–341.

Nimsky, C., Ganslandt, O., Kober, K., Möller, M., Ulmer, S., Tomandl, B., & Fahlbusch, R. (1999). Integration of functional magnetic resonance imaging supported by magnetoencephalography in functional neuronavigation. *Neurosurgery, 44,* 1249–1256.

Okada, Y. C., & Kyuhou, S. (1997). Genesis of MEG signals in mammalian CNS structure. *Electroencephalography and Clinical Neurophysiology, 103,* 474–485.

Oldfield, E. C. (1971). The assessment and analysis of handedness: The Edinburgh inventory. *Neuropsychologia, 9,* 97–113.

Orrison, W. W., Jr., Douglas, F. R., Blaine, L. H., Edward, L. M., Sanders, J. A., Willis, B. K., Marchand, E. P., Wood, C. C., & Davis, L. E. (1992). Noninvasive preoperative cortical localization by magnetic source imaging. *American Journal of Neuroradiology, 13,* 1124–1128.

Rezai, A. R., Hund, M., Kronberg, E., Zonenshayn, M., Cappell, J., Ribary, U., Kall, B., Llinás, R., & Kelly, P. J. (1996). The interactive use of magnetoencephalography in stereotactic image-guided neurosurgery. *Neurosurgery, 39,* 92–102.

Robinson, S. E., & Rose, D. F. (1992). Current source image estimation by spatially filtered MEG. In M. Hoke, S. N. Erné, Y. C. Okada, & G. L. Romani (Eds.), *Biomagnetism: Clinical aspects* (pp 761–765). New York: Excerpta Medica.

Segebarth, C., Belle, V., Delon, C., Masarelli, R., Decety, J., Le Bas, J.-F., Décorps, M., & Venabid, A. L. (1994). Functional MRI of the human brain: Predominance of signals from extracerebral veins. *NeuroReport, 5,* 813–816.

Simos, P. G., Breier, J. I., Zouridakis, G., & Papanicolaou, A. C. (1998). Identification of language-specific brain activity using magnetoencephalography. *Journal of Clinical and Experimental Neuropsychology, 20,* 706–722.

Steinmeier, R., Fahlbusch, R., Ganslandt, O., Nimsky, C., Buchfelder, M., Kaus, M., Heigl, T., Lenz, C., Kuth, R., & Huk, W. (1998). Intraoperative magnetic resonance imaging with Magnetom open scanner: Concepts, neurosurgical indications, and procedures: A preliminary report. *Neurosurgery, 43,* 739–748.

Stippich, C., Freitag, P., Kassubek, J., Sörös, P., Kober, H., Scheffler, K., Hopfengärtner, R., Kamada, K., Bilecen, D., Radü, E. W., & Vieth, J. B. (1998). Motor, somatosensory and auditory cortex localization by fMRI and MEG. *NeuroReport, 9,* 1953–1957.

Stippich, C., Kassubek, J., Kober, H., Sörös, P., & Vieth, J. (2000). Time course of focal slow wave activity in transient ischemic attacks and transient global amnesia as measured by magnetoencephalography. *NeuroReport 11,* 3309–3313.

Stippich, C., Kassubek, J., Sörös, P., Ganslandt, O., Kamada, K., Kober, H., Hopfengärtner, R., Steinmeier, R., & Vieth, J. B. (1996). Precise pre- and intraoperative assessment of functional cortex by magnetoencephalography (MEG). *Biomedical Engineering (Berlin), 41* (Suppl. 1), 306–307.

Vieth, J., Grummich, P., Kober, H., Ulbricht, D., Fenwick, P. B. C., & Claus, D. (1993). Localization of slow and beta wave MEG waves associated with epileptogenic lesions. *Epilepsia, 34* (Suppl. 6), 123.

Vieth, J. B., Kober, H., Ganslandt, O., Möller, M., & Kamada, K. (1999). The clinical use of MEG activity associated with brain lesions. *Biomedical Engineering (Berlin), 44* (Suppl. 2), 61–69.

Vieth, J. B., Kober, H., & Grummich, P. (1996). Sources of spontaneous slow waves associated with brain lesions, localized by using the MEG. *Brain Topography, 8,* 215–221.

Vieth, J., Kober, H., Grummich, P., Ulbricht, D., Brigel, C., Claus, D., & Fenwick, P. B. C. (1994). Localization of the epileptogenic lesion by focal slow and beta wave MEG activity. *Biomedical Engineering (Berlin), 39*(Suppl.), 133–134.

Vieth, J. B., Kober, H., Kamada, K., & Ganslandt, O. (1998). Normal and abnormal MEG activity in border zones of brain lesions. In Y. Koga, K. Nagata, & K. Hirata (Eds.), *Brain Topography Today* (pp. 39–46). New York: Elsevier.

Vieth, J., Kober, H., Weise, E., Daun, H., Moeger, A., Friedrich, S., & Pongratz, H. (1992). Functional 3D localization of cerebrovascular accidents by magnetoencephalography (MEG). *Neurological Research, 14,* 132–134.

Wada, J., & Rasmussen, T. (1960). Intracarotis injection of sodium amytal for the lateralization of cerebral speech dominance: Experimental and clinical observations. *Journal of Neurosurgery, 17,* 266–282.

Watanabe, E., Mayanagi, Y., & Kaneko, Y. (1993). Identification of the central sulcus using magnetoencephalography and neuronavigator. *No To Shinkei, 45,* 1027–1032.

Zanow, F. (1997). *Realistically shaped models of the head and their applications to the EEG and MEG.* Unpublished doctoral dissertation, University of Twente, The Netherlands.

Zentner, J., Hufnagel, A., Ostertun, B., Wolf, H. K., Behrens, E., Campos, M. G., Solymosi, L., Elger, C. E., Wiestler, O. D., & Schramm, J. (1996). Surgical treatment of extratemporal epilepsy: Clinical, radiologic, and histopathologic findings in 60 patients. *Epilepsia, 37,* 1072–1080.

# Epilogue

## Samuel J. Williamson

The idea for this book originated at a conference held in October 1999 to honor Samuel J. Williamson, Professor of Physics and Neural Science at New York University (NYU). Officially, he was being honored on the occasion of his 60th birthday; however, lurking in the background was the fact that Sam was ill—so ill that he could no longer carry out his duties as a professor. Out of affection and respect for Sam, several of the many conference participants prepared chapters for this book. Other chapter authors could not attend the conference but volunteered to contribute chapters anyway. These chapters reflect the personal as well as the scientific impact that Sam had on all of these authors. This epilogue will explain why they felt so strongly about Sam that they decided to devote a substantial amount of time to preparing this book, which is dedicated to Sam.

This brief biography has two authors. The first, Peter Levy, Professor of Physics at New York University, focuses on Sam's early career as a condensed matter physicist, before he became thoroughly involved in neuromagnetism. The second author, Lloyd Kaufman, Emeritus Professor of Psychology at NYU, was Sam's partner from the beginning of his career in neuromagnetism and for more than 20 years was codirector with Sam of the Neuromagnetism Laboratory of NYU's Departments of Physics and Psychology.

## Early Career

*By Peter Levy*

Born in West Reading, Pennsylvania, on November 6th, 1939, Sam stayed in the region of the Lehigh Valley until he went to MIT. Those who have been to his home in New York City can't miss the large bell from one of the Lehigh Valley's steam engines. This was a memento of his father's career as a railroad man. In 1961, Sam received a SB and, in 1965, a ScD, both in physics, from MIT. He was on a science scholarship as an undergraduate and received the Karl Taylor Compton Award on graduating. During the summer of 1960 he was an intern at Sandia Laboratories in New Mexico; he evaluated the seismometry performance around the Nevada test site to help justify the United States signing the nuclear bomb test ban treaty. The United States signed the treaty. It was during the completion of his thesis that he started working at the Francis Bitter National Magnet Laboratory, under the guidance of Si Foner and Mildred Dresselhaus on the effects of magnetic fields on the electronic structure and electron spin resonance in metals and semiconductors (e.g., the electronic properties of graphite by using the deHass–van Alphen effect). After earning his ScD Sam stayed on at the magnet lab as a staff member and he started his work on superconducting materials; he continued this work as a National Academy of Science-National research Council postdoctoral research fellow at the Laboratoire de Physique des Solides at the Université de Paris-Sud in Orsay, France.

Sam returned to the States in 1967 and was appointed a member of the technical staff at the newly formed North American Rockwell Science Center in California. There he continued to work on superconductivity, particularly on the effects of magnetic fields. These two themes—magnetism and superconductivity—were to be the focus of his work in physics. His interest in civic affairs led him to become chairman and spokesperson for the Ventura County Citizens Committee for Clean Air. When he was working for the Science Center of Rockwell the Sierra Club asked him to advise them regarding whether a new electrical power generating station planned for installation by the local power company would impose an air pollution threat. Up to that time, the criterion set for a pollutant of concern was a limit on the concentration (e.g., so many parts per million). Companies could meet these criteria simply by forcing more clean air into the bottom of the smokestack to mix with the air and gases coming out of the boiler. That certainly reduced the pollutant concentration within the stack, but once the gases left the stack, the same amount of pollutant remained in the communities' air! Clearly, it was more meaningful to control the quality of community air by imposing a maximum limit on the number of tons per day of the pollutant.

Indeed, with the help of the Sierra Club, Ventura County, California, was the first entity in the world to impose such a maximum mass-emission rate of a pollutant. Within 4 months, Ventura County, Orange County, and the Los Angeles Air Basin imposed such a criterion. The news was even better than Sam anticipated, because the governmental entities within the Los Angeles Air Basin imposed more stringent limits, one after the other, because no entity could afford politically to be less stringent than the others! That criterion now forms the backbone for improving the air quality in many other counties in California and in many other states. It was a simple concept for a physicist but heretofore no one had asked for a physicist to look at this problem. An article on this experience, titled "Local Politics and Air Pollution" appeared in MIT's *Technology Review*, and to Sam's surprise, three other publishers reprinted that article.

The Rockwell Science Center was in crisis as early as 1970, so Sam spent that year as a lecturer at the University of California, Santa Barbara. It was during this period that Sam gave a lecture course on air pollution and wrote the major text on this subject: *Fundamentals of Air Pollution*; which was published in 1973. In 1971, Sam joined NYU as an associate professor of physics. He immediately started work on "high temperature" A-15 superconductors, for example, $V_3Si$, (in those days, "high" meant $T_C = 20\text{-}23K$), and the magnetic and transport properties of the rare-earth pnictides; both topics were of interest to other individuals in the physics department (Joe Birman and myself). Sam readily lent his broad interests to developing new popular courses that attracted liberal arts majors. In addition to continuing his interest in "Weather and Man," Sam joined forces with Herman Cummins to teach "Light and Color in Nature and Art"; their textbook of the same name grew from the course and was published in 1983. It is noteworthy that this book is still in print. Its illustrations are extremely attractive and no doubt some reflect Sam's enormous skill as a photographer.

In 1972, at a lunch to celebrate the results of a National Science Foundation Excellence award to the Departments of Physics and Psychology at NYU, Sam met Lloyd Kaufman; with Sam's knowledge of superconducting quantum interference devices (SQUIDs) and Lloyd's knowledge of visual perception, they gave birth to the new area now known as neuromagnetism. Before we follow this major development let us continue to follow Sam's trajectory in physics, the time-dependent dynamic properties of condensed matter. He joined forces with Bob Richardson, a professor in the physics department, and Elliott Flowers in a study of transverse zero sound in normal $^3$He, an exotic quantum fluid that displayed some of the properties of superconductors. With his nearly unique ability to measure magnetic responses in very weak fields, in 1977 Sam started work on "spin glasses," magnetic systems whose properties are altered by the fields used in measuring its properties. In the early 1980s he started work on the magnetoelastic properties, or stress-induced changes, of rare-earth intermetallic compounds with Pierre Morin, a visitor from Grenoble, France. By the mid-1980s, Sam's involvement in neuromagnetism was so overwhelming that he had to stop his research in conventional physics. In 1987, he published his last physics article in the *Physical Review Letters:* "Evidence for a Phase Transition in the Spin Glass $Eu_{0.4}Sr_{0.6}S$ by Dynamic Susceptibility Measurements."

Sam's collaborators and co-authors over the 20 years during which he studied the electronic, magnetic, and superconducting properties of condensed matter included: Si Foner, Milli Dresselhaus, Haskell Taub, myself, Myriam Sarachik, Marvin Milewits, Bob Richardson, Elliott Flowers, Joe Birman, Lia Krusin, Frank Milliken, David Osterman, Carley Paulsen, Pierre Morin, and Hans Maletta.

## Career In Neuromagnetism
### *by Lloyd Kaufman*

As mentioned in the preceding section, Sam and I met at a luncheon to celebrate the move of the Departments of Physics and Psychology into new laboratories and offices in the same National Science Foundation-funded complex at NYU. Actually, George Sperling, then professor of psychology at NYU, and a contributor to this book, introduced us. In a casual conversation, George discovered that Sam was intrigued by the idea of using his superconductor sensors (SQUIDs) to study the brain's magnetic field. George knew that I had a strong interest in the electrical activity of the brain, especially as it relates to visual perception. In point of fact, in the 1960s I had conducted an amateurish experiment using an induction coil to see if I could detect the brain's magnetic field. This effort was a miserable failure, so I was very pleased that Sam was interested in same phenomenon and seemed to have the tools, knowledge, and skills to carry it out. We decided then and there to spend no more than 3 months in a joint effort to detect a visually evoked magnetic field.

Sam recruited his graduate student Douglas Brenner to work with us in the low-temperature physics laboratory. Needless to say, this was not a 3-month project. With direction from Sam, Doug built his own point-contact SQUIDs and constructed second-order gradiometers wound on phenolic rods. I contributed my own guess as to the baseline dimension of the gradiometer (I think it was 8 cm) and participated in designing and conducting most experiments. We knew that the ambient magnetic noise about 40 m above the subway line directly under our building would be an imposing source of interference. We did not have the financial resources to construct a magnetically shielded room, so we had to rely on the gradiometer. However, we made many mistakes. Our first dewar, which was already available in the laboratory, was made of stainless steel. Eddy currents set up by ambient fields in the walls of the dewar made it impossible to detect signals that we hoped to study. Somehow we found sufficient funds to purchase a fiberglass dewar, thus eliminating the offending noise source, and made various changes in the gradiometer that enabled us to sufficiently cancel out effects of uniform fields and fields with uniform spatial gradients, such as might arise from distant sources. Finally, using our seventh system, we had Sam lie on a platform and look down at the face of an oscilloscope displaying a visual stimulus—a changing pattern rather than a flashing light. The tail section of the dewar was placed near the occipital portion of Sam's skull, just over the visual cortex. Signal averaging enabled us to pick up a response that was in step with changes in the visual pattern. This was the first detected field evoked by a sensory stimulus. When the display was occluded by a piece of cardboard, the response disappeared. This, our first recorded response, was not detected until 1974, after 2 long and frustrating years of work. The results are described in Brenner et al. (1975), which is cited in chapter 1.

Sam and Doug alternated as subjects in a long series of experiments. We usually worked at night to minimize effects of ambient noise, often until 4:00 AM. Unfortunately, as soon as I lay down on the platform I tended to fall asleep. When I could stay awake, I too presented an evoked magnetic field, so Sam and Doug concluded that I had a brain after all. Even so, it was far better that I be assigned the job of operating miscellaneous electronics to produce and control the visual stimuli and process magnetoencephalography signals. In those days I worked with a venerable analog averaging computer that I had contributed from my own laboratory. These were very happy days for all of us. There was that wonderful camaraderie but, mostly, we began to make discoveries! If anything motivates a scientist, it is the thrill of discovery.

George Sperling remembers,

When Sam Williamson and Lloyd Kaufman established their partnership, their labs were in different buildings. The Physics and Psychology buildings were adjacent to each other, so Sam and Lloyd broke through the exterior wall of Sam's MEG lab and through the adjacent exterior wall of the Psychology building into Lloyd's lab. The floors in the two buildings didn't line up exactly so that there were several steps in the passageway between the two labs. The Williamson-Kaufman joint MEG lab literally broke down the walls between Physics and Psychology. (personal communication, May, 1999)

We went on to make many astonishing discoveries. I recall an experiment in which the little finger and thumb of one of Doug's hands were stimulated with mild electric shocks. We moved the dewar so that the pick-up coil of the gradiometer was at different positions along the scalp on different trials. Afterwards, Sam plotted field strength as a function of position across the scalp and noticed that the locations where the fields that emerged and re-entered the head when the thumb was stimulated differed from the locations of the similar field extrema when the little finger was stimulated. Sam immediately recognized that this is precisely what would happen if the sources were current dipoles in different positions along the posterior bank of the central sulcus of the brain. These results culminated in a 1978 article published in *Science* (cited in chapter 1) as well as several follow-up studies with a growing number of students and postdoctoral fellows. Sam also had an amazing insight. If the source is modeled as a current dipole, then one can compute the depth of the source beneath the skull merely from the distance along the scalp between the two extrema and a measure of the radius of curvature of the sphere that best fit the skull in that region. From that time on, we never conducted an experiment without mapping the field at many different places. Wherever possible we plotted isofield contour maps and estimated the locations of the sources within the head of each subject.

Sometime in the late 1970s we realized that our homemade system was not sufficiently sensitive to detect weaker signals, especially those at low frequencies where the noise levels were high. Also, the system's dimensions were not stable when the dewar was warmed up for some repair or other and then refilled with liquid helium to bring it back to the superconducting state. By then we had managed to obtain a small grant from the Office of Naval Research (ONR), thanks to the efforts of Dr. Don Woodward of ONR, one of our strongest supporters. We used some of the funding to purchase a specially designed system similar to our System 7 but with a lower noise thin-film SQUID and a niobium gradiometer wound on quartz rather than on a phenolic rod. Sam worked with Duane Crum, then of Superconducting, Helium and Electronics, Inc. (SHE) to design a better system. Gene Hirschkoff, coauthor of one chapter, worked for SHE at that time. He wrote, "One of us (GH) recalls hand carrying a pickup coil lashed to the bottom of a SQUID on a thin transmission line as a special order for Sam in the mid-1970's so he could try detecting these minute fields in his NYU lab" (personal communication, April 2002). Sam worked with SHE on the design of a 5-channel system, which we purchased with funds from ONR and from the Air Force Office of Scientific Research (AFOSR). Al Fregly, our project officer at AFOSR, was a staunch supporter of our work then and for many years afterward. This 5-channel system made it possible to map the field outside the head with much greater efficiency and was the mainstay of our laboratory. It was the basis for the design of a 7-channel system built for the NYU School of Medicine. In 1984, Sam, together with myself and with Charles Nicholson and Rodolfo Llinas of the medical school, helped with the design of a 37-channel system that was installed at the medical center. At the same time, we envisioned a whole-head system so that MEG could be a truly useful instrument for medical diagnostic procedures. Such a system is installed and in use at the NYU medical center.

In 1979, Yoshio Okada, a graduate student of William K. Estes at Rockefeller University, heard Doug Brenner talk about his PhD. Yoshio was struck by an article in *Vision Research* (Williamson, Kaufman, & Brenner, 1978) that reported a striking similarity between the reaction time in a simple detection task to the onset of a grating and the latency of the visually evoked field to the grating stimuli. Moreover, both the reaction time and the latency of the evoked field changed in the same way with the spatial frequency of the grating. Yoshio stated, "I became immediately very excited as I realized that MEG is a tool for relating physiological functions of the human brain to the structure and function of human mind.

"In the summer of 1979, I started working in the Neuromagnetism Laboratory while writing my doctoral thesis. In the next several years, we carried out some of the first studies of the sensory and motor cortices of the human brain with MEG" (personal communication, May 2002).

Yoshio went on to become a major contributor to the work of the Neuromagnetism Laboratory, and today he is one of the pre-eminent workers in the field. His chapter is one of the most important in this book.

In 1980, Yoshio was joined by Marco Pellizone, a PhD in physics from Switzerland. They worked closely together on the installation and shakedown trials of our new 5-channel system, named "Freddy." Physicists and psychologists worked together throughout the lifetime of the Neuromagnetism Laboratory. They learned from each other. Doug Brenner, a physicist, taught me how to transfer liquid helium from a storage dewar to the dewar housing our SQUID. I helped Doug develop a strong interest in vision. Yoshio Okada, a cognitive and mathematical psychologist, went on to become a neuroscientist. Our predoctoral students were a mix of several different disciplines, and they educated each other. Regardless of discipline, they all developed computer skills, took turns at transferring helium, and helped out in the many truly major construction projects designed by Sam. With apologies to those I forgot, I list at the end of this biography the names of as many of our pre- and postdoctoral students as I can remember.

Sam's collaborations with visiting colleagues and postdoctoral students were among the most fruitful of all. Professor Gian Luca Romani tells the story of his work with Sam in his chapter with Cosimo Del Gratta for this volume. Professor Olli V. Lounasmaa, a very distinguished physicist and then the Director of the Low Temperature Laboratory (LTL) and its Brain Research Unit at the Helsinki Technological University, worked with Sam at NYU for 9 months. He spent some time working on visual problems. Mostly, however, he interacted with Sam. This was part of a long-standing relationship that was of great benefit to both the laboratory in Helsinki, and our laboratory in New York. Since 1980, Sam made eight short visits to Helsinki, and spent a 5-month sabbatical there in 1994. He collaborated on several projects with LTL scientists, including M. A. Uusitalo, M. T. Seppli, M. Sams and, most frequently, Risto Ilmoniemi, a PhD in physics. Risto came from the LTL to spend 2 postdoctoral years at NYU. He collaborated with many of our psychology students as well as his physics peers. Today Risto is director of the BioMag Laboratory of the University of Helsinki, the Helsinki Central Hospital, and the Helsinki Technological University. Lounasmaa made many short visits to NYU, as did Professor Riitta Hari, now Director of the Brain Research Unit of the LTL. Sam's work with Uusitalo and Deppli on the lifetimes of activation traces evoked by visual stimuli was part of Sam's major research interest in his last years in neuromagnetism. This area is now of central importance to cognitive scientists, as evidenced by the chapter by Zhong-Lin Lu and George Sperling in this volume. Nevzat G. Gençer, a PhD in biomedical engineering, spent the entirety of 1994 at the Neuromagnetism Laboratory as a postdoctoral student. He wrote, "I remember Sam working alone in the lab with an endless motivation and enthusiasm. He was full of ideas and never stopped learning (so that he could explore) the human brain using Magnetic Source Imaging" (personal communication, May 10, 2002). Nevzat contributed a chapter to this volume.

I believe that Dr. Christoph Michel spent the year of 1991 in our laboratory. He too came from Switzerland, and was already an expert in electroencephalography and evoked potentials. I suggested a project on mental rotation, and he and Sam collaborated with me to produce a wonderful article cited in chapter 1 of this volume (Michel et al., 1993). The correlation between variation in reaction time with difficulty of task rotation and the duration of suppression of alpha-frequency magnetoencephalography signals over the occiput was truly impressive. The two functions mimic each other.

One person deserves special treatment here. Jia-Zhu Wang, a fresh PhD from the NYU Physics Department, took the job of computer systems manager of the Neuromagnetism Laboratory. This must have been in 1983 or thereabouts. Jia-Zhu became increasingly involved in the ongoing work of the laboratory. She saw to it that all of the students kept to their schedules for maintaining our systems, and began to develop software that made all of our jobs possible. She attended all of the laboratory meetings and related colloquia and, in her quiet way, became a major force in the laboratory. In 1990, I asked her to collaborate with me on a study that James H. Kaufman of IBM Research and I had begun concerning how the shape of the cortex might affect the extracranial magnetic field. She became an equal partner in this work and proved herself to be a creative thinker. By now all of us were so very impressed with Jia-Zhu that Sam and I decided that she should be given the title of Research Scientist. She went on to do some enormously creative work on the inverse problem. This is summarized in her chapter in this volume. I am very proud of the fact that I asked Sam to pay careful attention to Jia-Zhu's ideas about the inverse problem. In his inimitable fashion, Sam recognized the importance of these ideas and threw himself into a rich and rewarding collaboration with her. She continues to be a good friend to both of us.

Many other people passed through the Neuromagnetism Laboratory as students, collaborators, and visitors. Most offered moral support, and both Sam and I express our appreciation for that support. Sadly, we were unsuccessful in obtaining sufficient grant support for our work. Ultimately, owing to a shift in priorities, ONR stopped supporting us, but AFOSR (thanks to Dr. Fregly) kept us going for several years. However, we failed to win needed support. Sam took these defeats with great equanimity, and tried to go it alone even though he lacked the funds. I retired at the end of 1994. It was clearly time to go. Sam continued to work with his last student, Wei Yang, in an effort to study the lifetime of the activation trace of visual stimulation. Sam used his own money to purchase needed equipment. Freddy was no longer functional, he could not purchase liquid helium, and our powerful computers succumbed to age and disuse. However, our old electroencephalography machine was still functional, and Sam's support enabled Wei to win his PhD in psychology. Perhaps this may have been the first time that a physics professor was thesis advisor to a psychology student but, to be honest, Wei had some generous help, especially from Marissa Carrasco, now the Chair of the Department of Psychology. Wei was Sam's last student.

Sam was enormously proud of his work on the decay of sensory memory, which inspired his project with Wei. This work was the product of work with his physics student Zhong-Lin Lu, who is the first-listed editor of this book. Zhong-Lin wrote to me as follows: "Sam used to tell me that the true value of a PhD education is in the confidence one obtains through the dissertation work: A successful dissertation proves that one can make some substantial progress on perhaps a small set of scientific problems; However, the problem solving skills and the confidence one obtains in the process are invaluable in facing any new problems, both in science and in daily life" (personal communication, May, 2002). Based on his experience in the Neuromagnetism Laboratory, Zhong-Lin's interests slowly shifted from physics to cognitive neuroscience, perception, and cognitive psychology. He even confesses an interest in clinical neuroscience. He has been enormously successful in all of these endeavors, especially since he took a postdoctoral position with George Sperling, as this solidified his dedication to cognitive science. Sam is most proud of Zhong-Lin.

Sam received many awards and honors, but this volume is sufficient testimony to the high regard in which he is held. He was a wonderful citizen of the university and played a significant role in the establishment of NYU's Center for Neural Science. He will surely be remembered fondly, and with some awe, by all who knew and worked with him.

### Predoctoral Students of the Neuromagnetism Laboratory

Douglas Brenner, physics PhD
Sarah Curtis, psychology PhD
Yael Cycowicz, psychology PhD

Dan Karron, applied science PhD
Gladys Klemic, physics MS
Zhong-Lin Lu, physics PhD
Bruce Luber, psychology PhD
Ed Maclin, psychology PhD
Wei Yang, Psychology PhD
Postdoctoral fellows
Seline Cansino (psychology)
Nevzat G. Gençer (biomedical engineering)
Risto Ilmoniemi (physics)
Christoph Michel (psychology)
Yoshio Okada (psychology)
Marco Pellizone (physics)
Paolo Costa Ribiera (physics)
Carlo Salustri (physics)
Barry Schwartz (psychology)
Jia Zhu Wang (physics)

## POSTSCRIPT

Note from Gerhard Stroink to Peter Levy on the occasion of the conference honoring Sam.

> I couriered some smoked salmon over for the Sam-fest. Lloyd suggested I send it to you, to give as a present to Sam.

> The story behind this is that in the early 80's Sam came here (Dalhousie University) to give a series of lectures on Biomagnetism. In between lectures, he kept talking about this particular place where they prepared smoked Salmon. Apparently the quality and taste was described in detail in the NY Times and he wanted a taste of it. So on the day of his departure I committed myself to go there and buy some. However, I did not realize that this fishing village was a 2 hour drive from Halifax and that, despite what the maps said, a lousy dirt-road went from there to the airport.

> In any case we got to the salmon place, Sam got the salmon and I raced over this dirt-road with Sam and the salmon to the airport where we arrived just in time for him to catch the plane. With his one jacket for all opportunities, his little shoulder bag containing all needed (for 1 day or two weeks) and the stinking salmon wrapped in news papers he disappeared into the sun-set.

> So, I hope you find an opportunity to present this to him.

A toast to Sam and that he may enjoy this salmon, that even made it to the culinary pages of the NY Times.

Greetings,
Gerhard Stroink

Another comment by George Sperling is worth noting:

When Sam first started recording human MEG, he had very little background in psychology and physiology. His penchant for skiing provided a wonderful opportunity for self education. Between 1988 and 1998, he attended eight week-long meetings of the Annual Interdisciplinary Conference held in the last week of January at the base of the ski slopes in Jackson, Wyoming. Each year, he faithfully attended the 30-odd lectures at the conference (which were devoted mainly to current topics in cognitive and neuroscience; I believe he learned a lot). He always presented an interesting account of his own recent work and thoughts. He was a excellent speaker, skilled in communicating to a diverse audience. His talks and comments were always highly stimulating and from a different perspective. We're hoping he'll be able to return. (personal communication, May, 2002)

## REFERENCES

Williamson, S. J. (1972).Local politics and air pollution. *MIT Technology Review, 74,* 50–53.

Williamson, S. J. (1973). *Fundamentals of air pollution.* Reading, MA: Addison-Wesley Publishing Company.

Williamson, S. J., Kaufman, L., & Brenner, D. (1978). Latency of the neuromagnetic response of the visual cortex. *Vision Research, 18,* 107–110.

Williamson, S. J., & Cummings, H. Z. (1983). *Light and color in nature and art.* New York: Wiley.

# Author Index

# Subject Index

## M